Economic Evaluation in Health Care
Merging theory with practice

Economic Evaluation in Health Care
Merging theory with practice

Michael Drummond
University of York

Alistair McGuire
City University, London

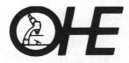

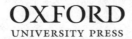

OXFORD
UNIVERSITY PRESS

Great Clarendon Street, Oxford OX2 6DP

Oxford University Press is a department of the University of Oxford.
It furthers the University's objective of excellence in research, scholarship,
and education by publishing worldwide in

Oxford New York

Athens Auckland Bangkok Bogotá Buenos Aires
Cape Town Chennai Dar es Salaam Delhi Florence Hong Kong Istanbul
Karachi Kolkata Kuala Lumpur Madrid Melbourne Mexico City Mumbai
Nairobi Paris São Paulo Shanghai Singapore Taipei Tokyo Toronto Warsaw

and associated companies in Berlin Ibadan

Oxford is a registered trade mark of Oxford University Press
in the UK and in certain other countries

Published in the United States
by Oxford University Press Inc., New York

A catalogue record for this title is available from

the British Library

Library of Congress Cataloguing in Publication Data

Drummond, M. F.
Economic evaluation in health care: merging theory with practice/
Michael Drummond, Alistair McGuire.
Includes bibliographical references and index.
1. Medical economics. I. McGuire, Alistair. II. Title.

RA410.5 .D768 2001   338.4'33621–dc21   2001033912

ISBN 0 19 263177 2 (Hbk)   ISBN 0 19 263176 4 (Pbk)

Typeset in Minion
by Florence Production Ltd, Stoodleigh, Devon
Printed in Great Britain
on acid-free paper by
Biddles Ltd., Guildford & King's Lynn

To Elspeth, Finn, Kate and Tom

Foreword

Economic evaluation is playing an increasing role in the allocation of health care resources. The National Institute for Clinical Excellence (NICE) in the UK is, perhaps, the best known of a number of recent European initiatives. These follow in the path of the Pharmaceutical Benefits Advisory Committee in Australia, the Canadian Co-ordinating Centre for Health Technology Assessment, and Provincial Formulary Committees in Canada, in seeking to make formal assessments of the value of health technologies. Health Maintenance Organisations in the USA are also showing greater interest in the cost-effectiveness of treatments, particularly new pharmaceuticals, as shown by the Association of Managed Care Pharmacists' development of guidelines for economic submissions. At local level in many health care systems, budget holders in hospitals and doctors' offices are seeking to identify whether more expensive but more effective treatments represent value for money.

This partner book to the Drummond *et al. Methods for the economic evaluation of health care programmes* is designed to give those involved in planning, undertaking, and reviewing economic evaluations of health technologies a clear understanding of the theoretical underpinning of the science of economic evaluation and of how to apply theory to practice. In particular it examines:

- the value judgements and theoretical assumptions that underpin different outcome measures and which need to be understood by users of these tools;
- options for measuring resource use and for pricing such use, including the treatment of learning curve effects, informal medical care, unrelated medical costs, and productivity effects;
- choice of decision analytic modelling technique, and the handling and reporting of uncertainty;
- theoretical and practical aspects of collecting and analysing resource use data in clinical trials;
- theory and evidence underlying the different approaches to choosing discount rates to value health benefits and costs over time;
- transferability of economic evaluation results from one setting to another and the implications for designing clinical trials and other studies.

This collection of papers written by the leading health economists in the field provides an invaluable guide to the current state of economic theory as applied to health technology assessment, and to the practical implications of this theory for the conduct, reporting and understanding of economic evaluations in health care.

Adrian Towse
Director of the Office of Health Economics
August 2001

Contents

Chapter 1

Theoretical concepts in the economic evaluation of health care

Alistair McGuire

1.1 Introduction

The traditional theoretical base of economic evaluation rests on welfare analysis. Individuals are said to maximize utility and societal welfare is defined as an aggregation of utility across all individuals. Governments, in taking societal decisions, do so in a completely benevolent manner; they have no additional objective other than to maximize welfare. Under idealized conditions certain institutions, including perfectly competitive markets, will allocate resources in a manner consistent with this aim. Where markets do not exist the technique of cost-benefit analysis can be used as means of mimicking market allocations to ensure welfare maximization.

While there is a long history in economic analysis of attempting to value health care benefits through the use of monetary measures, economic evaluation based on cost-effectiveness remains the most popular approach. It is not difficult to understand why this is the case: the growth in evidence-based medicine has provided a number of useful measures of effectiveness and the extension to cost-effectiveness is relatively straightforward. Moreover, cost-effectiveness has become a pragmatic tool given increasing technologies competing for limited budgets. At the same time individuals and decision-makers generally find it difficult to apply monetary measures to the benefits of health care for a variety of reasons; it is intrinsically difficult although not impossible.

Attempts to value health states face a multitude of difficulties. Individuals, even if they have adequate information find it problematic attaching value to something as fundamental as health. Even if this is overcome, there is a potential preference revelation problem when individuals do not finance their health care directly. Indirect methods, such as contingent valuation methods, rely on an appropriate specification of the characteristics to be valued. Given the range of potential characteristics which may play a role, aggregation techniques must be used to reduce the dimension of the issue to a manageable scale. Nonetheless economic evaluations of health care interventions continue to play a role in resource allocation decisions. The aim of this book is to provide some justification for that role and an assessment of the techniques and processes that may be used when undertaking an economic evaluation of health care.

This is a fairly limited objective, but even so is a difficult one to meet. The field is progressing rapidly, intellectually as well as on a pragmatic level. As an emerging tool, disagreements over its precise specification and utilization have emerged.

In this opening chapter the background to the general conceptual basis of cost-benefit and cost-effectiveness analysis is outlined. Within this chapter we consider the theoretical foundation arguing that at least two defences may be mounted for the use of such analysis. There is then a brief discussion of what is meant by cost-effectiveness analysis in the health care sector.

1.2 The conceptual basis of economic evaluation

There are many ways in which resources can be re-allocated including robbery, theft and fraud. Generally few would condone these particular methods. A number of other methods, fortunately, also exist and a related normative question arises as to which allocation or resources is best (optimal). The answer to this question obviously depends on the objective being pursued. Amongst these, economists have shown that, if there is a concern with efficiency in re-allocation, a competitive general equilibrium can be described which satisfies this concern. This equilibrium, moreover, is attained under a relatively weak set of conditions. The formal presentation of these conditions was outlined by Arrow–Debreu (1954). This Arrow-Debreu economy presents the basis of the welfare conditions that justify the claims made over efficient outcomes and their tie to competitive markets.

The Arrow–Debreu economy is concerned with exchange primarily between consumers and producers. Consumers have initial endowments of commodities while producers own inputs which produce commodities under known technologies. Each consumer attempts to maximize utility and has a utility function that represents their preferences for commodities. For these preferences to aid establishment of the equilibrium set of prices they must be reflexive, transitive, complete and continuous. They are assumed to be convex. Such restrictions impose useful functional form. Even adopting such well behaved preference functions, a major unresolved problem, to which we return below, is that of inter-personal comparison. This problem essentially recognizes that strength of preference, as well as equity concerns, may impact on outcome.

Producers maximize profits all of which are distributed to shareholders. The production set, which determines the supply of commodities, is assumed to be convex. Trade takes place simultaneously and is only undertaken at the established equilibrium prices. There are a finite number of commodities. Prices are taken as given by consumers and producers. That is no individual can affect the observed prices; they are said to be parametric. This assumption ensures no distortion through monopoly power.

Equilibrium is established when market demands equal market supply. Alternatively equilibrium can be defined as the position attained when excess demands are less than or equal to zero. This is related to as Walras' law, which states that the aggregate value of excess demands must be less than or equal to zero. The less than zero component encompasses situations where the economy may have endowments of commodities not demanded by any consumer, in which case the price will be zero. This condition of equilibrium is established by any set of prices that are consistent with excess demands being non-positive. Indeed, as may be suspected, there are many equilibria which may emerge depending on the initial endowments and the clearing prices.

With this remarkably small number of weak assumptions the Arrow–Debreu equilibrium is established. The beauty of which is that a complete economic system is specified which attains market clearing, that is equilibrium of demand and supply. Moreover, it is equilibrium attained through the individual actions of consumers and producers and, therefore, consistent with a long heritage of economic thought going back at least to Adam Smith. The equilibrium can be embellished to include uncertainty and can also be brought about through coalitions between the individual households; such outturns are referred to as being in the core of the economy.

1.2.1 Pareto optimality and welfare economics

Consistent with this equilibrium is the notion of Pareto optimality. Pareto optimality encompasses at least two concepts: Pareto improvement and Pareto efficiency. A Pareto improvement occurs if a re-allocation of resources increases the utilities of all individuals in an economy. A weaker version states merely that some individuals must gain from the re-allocation. If there are some gainers and some losers then it is not possible to rank the re-allocation outcomes with reference to the Pareto improvement criteria; the states are said to be Pareto non-comparable. This is shown in Figure 1.1 where the hypothetical utility levels of two individuals are plotted against each other. Consider the starting point as position e. A movement from e to y is a Pareto improvement; a move from e to w is a Pareto deterioration. Whereas it is impossible to state whether movements from e to either x or z are improvements or deteriorations. All points in quadrant B are said to be Pareto superior to e, while all those in quadrant C are Pareto inferior. All the states in quadrants A and D are non-comparable as in both cases one individual gains while the other loses utility. As utility cannot be compared directly across individuals, all states A and D are said to be Pareto non-comparable. This is merely a re-instatement of the problem of interpersonal comparability which will be returned to below.

Pareto efficiency is a more powerful concept. It defines the central notion of efficiency as follows: a re-allocation of resources is said to be efficient if at least one individual in the economy is made better off and no other individual is made worse off. This definition turns out to be generally rather useful. It is weak, however, in the sense that many changes in economic circumstances in real life involve the suffering of some and, if this is the case, we require some means of inter-personal comparison to adjudicate over the optimality of the re-allocation. Again discussion of this issue is delayed until later. The Pareto efficiency conditions comprise three main elements: attainment of optimality between inputs; optimality between outputs; and optimality between inputs and outputs.

Optimality between inputs leads to an analysis of producers. Assume that more output, or conversely less use of any input, is deemed a good thing. If the organization

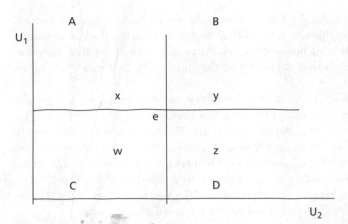

Fig. 1.1 Pareto comparable and Pareto incomparable states

of production is altered such that no further re-allocation would increase the output of one commodity without decreasing the output of another, holding inputs into the production process constant or, given the stock of commodities, decrease the use of one input without increasing the use of another input, such a situation is deemed Pareto optimal. The Appendix to this chapter outlines the technical conditions for this situation to be attained, showing it to be compatible with the marginal rates of transformation (MRT) between production inputs being equalized across all firms. Essentially this relies on re-allocating factor inputs across firms until at least one firm finds it is producing less than its maximum possible output.

Optimality between outputs can be thought of as the efficient distribution of commodities across consumers. It has already been noted a number of times that interpersonal comparisons of utility are, generally, unmanageable. It might appear, therefore, that we can say little about the distribution of commodities across individuals. In fact, Pareto optimality allows some statement of the distribution of commodities to be made. The Pareto criterion sanctions any change that makes one individual better off without making another worse off. So, if from any given distribution of resources such a re-allocation is possible, the given distribution must be sub-optimal. Again the Appendix gives the formal conditions that show that Pareto optimality is attained when the marginal rates of substitution (MRS) for commodities are equalized across consumers.

Optimality between inputs and outputs establishes efficiency between the consumption and production uses of resources. In this case concern is with the use of resources across consumers and producers. So if re-allocation is possible across the consumption and production sectors, which increases the utility of one individual without leaving another worse off this movement of resources, ought to take place.

The Arrow–Debreu economy and the definition of Pareto optimality gives rise to the First and Second Theorems of Welfare Economics. The first states that if a perfectly competitive equilibrium is attained, under the Arrow–Debreu assumptions, then this is also a Pareto equilibrium. The second is the corollary of the first and states that if a

Pareto optimum exists, under the assumptions consistent with Arrow–Debreu, then this is also a competitive equilibrium. These theorems lie at the basis of much of welfare economics. They are remarkable largely because they give rise to a definition of efficiency, Pareto efficiency, and of equilibrium states under relatively few assumptions and the seemingly innocuous ruling that the decision-maker is merely moving resources until no one individual can be made better off without someone being made worse off.

At least two damaging criticisms can be made of Pareto optimality, however. First the Pareto criteria are compatible with a large number of potential allocations some of which represent highly inequitable resource allocations. Pareto optimality is optimal only in one dimension; it is indifferent to the distribution of utilities across individuals. Second, note that we have already stated that Pareto optimality cannot rank all states; the Pareto improvement criteria are inconclusive across resources allocations where some gain and others lose. To adjudicate over these states would entail inter-personal comparison.

Hicks (1939) proposed an ingenious but ultimately flawed attempt to rank states which were Pareto non-comparable. Assume $u_i(y_a, z_a)$ is the utility of individual i under the circumstances described as 'a', with y_a being the individual's income and z_a being a vector of characteristics associated with the state 'a' which individual i values. For example state 'a' could be a state of ill-health and some of the z's could be associated with the individual's ability to work, rest and play in that state of ill-health. Let us introduce another state of the world 'a_1' where the individual's ill health is improved. Then we can define CV as the willingness to pay for an improvement in health:

$$u_i(y_a - CV, z_{a1}) = u_i(y_a, z_a)$$

This amount is referred to as the compensating variation (CV) and represents the maximum, permanent amount of income that may be taken from the individual leaving them as well off in utility terms as they were prior to the improvement in health. In the current case CV is a positive value which is subtracted from income. If the individual was made worse off by the change in the state of the world, CV would be negative and therefore would be added to income (two negative signs are positive remember) as the amount of money the individual would be willing to accept in compensation for the deterioration in health. Adding the compensating variation across individuals as we move from state of the world 'a' to 'a_1', we can see that $\sum CV > 0$ if the gainers place a higher monetary value on the move than the losers.

This is the so-called Hicks-Kaldor criterion that was proposed to overcome the Pareto non-comparability limitation. Looking back to Figure 1.1 it provides a means to state whether moves from e to x and e to z are 'good'. It appears to circumvent the need for inter-personal comparisons as individuals themselves place monetary value on the movement across different states, that is across the different re-allocations of resources. Aggregating these money values across individuals then easily attains the net gain or loss in consumer welfare. In fact four measures were proposed, of which we have outlined two, and the technique can be applied to situations where the relative prices of commodities change or, much more common in the public sector, where the relative quantities of the commodities supplied change (see Willig 1976 and

Randall and Stoll 1980 for further detail). These measures, all based on individual income gains or losses were initially assumed to give a very generalizable solution to the problem of comparing utilities across individuals. The criterion was often referred to as the potential Pareto criterion on the basis that the compensation measures were hypothetical; there was no true re-allocation of incomes associated with the resource re-allocation. It was a mind game.

This raises, at least, two flaws. First for the hypothetical compensation test to operate while avoiding direct inter-personal comparisons implies that all individuals have the same marginal utility of income; all individuals must place exactly the same value on a $1 income regardless of their initial level of income. Second, it is possible, although it must be said unlikely, for the Kaldor-Hicks criterion to suggest a given re-allocation increases social welfare but also, after the change, that a movement back to the original allocation also increases welfare (see Johannson 1991 for details). This leads to a third criterion, the so-called Scitovsky reversal criterion which states that a re-allocation is a potential Pareto improvement if, and only if, after the re-allocation a movement back to the original allocation is not supported by the Kaldor-Hicks criterion. The reversal criterion does not overcome the first flaw.

A number of studies have adopted this general approach to value the health benefits gained from health care interventions. Early studies relied on direct questionnaire approaches. These were fraught with difficulties, including the framing of the questions, the reliance on appropriate specification of the health benefit to be gained and the true revelation of preferences defined over health states by individuals. Johansson (1991) gives a full description of the difficulties faced. Latterly indirect methods have been relied on to value health benefits. For the most part these rely on methods that attempt to proxy such values through statistical models. Contingent valuation models, where the health benefits are valued contingent on a given experimental design, and the related conjoint analysis, where differing aspects which characterize the health state to be valued are considered jointly are the most common of such methodologies.

A number of methodological and practical issues accompany conjoint analysis. First there is the issue of what ought to be measured. In a number of studies the end-point addressed lacks justification. At least three alternatives are possible; valuation of the actual health outcome, valuation of an uncertain health outcome or valuation of a new health care technology where both the treatment benefit and the health outcome are uncertain. The valuation itself may be based on willingness to pay (WTP) or willingness to accept (WTA) premises. There is no theoretical reason to accept one measure over the other although income effects will mean that the estimates will differ. Shogren et al. (1994) show that there is convergence of WTP and WTA for market based goods but for non-market based goods (such as changes in health outcome) the estimated values based on WTP and WTA do differ in a persistent manner. As Deiner et al. (1998) note contingent valuation studies are, in any case, seldom clear as to whether their concern is with WTP or WTA and, in a related manner, whether compensating or equivalent variation is being measured. It is likely that the WTP measure is more practical as it is bounded by the income constraint. The valuation instrument also varies across studies with choice being largely defined by the alternatives of open ended and closed questionnaires versus bidding rounds. Johansson

(1995) outlines a number of practical concerns surrounding all forms of contingent valuation, including the framing reference for the questions, the incentive to misrepresent preferences and the potential to misrepresent the scenario being tested. Such issues raise concerns over the way in which such studies are designed. At almost every stage there is a potential for bias to be imparted.

It is important to recognize that, regardless of the method employed, the theoretical basis of cost-benefit analysis relies directly on the notion of the potential Pareto improvement and the Kaldor-Hicks criterion. That is, the case for cost-benefit analysis relies completely on a buy-in to the Pareto optimality concept. Individual utility is what is being maximized and to overcome the problem of inter-personal comparison monetary weights are placed on competing resource allocations. Consumers reveal their true preferences through their willingness to pay. There is no concern with distributional notions; compensation need not and, in general, will not be paid.

There have been two reactions to these limitations of the welfare economics approach. First some have advocated the formalization of interpersonal comparability within the welfare criterion (see Ng 1985). This has not occurred to any significant degree. More importantly there was an increasing reliance on the use of explicit welfare functions to aggregate individual preferences and to explicitly address the issues of resource distribution across individuals. The Bergson-Samuelson welfare function was one of the first to address this issue (Bergson 1938; Samuelson 1947). While welfare functions can, and generally should, encompass more than information confined purely to utilities, this form of welfare function tends to be specified such that it is no better than neutral towards all non-utility characteristics of the social preferences it is ordering and is explicitly derived solely from the utility levels of individuals. A particular re-allocation of resources is said to be beneficial if societal welfare, defined across the utility levels of individuals, increases. Explicit weighting of particular individuals' utilities may overcome the potential compensation requirement; essentially decision-makers reveal their trade-offs between efficiency and equity under the social welfare approach. In other words, comparisons across individuals with regard to resource allocation have to be made.

This approach has admittedly been difficult to implement. Arrow (1951) showed some time ago that under a weak set of assumptions it is impossible to aggregate individual preferences in a coherent fashion. Arrow's assumptions included Pareto efficiency; non-dictatorship; independence of preferences such that any social choice concerning a set of social outcomes only depended on the preferences relating to those outcomes; and complete and transitive preference ordering. Each of these assumptions has been closely examined to try to break the Arrow Impossibility Theorem. The conclusion being, from a long literature, that only if interpersonal comparisons are accepted, and convexity is imposed, does the Bergson-Samuelson social welfare function remain a valid criterion for the acceptance or rejection of re-allocation patterns. It is also normally assumed, although this is not necessary, that this form of welfare function satisfies the Pareto criterion such that if a utility ordering of states of the world places state 'a' above state 'a_1' then the social welfare function will also place the social welfare, which is purely defined across utilities, associated with state of the world 'a' above state 'a_1'.

Thus the highest criterion for welfare assessment is a welfare function that is defined purely across utilities and adopts, at least implicitly, some form of interpersonal comparability across individual utility. In other words, the ultimate decision-maker has to make some distributional judgement over which utilities should count higher than others. While other forms of social welfare function can be constructed again defined purely over individual utilities, all are based on a notion of interpersonal comparison (see Boadway and Bruce 1984).

1.2.2 An extension beyond welfarism

A number of investigators, most notably, Sen (1999) have argued that interpersonal comparisons are central to the breaking of the Arrow Impossibility Theorem. In his writings Sen has shown the conditions under which a social welfare function can remain a useful criterion for social decision-making. The conclusions are rather interesting. As he states 'It can be shown that admitting cardinality of utilities *without* interpersonal comparisons does not change Arrow's impossibility theorem at all ... In contrast even ordinal interpersonal comparison is adequate to break the exact impossibility ... But it turns out that even weaker forms of comparability would still permit making consistent social welfare judgements, satisfying all of Arrow's requirements, in addition to being sensitive to distributional concerns' (Sen 1999, p. 357).

The weaker forms of comparability referred to enter the decision-making process when the social welfare function is defined across a wider range of arguments than mere utilities. Sen, amongst others (see Culyer 1990 and Wagstaff 1991 for similar arguments as applied to health care), argues that other types of interpersonal argument are as important as the consideration of interpersonal comparison of utilities. Indeed they may be more important than utility measures. If these other forms of interpersonal comparison can be separated from utility measures then they may even be considered in isolation from the interpersonal comparison restricted to utility measures alone.

Building on these insights it has been argued by some that health in particular is an important independent argument in the welfare function (Culyer 1990). An obvious measure for interpersonal comparison in the health care sector would be based on a quantifiable, commensurate measure of health benefit. In other words, some notion of effectiveness that is quantifiable and amenable to comparison across individuals would be a suitable starting point. An immediate candidate is the QALY measure largely as it may be used as a commensurate instrument that may be applied to any health care intervention. This raises an important question what is the QALY measuring? Is a QALY to be regarded as a measure of health benefit alone (i.e. health outcome) or is it, as some would argue, a measure of preference or utility associated with a given health outcome? Historically, the QALY has been used as a measure of preference, but the implication of doing so is that it adheres to the underlying axioms of expected utility theory and there is a literature defending this use (Pilskin *et al.* 1980; Garber and Phelps 1997; Garber 2000).

First let us be clear that expected utility theory is an approximation to behaviour under uncertainty, has a number of rival theories which are held to be better descriptions of actual behaviour (see Machina 1987 or Schoemaker 1982), and stipulates that preferences be specified in such a way that they have desirable mathematical properties and meaningful economic interpretations. Within expected utility theory individuals are assumed to choose amongst different options (health states for example) in a mathematically convenient and consistent manner – in short they are logical. The axioms of the theory define the logic. The important axioms include the following: Completeness; individuals must be able to judge utility across different health states. Transitivity; individuals must choose in a consistent manner such that if outcome H_1 is preferred to outcome H_2, and H_2 is preferred to H_3, then H_1 must be preferred to H_3. Continuity; which implies that each preference set of the same utility level is bounded (i.e. indifference curves cannot cross). Strong independence or the 'sure-thing principle'; states that the utility an individual attaches to an action (e.g. treatment choice) which results in a given outcome (e.g. health state) is independent of the utility attached to any other act if the outcomes are mutually exclusive. If QALYs are measured across different health attributes or characteristics, as most are, then, as Pilskin et al. (1980) show, a further axiom is needed concerning the independence of utility across the attributes (see Drummond et al., 1997). The last two axioms give rise to a particular structure of preferences, namely they are said to be additively separable implying that the utility attached to the quality-of-life attained by an individual in any given time period is independent of the quality-of-life realized by that individual in any other time period.

Two further assumptions are necessary before QALYs can form the basis of well-behaved preference structures. First, individuals must adhere to constant proportional time trade-offs. That is, an individual must be willing to sacrifice a constant proportion of their remaining years of life to achieve a given improvement in their health status. Second, individuals must also exhibit risk constancy such that their risk preference is independent of their health state and their utility function is characterized by constant proportionality with respect to risk. If all such assumptions were adhered to then the QALY would be a true representation of individual preferences over health states, holding everything else constant. They would be a cardinal measure of utility in a rather limiting sense; they would not allow direct comparison across individuals but any individual utility function could be linearly transformed. Such utility functions demonstrate that cardinality, in itself, does not imply interpersonal comparison. Bleichrodt (1997), drawing on the work of Sen (1977) shows that only under certain further conditions, essentially that the QALY reflects a cardinal ratio scale, would it become a measure useful for interpersonal comparison. Although the conditions under which a cardinal ratio scale exist are extreme this would make the QALY capable of comparison of levels and gains and losses arising from health care resource allocations.

As noted, there is extensive empirical evidence that suggests that expected utility theory is not an adequate description of how individuals actually behave under conditions of uncertainty. While this is a harsh criticizm in itself it is even more devastating when applied to QALYs. The quality-of-life weights in the QALY are normally gained through instrument measures based on simulated or experienced circumstances. If individual respondents to these instruments do not base their responses on the logical structure (i.e. the assumptions) demanded by expected utility theory then the use of the resulting QALY measures as representations of preferences, and therefore their use as measures of utility within a Paretian framework is violated.

Indeed for many the axioms surrounding expected utility theory and Pareto optimality are too strong, and violated too often in reality, for them to accept this as a conceptual basis for using economic evaluation based on a cost per QALY calculation.

This leads back to the alternative interpretation of the QALY as a measure of health benefit unrelated to individual preferences over health states. The most thorough assessment of QALYs under this interpretation is given in Broome (1993). There Broome sets out examples of how QALYs fail generally to meet the axioms of expected utility theory and gives an interpretation of QALYs as a measure of health benefit. As he, and Culyer (1990) point out this interpretation is not de-limiting. Defining QALYs in this way leaves open the possibility that QALYs are cardinal measures of health benefit defined in some quantitative manner, or expressions of the value individuals attach to this health benefit or, even again invoking the assumptions of expected utility theory, expressions of the utility attached to this health benefit.

Ironically, accepting the QALY in terms of the lowest degree of preference revelation, which is simply as a cardinal measure of health benefit, gives the greatest power in terms of interpersonal comparison which is unrestricted by the axioms of expected utility theory. It is, therefore, consistent with the social welfare basis of resource allocation, outlined above, advocated initially by Sen based on arguments other than utility entering the social welfare function.

Adoption of this approach entails a move away from the Paretian definition of efficiency to some other notion of efficiency, the most obvious being that of, assuming separability in the welfare function, maximizing health or maximizing QALYs. This has been discussed by Wagstaff (1991) who points out that pure maximization of QALYs gives rise to a social welfare function which resembles a utilitarian welfare function (i.e. Σ_i QALY = summation of QALYs across individuals). While this meets the requirement of inter-personal comparability, as he points out it seems to lead to definitions of efficiency which ironically turn out to be more restrictive than the Pareto criteria. If QALYs are gained more by the young, merely because they have more life to lead than the elderly, an efficiency criteria which states maximize QALYs would redistribute health care resources from the elderly to the young.

Of course, this raises distributional concerns. A different conceptual version of the social welfare function would retain the QALY as a health benefit measure but also incorporate explicit weights to be attached to individual QALYs to reflect distributional concerns. In fact the introduction of explicit weights gives rise in theory to a wide range of possible welfare functions (see Williams and Cookson 2000). In practice it may mean maximizing the distributional weights assigned by policy makers. In this respect note that the role of the QALY becomes akin to the health benefit measures used in the Oregon experiment.

The extensive use of cost-effectiveness, and the calculation of cost-per-QALY is included in this definition, can therefore be justified on at least two grounds. First, traditionally, but with difficulty, through recourse to Paretian welfare economics. Second, through adoption of the QALY as a measure of health benefit, and the pursuit of some extended form of social welfare function. Within the Paretian framework Mishan (1971) has stated that 'To be rather rude about it, the analysis of cost-effectiveness can be described as a truncated form of cost-benefit analysis'. As he details cost-effectiveness is concerned with resource allocation issues *after* the overall budget has been allocated to a particular activity, while cost-benefit analysis provides information necessary to determine the overall budget consistent with efficient resource allocation. In this sense it is implied that cost-effectiveness is piecemeal and operates on efficiency grounds within constraint. Such piecemeal approaches are more consistent with the second, more general justification. Acceptance of a more general justification is also consistent with cost-effectiveness analysis being complementary to cost-benefit analysis. Either way cost-effectiveness analysis remains concerned with the process of allocating resources efficiently; all that is being discussed is what definition of efficiency is appropriate. Yet if the definition is not explicitly detailed then the cost-effectiveness of an intervention cannot be anything other than flawed.

1.3 Cost-effectiveness analysis

Assuming that the definition of efficiency has been agreed upon, difficulties remain in implementation. The application of cost-effectiveness analysis follows directly from the attribution of relevant costs to relevant effects. A large component of this book is concerned with the definition of what is deemed relevant. In this section an overall introduction to the practical use of cost-effectiveness is given.

Generally cost-effectiveness is pursued to test the null hypothesis that the mean cost-effectiveness of one health care intervention is different from the mean cost-effectiveness of some competing intervention. It is calculated as a ratio:

$$R = \frac{C_a - C_b}{E_a - E_b} = \frac{\Delta C}{\Delta E}$$

defining the incremental cost per unit of additional outcome. This calculation can be undertaken in a number of ways reflecting both the available data and the preferred methodological approach.

Ideally data should be available from a true random sample of the patient population under study. If this is the case, estimation of the incremental cost-effectiveness ratio (ICER) follows the notion of statistical inference based on sample means. In other words the ICER becomes:

$$R = \frac{(\mu_{CA} - \mu_{CB})}{(\mu_{EA} - \mu_{EB})}$$

where μ is the expected value of the true population cost of treatment A (μ_{CA}), the expected value of the cost of treatment B (μ_{CB}), etc. O'Brien *et al.* (1994) noted that four states of the world could be observed based on the relative magnitude of the incremental costs and effects:

1. $\mu_{CA} - \mu_{CB} < 0$; $\mu_{EA} - \mu_{EB} > 0$; which is defined as a dominant outcome for intervention A as it is both less inexpensive to implement and more effective than treatment B.

2. $\mu_{CA} - \mu_{CB} > 0$; $\mu_{EA} - \mu_{EB} < 0$; which is defined as a dominant outcome for intervention B as it is both less inexpensive to implement and more effective than treatment A.

3. $\mu_{CA} - \mu_{CB} > 0$; $\mu_{EA} - \mu_{EB} > 0$; which defines a trade-off in which the higher cost of treatment A must be compared in terms of its higher effectiveness.

4. $\mu_{CA} - \mu_{CB} < 0$; $\mu_{EA} - \mu_{EB} < 0$; which defines a trade-off in which the lower cost of treatment A must be compared in terms of its lower effectiveness.

Note some important points here. First, these comparisons apply to where the decision-maker is already faced with a budget and mutually exclusive projects. Under these circumstances the objective is to maximize the level of health effects or the preferences attached to these health effects, depending on your persuasion, given the budget. ICERs are ranked with the least cost per unit of health effect (least cost per QALY produced) being the most desirable and the decision-maker then works down the list until the budget is exhausted. If there are really only two interventions to be compared then given dominance and a desire to maximize health the fourth situation is automatically redundant. If there are other interventions against which these two interventions are to be compared, in as much as they are competing for the same budget, as Weinstein and Zeckhauser (1973) note linear programming approaches may be adopted to find the optimal ranking of projects. Even in these wider circumstances if the desire is to maximize health effects, unless the true resource use of readily transferred resources from one treatment intervention to another can be established, it is unlikely that the fourth situation warrants much attention.

Dominance and trade-offs may not be clear-cut, however. This can be seen by concentrating on the third situation above ($\mu_{CA} - \mu_{CB} > 0$; $\mu_{EA} - \mu_{EB} > 0$), which is commonly the one of greatest interest. Figure 1.2 is illustrative. Note first that any cost-effectiveness ratio lying on a straight-line drawn from the origin will be the same; that is the value of the cost-effectiveness ratio for treatment A is equal to the cost-effectiveness value of treatment C; although obviously the budgetary implications differ.

Dominance exists when an option is both more costly and less effective than an alternative. Thus, starting at A, any point to the north-east (in the area labelled D) is dominated by A. However, extended dominance exists when an option is less effective and more costly than a linear combination of two other strategies with which it is mutually exclusive. Assuming constant returns to scale and perfect divisibility of projects, any combination of treatments A and C along the heavily shaded portion of the line joining them will be more cost-effective than Option B, as this will be provided at lower cost with more effect. However, an implication of this is that some proportion of the treated population will be receiving the less effective treatment (A). In practice ICERs should compare each intervention to the next most effective option, after eliminating options that are dominated.

Given that the expectations which generate the ICER (the means, μ are drawn from a random sample of the true population of the individual costs and effects they will have other distribution defining moments associated with them, such as variances, levels of skewness and so forth. This allows the possibility of hypothesis testing and most obviously a null can be formulated as $R = 0$, to be tested against an alternative

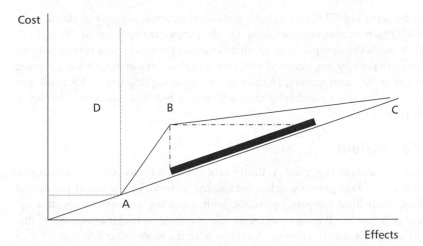

Fig. 1.2 Dominance and extended dominance

that $R \neq 0$. A major difficulty arising here is that as a ratio the ICER itself will have undefined moments as the denominator tends to zero. In particular the variance may be undefined rendering such hypothesis testing impossible. A number of methods for overcoming this problem have been proposed and are discussed in the chapter by Andy Briggs (see also O'Brien *et al.* 1994; Wakker and Klaassen 1995; Chaudhary and Stearns 1996; Willan and O'Brien 1996; Gardiner *et al.* 2000; Heitjan 2000). One of the most fruitful is the net-benefit approach (Tambour *et al.* 1998; Stinnett and Mullahy 1998). The net-benefit of treatment A is defined as:

$$\text{NB}_A = \mu_{\Delta E} - \frac{\mu_{\Delta C}}{\lambda}$$

where $\mu_{\Delta E}$ incremental health effects, $\mu_{\Delta C}$ measures the incremental costs, and λ is a threshold cost-effectiveness ratio measuring the marginal rate of substitution between money and health effect at which the decision-maker is just indifferent. The advantage of this approach is that standard errors can be easily attained and that higher values are always better. The major difficulty being the explicit use of a threshold cost-effectiveness level. Other solutions include direct transformations of the ICER (see Chapters 8 and 9).

Once the hypothesis to be tested, which essentially involves defining the appropriate comparator treatment, has been set out a whole myriad of issues is raised regarding the appropriate costs and outcomes to consider. The appropriateness or otherwise of which costs and outcomes to include, while the subject of a growing literature (e.g. see Meltzer 1997), rests on the underlying welfare function being maximized. For example, if a study is limited to a payer or provider's perspective then it may be that consideration of indirect costs is inappropriate (see Schulpher's chapter for more on this issue). Indeed the welfare maximand and perspective will also dictate the treatment of producer's surplus. In the some cases it may be assumed that the producer's surplus is negligible, technically zero with the price paid equal to the marginal cost of resource use. This can only be justified if treatment supply is elastic, fully responding to new treatment demands. Or the perspective may not be societal but limited to the health care producer, in which case that producer's rent may be ignored and the price paid for any inputs should reflect the market purchase price assuming inelasticity in the factor market. The aim of the remaining chapters in this book is to highlight and discuss a number of these and related practical issues, without being unduly prescriptive.

1.4 **Conclusions**

Economic evaluation as applied to health care has been dismissed on a number of occasions on various grounds: it has been stated to be lacking a sound theoretical foundation, unethical, too prescriptive, too limited and too narrow. On a great many of these occasions no alternative decision rule is offered. A major advantage of this form of analysis is that it serves to illuminate both the issue (what is it that is being maximized?) as well as the arguments to be considered when addressing the issue at hand. Indeed there are few occasions when even a rudimentary back-of-the-envelope calculation of critical costs and effects will not serve to guide decisions. Economic evaluation remains a useful tool that focuses attention on the necessary choices relating to the allocation of resources and is capable of application in various degrees of sophistication. For some the flexibility inherent in the technique reflects a robustness that is all too often dismissed as a lack of rigour. This is simply not the case. One of the major attributes ought to be that the stated hypothesis and the assumptions concerning perspective serve to define the parameters of the model.

What is clear is that the welfare basis of economic evaluation generally, and cost-effectiveness in particular, is only supportable under specific, restricting conditions. If these conditions hold then the link between cost-benefit and cost-effectiveness analysis is clear-cut. Under this justification the link between the differing forms of evaluation is to traditional welfare economics, with all its attendant limitations. If, on the other hand, cost-effectiveness is interpreted as an instrument accompanying the more general objective of maximizing health *per se* it becomes conceptually distinct from cost-benefit analysis. In this instance cost-effectiveness is a means of ensuring that the least cost interventions are utilized given the allocated budget. Either way the application of economic evaluation to the health care sector remains a useful means of considering the fundamental problem of how to allocate scarce resources. Such evaluation will not solve this problem. For some, the role of economic evaluation is merely to highlight the efficient use of such scare resources, leaving distributional concerns to the politicians. For others, economic evaluation will always be unsatisfactory, either because they do not understand its role, misunderstand the techniques or have their own agenda. For yet others there is general support for such evaluations but little understanding of its limitations.

Acknowledgement

I wish to thank Maria Raikon for her comments on this chapter (as well as on life generally). Errors, in their entirety, remain mine.

Appendix

The aim of the appendix is to show how Pareto optimality is derived formally and how this relates to a general specification of the welfare function. Assume an economy with a production and consumption sector. Pareto optimality rests on trades within each sector and across the two sectors being consistent with the allocation of the economy's resources such that any further re-allocation cannot make anyone better off without making someone else worse off. Let us start with the conditions for production. The objective here is to outline conditions under which it is impossible to produce more at any output (or use less of any input) without increasing the volume of factor input (or reducing the total supply of output). Assume we have n goods (goods can be either inputs or outputs). Assume also a large number of firms such that no firm has market power; all are price takers. Each firm (i) has a relation between inputs and outputs, remembering that goods are both inputs and outputs, specified by an implied production function:

$$f_a(x_1^a, \ldots, x_n^a) = 0 \tag{1.1}$$

where x_n etc., is the volume of the nth good produced or used by firm a. The total volume of any good, say n, summed over all firms is given by X_n.

We can formalize our problem by setting the total levels of all inputs and outputs (i.e. all goods) except one, say X_1, at fixed levels denoted by X_2^*, X_3^*, etc. This restriction means that when we arrive at a solution to our problem the total of good 2, summed over all firms must equal X_2^*. In other words, $x_2^1 + x_2^2 + x_2^3 + \ldots + x_2^v = X_2^*$. Our problem then becomes one of maximizing X_1 subject to this restriction and the restriction imposed by the production function. The solution would indicate an outcome where it is not possible to produce more of any one good without producing less of others or more inputs.

We can look at this problem using a particular mathematical technique that is useful in analysing problems of maximization or minimization. The approach is based on a Lagrangean expression:

$$L = X_1 - \sum_{j=2} \Phi_j(x_j^1 + x_j^2 + \ldots + x_j^v - X_j^*) - \sum_{a=1} \lambda_a f_a(x_1^a, \ldots, x_n^a) \tag{1.2}$$

Which merely states that our maximand (L) is given as the maximum value of total goods described by X_1 which is consistent with our two constraints – the fixed levels of all other goods and the production structure of the firms in our economy. The ϕ's and the λ's are, as yet, undetermined multipliers which help define our solution.

The first order conditions, which are the first set of conditions which help solve the maximization problem, are given by noting that at a maximum the rate of change of L (δL) relative to the rate of change of $x_j^a(\delta x_j^a) = 0$ (i.e. ($L/\delta x_j^a = 0$). Also $\delta L/\delta \Phi_j = 0$ and $\delta L/\delta \lambda_a = 0$. (For the non-mathematically inclined, if you have got this far, imagine you have reached the top of a hill. At this maximum point the rate of change in the incline is zero; the hill has flattened off. Mathematically speaking we are at the same point in our solution.)

Concentrating on $\delta L/\delta x_j^a = 0$, this solves to the following expression:

$$\frac{\delta L}{\delta x_j^a} = (-)\Phi_j = \frac{\lambda_a \delta f_a}{\delta x_j^a} = 0 \quad a = 1, \ldots, v; j = 1, \ldots, n \tag{1.3}$$

As the number of individual firms, a, sum to v, and the number of goods sums to n, there will be n such equations for each of the v firms. We have expressed the solution in terms of X_1 but the same general expression would result if any of the other goods had been used to define the maximand. Leaving the definition of the multipliers (the ϕ's and the λ's) to one side for the moment we can draw an important conclusion from this result.

From Equatation (1.3) for good number 1, let us re-name $\delta f_a/\delta x_j^a$ as F_j^a. This expression indicates what has to be given up in firm a if more of good j has to be produced; it is the rate of change incurred in other goods which involves releasing resources for more of good j. From Equatation (1.3) we have:

$$\lambda_a = \frac{1}{F_1^a} \quad \text{for } a = 1, \ldots, v \tag{1.4}$$

It follows that:

$$(-)\Phi_j = \frac{F_j^a}{F_1^a} \quad \text{for } a = 1, \ldots, v; j = 1, \ldots, n \tag{1.5}$$

Finally, re-arranging Equation (1.5) across all goods and firms gives the main result:

$$\frac{F_j^a}{F_k^a} = \frac{F_1^b}{F_k^b} \quad \text{for } a, b = 1, \ldots, v; j, k = 1, \ldots, n \tag{1.6}$$

The ratio F_j^a/F_k^a represents the rate at which one unit of good k can be transformed into good j in firm a. In other words Equation (1.6) represents the marginal rate of transformation of good k for good j (the $\mathrm{MRT}_{k,j}$). Thus the main result can be expressed as follows:

$$\mathrm{MRT}_{k,j}^a = \mathrm{MRT}_{k,j}^b \tag{1.7}$$

This merely states that for Pareto optimality to exist, such that it is impossible for any one firm to produce more output without another firm decreasing their output, the rates at which each firm transforms one good into another must be equal. The logic being that if one firm was transforming one good into another at a higher rate than all other firms the economy would gain by shifting resources to that firm, thereby increasing economy wide output. This transfer of resources would continue until no more gain could be made. This would happen when the marginal rates of transformation were equalized across firms.

This solution could be generalized for all the goods. The resulting solutions will determine a particular distribution of the various factor inputs between uses. Taking different levels for the X_j^*'s or choosing different goods for the maximand will not alter the character of the derived first order conditions (Equation (1.7)). If we repeat this maximization process for different levels of the X_j^*'s each solution would determine the maximum value for X_1 given the levels of the other good. This process could be carried out indefinitely and the sum of the total results would provide information on the maximum value any given output can take, given the values of the other goods.

This is the definition of the production possibility frontier of the economy – the technically efficient boundary of feasible production opportunities associated with a given known technology as represented by the production function of the firm. The general specification of which may be given as:

$$F(X_1, \ldots, X_n) = 0 \qquad (1.8)$$

Which states that the production possibility frontier is derived from both inputs and outputs.

To complete our analysis of production let us return to the definition of the multipliers, Φ_j and λ_a. These were used to help specify the constraints placed upon our production process and may be thought of as the cost of these constraints. Φ_j may be thought of as the cost of extra output j in terms of what would have to be given up in the maximand for good 1. If j is an input then Φ_j is the marginal social product of j stated in terms of the extra amount of good 1 that can be produced. The λ's define the cost of the constraints imposed by the individual firm's production functions. They may be thought of as the marginal cost of extra output in terms of input 1.

Turning to the consumption conditions we find a similar approach can be adopted. Assume the economy has a large number, m, of individuals. Each has a utility function specified across goods:

$$U_i = U_i(x_1^i, \ldots, x_n^i) \qquad (1.9)$$

Where x_n^i is individual i's consumption of commodity n, or supply when n is an input, for example a labour input.

The solution is again determined as above by fixing the totals of goods at levels X_1^*, X_2^*, etc. We then set (some arbitrary indexes of) utility of all consumers except one at specific levels U_2^*, U_3^*, etc. We then maximize the utility of individual 1 subject to these constraints and the constraints imposed on the form of the utility function. This solution would then define the outcome where it is not possible to make one person better off without making another worse off. The appropriate Lagrangean expression is given as:

$$L = U_1 - \sum_{j=1} \lambda_j (x_1^j + x_2^j + \ldots + x_m^j - X_j^*) - \sum_{i=2} \Phi_1 (U_i - U_j^*) \qquad (1.10)$$

Where again we have Lagrangean multipliers, λ_j and Φ_1, but these have entirely different interpretations from those defined above. Let U_j^i denote $\delta U_i / \delta x_j^i$, etc., then the first order conditions for a maximum, analogous to those in the production sector, can be re-arranged to give:

$$\frac{U_j^i}{U_k^i} = \frac{U_j^d}{U_k^d} \qquad i, d = 1, \ldots, m; j, k = 1, \ldots, n \qquad (1.11)$$

As U_j^i etc., represents the marginal utility to an individual i from an extra unit of j, then the ratios in Equation (1.11) represent the individual's marginal rates of substitution between two goods. That is, the rate at which a person would switch out of good k and into good j while keeping utility at the same level. A given bundle of goods is optimally distributed only when such substitution rates are the same across all individuals. That is when:

$$\text{MRS}^i_{k,j} = \text{MRS}^d_{k,j} \quad i,d = 1, ..., m; j, k = 1, ..., n \tag{1.12}$$

The intuition being that if one individual could substitute consumption of one good for another at, say, a lower rate, while holding their utility constant, than any other individual then overall utility in the economy could be increased by the individual trading one good for the other with other individuals. Such trades would continue until the marginal rates of substitution were equalized. Note that we applied an arbitrary index to the utility functions to allow manipulation. This imposes additional constraint on the utility functions, but does not invalidate our general result.

So far we have specified Pareto optimality across production alone and consumption alone. Of course resources may be traded across the consumption and production sectors. So to complete this formalization we consider such trades. The maximization problem, for any given individual, can be specified this time with the constraints being the economy wide production function and the utilities of all other individuals:

$$L = U_1 - \lambda F(X_1, ..., X_n) - \sum_{i=2} \Phi_i(U_i - U^*_i) \tag{1.13}$$

The first order conditions are obtained by maximizing this expression with respect to each of the goods for each individual. Denoting $\delta F/\delta X_j$ by F_j etc., these first-order conditions can be re-arranged as:

$$\frac{U^i_j}{U^i_k} = \frac{F_j}{F_k} \quad i = 1, ..., m; j, k = 1, m ..., n \tag{1.14}$$

The left hand side expression is merely the common rate of marginal substitution applied to goods in the consumption sector under optimal conditions. The right hand side requires a bit more explanation. The F_j represents the partial effect (derivative) of the economies production possibility frontier with respect to a change in j; if the change in j represents increased output then the F_j represents the rate of change in inputs required to achieve this increase in output. The whole ratio therefore represents the economy's most technically efficient way of transforming k into j which, given the production conditions, is a common transformation rate to all firms. Equation (1.14) states that the rate at which individuals are prepared to switch good k for good j is equal to the rate at which it is technically feasible to transform k into j. This result can be expressed as:

$$\text{MRS}_{k,j} = \text{MRT}_{k,j} \quad k, j = 1, ..., n \tag{1.15}$$

That is the marginal rate of substitution for goods must equal the marginal rate of transformation of goods. Again the intuition behind this result is that, if this condition did not hold, output and utility in the economy could be increased, with no loss, by transferring goods from one sector to the other. This trade would continue until the marginal rates defined in Equation (1.15) were equalized.

The three set of results Equations (1.7), (1.12) and (1.15) combine to define an outcome where, if they hold, it is not possible, through any further redistribution of resources between or across firms and individuals, to make anyone better off without making some others worse off. If different goods, other than good 1, or different levels of the goods, other than X^*, were taken as a starting point the same Pareto conditions would ensure the same general result. Of course the actual solution bundles would be different, indicating that there is no unique equilibrium.

This reflects the weakness of the Pareto equilibrium. Another statement of this would be the recognition that different Pareto equilibria exist and each solution results in a different distribution of resources across individuals. This is, of course, why Pareto optimality can be consistent with some individuals living in poverty. While this will not necessarily be the case, it is nevertheless as possible as any other outcome.

Welfare functions relate to the prior analysis in as much as social welfare, W, is said to be a function of utilities of the individuals in the society. So we have

$$W = W(U_1, U_2, ..., U_m) \qquad (1.16)$$

Welfare, W, can take any level or form. However specified the maximization of W, subject to the constraint of the economy's production possibility frontier, will give a uniquely determined equilibrium in terms of resource allocation that is consistent with Pareto optimality. To be consistent with Pareto optimality the social welfare function, W, must have the property that $\delta W / \delta U_i > 0$, that is the welfare increases as the utility of any individual increases. The maximization process can be formalized as:

$$L = W - \lambda F(X_1, ..., X_n) \qquad (1.17)$$

If $\delta W / \delta U_i$ is given as W_i then the first order conditions which solve this maximization problem includes the following:

$$\frac{\delta L}{\delta x_j^i} = W_i U_j^i - \lambda F_j = 0 \quad i = 1, ..., m; j = 1, ..., n \qquad (1.18)$$

which gives

$$\lambda = W_i \frac{U^i}{F_j} \quad i = 1, ..., m; j = 1, ..., n \qquad (1.19)$$

If j is output then the interpretation of Equation (1.19) is that the social value of the extra utility derived from the use of any inputs, should be the same irrespective of which good is used to produce these inputs or which consumer receives that good. It can also be shown that

$$W_1 U_j^1 = W_2 U_j^2 = ... = W_m U_j^m \quad j = 1, ..., n \qquad (1.20)$$

which states that any good cannot be optimally distributed across consumers unless the net marginal social utility, which is derived from switching goods from one individual to another, is zero.

As long as the social welfare function, W, incorporates the characteristic that $W_i > 0$, then the Pareto conditions will be consistent with the maximization process. Notice that we have not given a specific form to W. We could go further, by giving different weights to different individuals in the economy to reflect equity concerns for example, and this would not necessarily invalidate the relationship to Pareto optimality.

If the social welfare function is not simply specified across individual utility levels, as it is in Equation (1.16) we cannot necessarily equate the maximization of the welfare function with Pareto optimality, indeed in general the consistency between the two concepts will not hold. It is the complications introduced by additional arguments in the social welfare function which leads to the competing analysis of 'extra-welfarism'. If, for example, we introduce an individual's health, H, into Equation (1.16) we have:

$$W = W(U_1, H_1, U_2, H_2, ..., U_m, H_m) \qquad (1.21)$$

Now the specific form of the welfare function does matter. If the utility levels and health levels are, somewhat unrealistically, assumed to be independent, that is if $\delta U_i / \delta H_i = 0$, then we might impose Pareto optimality as a normative goal on the goods sector and a competing maximand on the health sector, say health maximization. The complete optimal resource allocation solution is nevertheless complex given that resources will be drawn from the goods sector to be used in the health sector. On the other hand if utility and health interact then the complexity increases further.

References

Arrow, K. (1951). *Social choice and individual values*. New York, Wiley.

Arrow, K. and Debreu, G. (1954). Existence of equilibrium for a competitive economy. *Econometrica*, 22, 265–90.

Bergson, A. (1938). A reformulation of certain aspects of welfare theory. *Quarterly Journal of Economics*, 68, 233–52.

Bleichrodt, H. (1997). Health utilities and equity considerations. *Journal of Health Economics*, 16, 65–85.

Boadway, R. and Bruce, N. (1984). *Welfare Economics*. Oxford, Blackwell.

Broome, J. (1993). QALYs. *Journal of Public Economics*, 50, 149–63.

Chaudhary, M. and Stearns, S. (1996). Estimating confidence intervals for cost-effectivenss ratios: an example from a randomised trial. *Statistical Medicine*, 15, 1447–58.

Culyer, A. (1990). The normative economics of health care finance and provision. In: A. McGuire, P. Fenn and K. Mayhew, *Providing health care*, Oxford, OUP.

Diener, A., O'Brien, B. and Gafni, A. (1998). Health care contingent valuation: a review and classification of the literature. *Health Economics*, 7, 313–26.

Drummond, M., O'Brien, B., Stoddart, G. and Torrance, G. (1997). *Methods for the economic evaluation of health care*. Oxford, OUP.

Garber, A. (2000). *Advances in CE analysis*. In: A. J. Culyer and J. Newhouse (eds). *Handbook of health economics*, vol. 1B. North-Holland, Amsterdam.

Garber, A. M. and Phelps, C. E. (1997). Economic foundations of cost-effectiveness analysis. *Journal of Health Economics*, 16, 1–33.

Gardiner, M., Huebner, M., Jetton, J. *et al.* (2000). Power and sample size assessments for tests of hypothesis on cost-effectiveness ratios. *Health Economics*, 9, 227–234.

Hicks, J. (1939). *Value and capital*. Oxford, Clarendon Press.

Heitjian, D. (2000). Fieller's method and net health benefits. *Health Economics*, 9, 327–36.

Johannesson, M. (1996). *Theory and methods of economic evaluation of health care*. Kluwer, Amsterdam.

Johansson, P.-O. (1991). *An introduction to modern welfare economics.* Cambridge, CUP.

Johansson, P.-O. (1995). *Evaluating health risks, an economic approach.* Cambridge, CUP.

Machina, M. (1987). Choice under uncertainty: problems solved and unsolved. *Journal of Economic Perspectives*, 1, 124–54.

Meltzer, D. (1997). Accounting for future costs in medical cost-effectiveness analysis. *Journal of Health Economics*, 16, 33–64.

Mishan, E. (1971). *Cost-benefit analysis.* Allen and Unwin, Sydney.

Ng, Y.-K. (1985). *Welfare economics.* Macmillan, Basingstoke.

O'Brien, B., Drummond, M., Labelle, R., and Willan, A. (1994). In search of power and significance: issues in the design and analysis of stochastic cost-effectiveness studies in health care. *Medical Care*, 32, 150.

Pilskin, J., Shepard, D. and Weinstein, M. (1980). Utility functions from life- years and health status. *Operations Research*, 28, 206–24.

Randall, A. and Stoll, J.R. (1980). Surplus in commodity space. *American Economic Review*, 70, 449–55.

Samuelson, P. (1947). *Foundations of Economic Analysis.* Harvard University Press, Cambridge MA.

Schoemaker, P. (1982). The expected utility model: its variants, purposes, evidence and limitations. *Journal of Economic Literature*, 46, 529–63.

Sen, A. (1977). On weights and measures. *Econometrica*, 45, 1539–1572.

Sen, A. (1999). The possibility of social choice. *American Economic Review*, 89, 349–78.

Shogren, J. and Crocker, T. (1991). Risk, self-protection and ex ante economic value. *Journal of Environmental Economics and Management*, 20, 1–15.

Shogren, J., Shin, Y., Hayes, D.J. *et al.* (1994). Resolving differences in willingness to pay and willingness to accept. *American Economic Review*, 84, 255–270.

Stinnet, A. and Mullahy, J. (1998). Net health benefits: a new framework for the analysis of uncertainty in cost-effectiveness analysis. *Medical Decision-Making*, 18, S68-S80.

Tambour, M., Zethraeus, N. and Johannesson, M. (1998). A note on confidence intervals in cost-effectiveness analysis. *International Journal of Technology, Assessment*, 14, 467–471.

Wagstaff, A. (1991). QALYs and equity-efficiency trade-off. *Journal of Health Economics*, 10, 21–41.

Wakker, P. and Klaassen, M. (1995). Confidence intervals for cost-effectiveness ratios: an application of Fiellers thereom. *Health Economics*, 5, 297–305.

Weinstein, M. and Zeckhauser, R. (1973) Critical ratios and efficient allocation. *Journal of Public Economics*, 2, 147–157.

Willan, A. R. and O'Brien, B. (1999). Sample sizes and power issues in estimating incremental cost-effectiveness ratios from clinical trials. *Health Economics*, 8, 203–211.

Williams, A. and Cookson, R. (2000). Equity in health care. In: A. J. Culyer and J. Newhouse (eds) *Handbook of health economics*, vol. 1B, North-Holland. Amsterdam.

Willig, R. (1976). Consumers surplus without appology. *American Economic Review*, 66, 589-597.

Chapter 2

Welfare economics and economic evaluation

Aki Tsuchiya and Alan Williams

2.1 Introduction

It is said that there are two 'competing views' on economic evaluation in health care (see Brouwer and Koopmanschap (2000) for a critical overview). One is often seen as the 'theoretically correct' approach, that is based more firmly within the theory of welfare economics, whilst the other by comparison as some practical but not well formulated collection of rules of thumb. Another way to stylize the two approaches may be that although the first of the two may appear to have closer ties with accepted theory, it is less relevant to the particular context and background of health care resource allocation, where the objectives of the players do not entirely agree with those upheld by standard theory, whilst the second approach tries to reflect specific concerns of the health care sector.

In order to address these issues, the purpose of this chapter is to trace out the logical steps that health economists have taken as they move from economic evaluation based on classical welfare economics, using only individuals' self-assessed utilities, to economic evaluation based on Quality-Adjusted Life Years (QALYs) valued from a societal viewpoint, and to explain the reasoning behind the taking of each such step.[1]

Paretian Welfare Economics was developed to deal with a particular methodological problem, namely the recognition that utility is neither interpersonally comparable nor cardinally measurable. Yet economists wanted to be able to make judgements about whether one state of the world is better than another. Historically, classical utilitarians had done this by adding up people's utilities in each state of the world and seeing which yielded the largest aggregate amount of utility (without making any judgements about the fairness or otherwise of the *distribution* of utility within the society). Paretian Welfare Economics overcame the scientific objections to this simple procedure by assuming only that each individual is capable of ranking each state of the world in order of preference, and adopting the rule that only when no one is worse off (in their own judgement) from a movement from situation B (the Baseline) to situation A (the Alternative), can situation A be declared better than situation B. However,

---

[1] For a comprehensive exposition of the standard position, see for example, Boadway and Bruce (1984); Johansson (1991).

this very neat solution to the problem has two major weaknesses, one empirical, and one theoretical. The empirical weakness is that there are hardly any real-life situations that meet the strict Paretian conditions, so as they stand they do not constitute a very useful criterion for practical policy analysis. But even if we did find some such situations, the theoretical weakness is that the Paretian conditions start from the status quo and accepts that as value-neutral, ignoring any inequities embedded in it, so we are still left without guidance on distributional issues, except for the rule that no one shall be made worse off than they were before. A 'Pareto improvement' is not concerned with *who* is better off, or about the relative size of different people's gains, but only that there are no losers.

So the next methodological development was to introduce the possibility that the potential losers might be offered compensation (to be paid by the potential gainers) so that we once more get to a situation in which there are no losers. If, when all of the potential losers have been fully compensated, the gainers from a move from B to A still have some gains left, then, following the Paretian rule, we can safely say that situation A is better than situation B. But the widespread information gathering and policing necessary for such a 'market' in compensation to work efficiently for all social decisions ruled it out as quite infeasible. It would be necessary to motivate all affected individuals to reveal honestly the minimum sum of money that would compensate them for any losses that they would suffer (and so make them agree to the change) or be equivalent to any gains that they might enjoy (and so make then agree to remain with the status quo). This would be difficult if they believed (rightly) that the greater their estimated losses the more compensation they will get, and the greater their estimated gains the greater will be the sum 'taxed away' to finance the compensation payments to the losers. So what happens instead is that independent analysts estimate the money value of the gains and losses to all the affected people, to test whether the sum of the money value of the gains exceeds the sum of the money value of the losses. This was (and is) the role assigned to cost-benefit analysis as a technique of applied microeconomics. Note that it did not require that compensation actually be paid, but only that potential gainers could hypothetically compensate the losers and have some surplus left. Money values have replaced utility values as the maximand, implicitly assuming that each unit of currency carries the same social value (since the rich person's cash is not actually handed over to the poor person, and a loaf of bread is valued at the same price no matter who gains or loses it). Again no judgements are made about the actual distribution of money gains and losses, nor about the initial distribution of purchasing power. One way of rescuing this approach from the void concerning distributive justice is to assert that, so long as we ensure that every social policy action generates more gains than losses, then in the long run everyone will be a net gainer. But this assumes that the process by which social policy actions are generated, designed, evaluated and implemented is entirely neutral between the various interest groups in society, which seems highly unlikely, even in a democratic society (see Williams 1977). An alternative approach has been to try to derive some form or other of 'equity weights' or 'distributional weights' to apply to gains or losses depending on who gets them. Thus if reducing inequalities in the distribution of income and/or wealth is a major objective of social policy, gains or losses to rich people would be given a lower weight than gains or losses to poor people. See for example, Little and Mirrlees (1974); Ray (1984); Jones-Lee (1989).

The Paretian framework requires us to accept that each individual is the best judge of his/her own welfare, and that at the end of the day there must be no losers. One methodological innovation designed to enable it to deal with some rather persistent difficulties over widespread aversion to inequalities in the distribution of goods, income and/or wealth, has been the recognition of interdependent utilities (or caring externalities). There appear to be situations in which the rich care about the poor to such an extent that relieving poverty increases the utility of the rich, even though it reduces the amount of resources available to them (e.g. through income support payments financed by progressive taxes on income and wealth). This preserves the rule that each individual is the best judge of his/her own welfare and only those individual judgements are to be taken into account when making judgements about social welfare (which is the essence of the 'welfarist' approach), while allowing for some sense of social solidarity or social justice. But sometimes this methodological variant goes further, as when the 'donor' gets (dis-)utility from some specified aspect of someone else's welfare (e.g. their evident malnutrition) but wants to ensure that the transferred resources go on food rather than being used to buy some other good from which the recipient gets more satisfaction (e.g. gambling, alcohol, tobacco, illicit drugs) but of which the donor disapproves. Now there is a clash as to whose view of an individual's welfare is to dominate the situation. 'He who pays the piper calls the tune' breaches the absolute dominance of the individual's own judgements as the sole legitimate basis for judging changes in his/her own welfare.

It is against that background that the organization of this chapter has to be seen. Two broad themes emerge as fundamental: first, in Section 2.2, we consider what is to be taken as the appropriate basis for judging whether a particular individual is better off or worse off, and how is this to be measured and valued; and second, in Section 2.3, we consider what is to be the relationship between these measurements at individual level and broad social judgements about the welfare of the community of which that individual is a member (which we are calling the problem of aggregation). The term aggregation is used here to mean any use of *individual* data at the *societal* level, and not necessarily simply adding together such data. Throughout, the task is to compare two different outcomes: that under the baseline scenario (B) and that under the alternative scenario (A). The general line of argument is going to be that if the changes in individual welfare can be made cardinally measurable and interpersonally comparable, then the problems that have beset Paretian Welfare Economics (which include Arrow's Impossibility Theorem as well as the void about distributive justice) can be avoided.[2] There are of course other problems, and we shall come to

---

[2] For a detailed but accessible discussion of the different types of social welfare criteria with their informational requirements in terms of the different levels of cardinality in individual utility functions and the different levels of interpersonal comparability of utility, see Boadway and Bruce (1984), Chapter 5. Also see Ng (1983) as an example of a welfarist welfare economic theory explicitly based on cardinality and interpersonal comparability of utility functions.

those at the end, but they do not seem as inhibiting as those that face any analyst who, in the field of health and health care, tries to adhere to the more conventional method-ological line.

2.2 Different ways of measuring how well off an individual is

Individual wellbeing is not directly observable. What is done therefore is to look at the difference in something that the individual gets under the baseline scenario and the alternative scenario, and postulate some relationship between the observed item and the individual's wellbeing. Measurements can be made in three categories: natural units, subjective values and monetary values. In what follows, each of these types of measurement will be applied in turn to each of the three selected elements that might make an individual feel better off: goods, life- years, and health. The simplest way to describe the difference between scenarios is to give the facts in *natural units*, e.g. 'the amount of x will increase by 20 per cent'. This may be either good news or bad news, depending on whether or not the individual prefers more of x to less. Only by refer-ring to (or making assumptions about) *the value that the individual attributes* to these natural units (i.e. only by referring to the second category) can plain description be linked to judgements about changes in a person's wellbeing. At a minimum this requires the introduction of ordinal preference structures relating to the item in ques-tion. The extent to which an individual subjectively values a given outcome is a very general concept, and the unit in which this should be expressed is not predetermined. The most common and practical unit of value, however, is money, and therefore the last category taken up here is *valuation in monetary units*. The objective of expressing value in money terms, or in any other numeraire good, is to make other kinds of quan-tities commensurable with each other, with the additional advantage that money values are terms that people are generally familiar with.

Nevertheless, many people are very uncomfortable about assigning money values to (the postponement of) death and (the relief of) suffering, arguing that there are some subjective values that cannot be represented in monetary terms. However, if an indi-vidual is willing to sacrifice something that can be valued in monetary terms in order to pursue this source of wellbeing that is supposedly incommensurable, this then gives us some idea of the minimum monetary value to be attached to it. Further, by observing what the individual is not willing to give up in this pursuit, we can derive a corresponding maximum monetary value. At the end of the day, the only desirable item that is completely incommensurable with money is one for the pursuit of which no scarce resources are devoted. People *do* devote their scarce resources to a better life and to better health, which justifies regarding them as commensurable with money.

2.2.1 Goods

The typical transition here is to start with changes in quantities of goods and services measured in natural units, then by assuming them to enter (positively or negatively at the margin) into the person's preference function, to assign a subjective value to them in utility terms. The final stage is then to express that subjective value in money terms, since the measurement of changes in 'real income' is a more accessible concept than changes in an amount of utility.

Measurement in natural units

In standard economic analyses the natural unit is the quantity of a good as ordinarily measured (e.g. a number of items, their weight, their volume). There are three things to note. First, most goods can be measured on an absolute scale. Second, more or less of a given good does not by itself imply a better or worse outcome. Third, different quantities of goods cannot be aggregated into one measure. For example, how could one summarize the quantitative impact of a glass of beer, a haircut, and a new hat in a single natural unit?

The subjective value of different combinations of goods

The difference in value between the two scenarios will be the difference in individual utility under the baseline and the alternative consumption sets. Difference in utility can be conceptualized in two ways: ordinal and cardinal. The central assumption in mainstream economic theory is that individual utility can only be measured on an ordinal scale: ranking between any two outcomes can be determined, but not the extent to which the two are apart on any cardinal scale. The argument for this restrictive conceptualization of individual utility is that, since utility is a subjective phenomenon, it is not scientific and objective to treat individual utility as if it were cardinally measurable. There is much to be drawn from this limited conceptualization of individual utility under certainty. However, a large and important part of economic analyses that addresses individual choice under uncertainty requires that individual utility is cardinally measurable. This is because the concepts of expected utility and risk attitudes refer to the second derivative of individual utility functions. The implication is that the extent to which two different utility levels differ has meaning, and thus there is cardinality.

Monetary value of different combinations of goods

One major practical limitation of the concept of utility, both ordinal and cardinal, is that it is not directly observable. The most commonly used method to address that difficulty is to convert individual utilities into monetary values. If the individual regards situation *A* as preferable to situation *B*, there will be some sum of money that, if paid by the individual under the alternative outcome, will make him/her exactly as well off as he/she was at baseline. This is the compensating variation,[3] which is a cardinal measure that represents a change in utility, regardless of whether or not the underlying utility change itself is cardinal.

---

[3] A related concept, the amount of money that, if paid *to* the individual under the baseline outcome, will make him/her exactly as well off as under the alternative outcome, is called the equivalent variation. This is used less often in the literature.

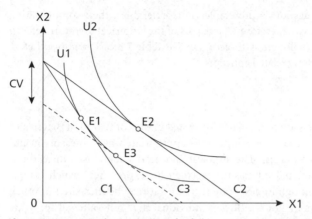

Fig. 2.1 Compensating variation of a fall in a 2-goods setting

Figure 2.1 is taken from Johansson (1991, Figure 4.6.b), and is an illustration of compensating variation in a 2-goods setting. The two axes are for quantities x of goods 1 and 2, and the straight line $C1$ is the initial budget constraint. The individual optimizes consumption at point $E1$, where the budget line $C1$ is tangent to indifference curve $U1$. Suppose the alternative outcome involves a fall in price of good 1 relative to the price of good 2, so that the new budget constraint is $C2$ and the individual's utility is maximized under a different consumption set: point $E2$. To derive the compensating variation regarding this change, a third budget constraint, $C3$, which is parallel to the new constraint and tangent to the original indifference curve is drawn. The point of tangency, $E3$, is a point where the relative prices are equal to those after the change and the individual is as well off as before the change. The distance marked 'CV' represents in terms of good 2 the amount of money that, taken away from the individual at point $E2$, will leave him/her as well off as at point $E1$: the compensating variation. For a more detailed discussion, see for example Boadway and Bruce (1984, Chapter 7), or Johansson (1991, Chapter 4).

The actual amount of compensating variation concerning the consumption of a single good can be derived in two ways. One is the 'revealed preference' approach, which is based on actual information on individual expenditures. An individual's behaviour of purchasing x units of a good at price p is here interpreted as evidence that he/she prefers this combination compared to both consuming $x-1$ and being richer by p, and consuming $x+1$ and being poorer by p. Therefore, compensating variation for x *at the margin* equals the price of the good. But this leaves open the possibility that the intra-marginal units yielded much higher utility than the marginal unit, so the money value of the marginal unit is a poor indicator of total utility from all units. This will not matter if the changes from B to A are small, but it will if they are very large. The second way is the 'expressed preference' approach, also known as the 'contingent valuation' approach. This approach does not rely on the existence of actual markets. The monetary value of a given outcome to an individual is elicited through a series of contingent questions that asks the respondent to picture him/herself in a hypothetical market-like situation.

When the change in question is preferable (not preferable), then compensating variation is positive (negative): therefore, a large part of the empirical literature refer to this as willingness-to-pay (willingness-to-accept).[4] See Table 7.8 of Drummond *et al.* (1997) for a summary of these related concepts.

2.2.2 Life years

Naturally, health economists are particularly interested in the contribution that health makes to an individual's sense of wellbeing, so the appropriate way to measure health in this context is a central concern. The simplest and most widely used measure of health is how long an individual still has to live (their life expectancy) which is typically measured in years (though in desperate situations it may be measured in much smaller units, such as days or hours). But an individual may not value all life years equally, depending for instance on the stage of life that the individual is at. Life years may also be valued differently according to how healthy that life year is going to be, but that will be dealt with in Section 2.2.3.

Life years as a natural unit

Many analyses in environmental and transport economics use life years as the outcome measure. It is also used in health economics, when the dominant gain from a change is in extra life expectancy rather than the relief of pain or disability. The natural unit can take two forms. One is the difference in the average number of years an average individual from a given population is expected to live, under the baseline and alternative scenarios. This is based on the change in the relevant mortality rates. Thus, the change in risk of death over a given period of time, say in the next 12 months, is another way of expressing this change in the expected number of life years to be enjoyed by the individual. But if not all extra (healthy) life years are regarded as of equal value by the individual, we have to go a step further.

The subjective value of life years

Most individuals will prefer a longer life to a shorter one, or a lower mortality risk to a higher one, and thus, they derive utility from life years. However there is no straightforward concept that embodies the concept of the subjective value to an individual of his/her life years. Both theoretical and empirical studies concerning life years move straight from natural units to monetary values.

Monetary value of life years

Since there is no explicit market in which individuals can buy or sell extra life years, Figure 2.1 needs to be amended to express the monetary value of life years. An illustration is given in Figure 2.2, taken from Johansson (1991, Figure 3.2). The vertical axis shows income and the horizontal axis shows life years measured in some appropriate

---

[4] The relationship is reversed for equivalent variation. It is when the change in question is *not* preferable that equivalent variation is positive, and individuals will be willing to pay positive amounts to *avoid* the alternative outcome.

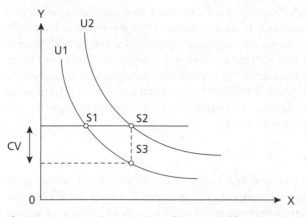

Fig. 2.2 Compensating variation of increased life years

way (e.g. life expectancy at present age). The initial state is indicated by point S1 and the change in question involves a move from there to point S2: an improvement in life years with no change in income. The amount of money that can be taken away from the individual and leave him/her as well off as at point S1 corresponds to the vertical distance between point S2 and the initial indifference curve U1. An important difference between this and Figure 2.1 above is that here, there is no reference to relative prices or to individual optimization. The gradient of the straight line (not drawn) through points S1 and S3 approximates the implicit exchange rate between money and life years for the individual. As is clear, the larger the difference between S1 and S2, the less precise this becomes (unless the nature of the indifference curves is such that a unit change in health leads to a constant compensating variation, which is a highly restrictive assumption).

In order to elicit the value of a change in mortality risks through the revealed preference approach, suppose an individual is indifferent between a safer job with a lower wage (S3) to a less safe job with a higher wage (S1) then, other things being equal, the decreased money wage will be his/her compensating variation for the additional safety in the first job. Alternatively, the expressed preference approach will look at individual willingness-to-pay (S2−S3) for a given mortality risk reduction (S2−S1), say a reduction of 1 in 100,000 over the next 12 months. For a critique of these techniques, which involve equating finite money amounts with the change in the probability of losing something to which most individuals are likely to assign an infinite value were it about to be lost for certain, see Broome (1978).

2.2.3 Health

In the discussion in the preceding section, no account was taken of the fact that the extra life years being offered to the individual might not be healthy ones. Indeed they might be so bad that the individual would rather not have them. So the (health-related) quality of a life year needs to be considered alongside the number of life years.

It is quite possible to do this without integrating the two measurements, i.e. measuring changes in life expectancy separately from, say, changes in disability status. But within the present context these separate measures cause problems if they are left incommensurable, just as was the case with goods measured in different natural units (beer, haircuts and hats). So the obvious next step is to find ways of eliciting the subjective value of each component of health to the individual, so that some utility-type measure can be used. And from that it is but a short step in principle to derive a monetary value for it. That is what this section is all about.

Is there a natural unit?

The closest we can get to a natural unit in the measurement of unhealthiness (as distinct from life expectancy) is the presence or absence of disease (morbidity) or the presence or absence of some manifestation of disease, such as physical or mental disability, pain, depression, requiring others to care for you, etc. In this vague sense very few of us are 'healthy', as reflected in the old joke that the only healthy people are those who have not yet been adequately investigated! In general, counting the number or persistence of symptoms gets us into the same difficulties over incommensurability as with beer, haircuts and hats, so it does not seem productive to linger at this level of measurement.

The subjective value of health

In general terms the counting of diseases is less useful in reaching the subjective value of changes in health than assessing the severity of the consequences of diseases as they impact on the aspects of health that mainly concern people. These are such characteristics as pain and disability. It is quite feasible to measure these instantaneously (present or absent at this moment), and that is typically what many instruments used to assess health-related quality-of-life do. Such instruments rely on repeated assessments to be taken over time to estimate the duration of the phenomenon in question. Methods such as rating scales, standard gamble, and time-trade-off can be used to discover how an individual rates the relative severity of different health states in subjective terms. But it makes more sense to assign states a specified duration before eliciting a subjective value for them, since this may affect that value.[5] If the subjective value of a health state is expressed on an interval scale anchored at Dead equals zero and Healthy equals one, then it can be integrated with life expectancy data for that individual and, by building up a profile representing the time spent in each state, we could generate a measure of quality-adjusted life expectancy measured in Quality-Adjusted Life Years (QALYs) using values that are specific to that individual. In that

---

[5] Another theoretical possibility is to first describe entire health profiles by identifying different health states through time and the duration of each state, and to have these profiles valued in terms of 'healthy-years equivalents'. The practical difficulty of such an approach is that the number of combinations of all possible health states, varying as they will in their order of occurrence and their respective durations, will be far too large for each of them to be individually evaluated and be matched to each individual's circumstances.

respect it remains compatible with the earlier postulate that individuals are to be regarded as the best judges of their own (health-related) welfare.[6]

The monetary value of health

The monetary value of different health states to a particular individual can also be elicited using contingent valuation methods. If the QALY concept is used to describe the health state to be valued, then since 1 QALY implies 1 year in full health, its monetary value is conceptually equal to the monetary value of a life year (providing that this was assumed to be a healthy life year).

2.3 Different ways of measuring how well off a group is

Each of the above ways of measuring changes in individual welfare could be used (with varying degrees of difficulty) to measure changes in the welfare of the social group to which that individual belongs. But this requires two key issues to be addressed in each case: the first of these is whether the measure is ordinal or cardinal, and the second is whether (and in what way) the measure is interpersonally comparable (or can be made so). At a societal level there is another important consideration which did not arise at individual level, namely, does it matter to that society *who* are the gainers and/or losers from any change? If it does, then the nature of this concern with the distribution of gains and losses needs to be made explicit. For that reason we shall now consider different rules for making social judgements using whichever of these individual data are selected as the main focus of policy interest.

But before doing that there are some contextual matters that need to be noted. It is here assumed that a prior decision has been made as to precisely who comprises the community of individuals about whom the judgement about a change in welfare is being sought. It could be patients with a particular condition being treated by a particular doctor at a particular time, or the whole of humankind, or any policy-relevant subset in between these two extremes. In health economics, evaluation is often conducted from the perspective of a health service, and the relevant community then becomes its actual and potential users and those who finance it. The second contextual matter turns on how the performance of the relevant organization (e.g. a health service) is actually measured. If it is expected to report primarily on its impact upon the health of the relevant community (given its budget constraint) then it will focus on measures of health rather than measures of general welfare. Costs which do not fall on its budget, and benefits which do not show up as health gains, will not be a major concern (indeed sometimes get ignored altogether). Although it may be justifiable in certain circumstances for people to limit the perspective of the analysis to that of a specific institution or budget, it is advisable for this to be made explicit.

---

[6] The concept of the QALY per se does not prescribe how the health state should be described or whose values it should reflect. For instance, Broome (1993) argues for an alternative interpretation of the QALY concept, not based on individual preference satisfaction, but on the good for an individual.

In what follows it will be assumed that these strategic decisions about what perspective to adopt have been made appropriately for the decision in hand, so that we can concentrate upon the measurement and valuation issues that are thrown up in each case. The important attributes of each variant of each rule are its implied individual value function, its implied social maximand, and its implications for the weight to be given to distributional considerations of one sort or another.

2.3.1 Simple maximization

A very common decision rule is to calculate the sum of the item that is of policy interest, and to choose the alternative social situation that will give the largest sum. The necessary conditions for this to work are that the unit of measurement is on an interval scale with a unique zero, and that each unit is of equal social value across different individuals.

Classical utilitarianism assumes that individual utilities satisfy all of these requirements, and that the social decision rule is the maximization of the sum of individual utilities. In other words, if the alternative scenario involves a decrease in individual i's utility and an increase in individual j's utility, and if the latter is larger than the former, then the loss incurred to i is more than compensated for (at the aggregate level) by the gain to j. Therefore there is an increase in overall utility and the alternative outcome is better than the baseline. Figure 2.3 illustrates this 2-person example. The axes represent cardinal and comparable utilities of individuals i and j. Points B and A stand for the outcomes of the baseline and alternative scenarios. The straight line through point B has a gradient of -1, and this is the locus of points under which the sum of individual utilities is constant. If point A lies to the north-east of this line, then the alternative scenario is better than the baseline scenario. Since the assumption is that a unit of utility is of equal social value no matter who is enjoying it, the implication is that it does not matter whether the person who gets the additional utility is well off or badly off. Some classical utilitarians, unhappy about this, have argued for the 'law' of diminishing marginal utilities to be adduced as well, so that an extra unit of a good will produce more utility if given to a worse off person than to a better off person, and therefore the maximization of the sum of individual utilities will reflect concerns for distribution. However, this concern for distribution is not incorporated in the social decision rule, but in the manner in which individual utility is expressed numerically. The introduction of 'caring externalities' into the analysis (as outlined in the introductory section of this chapter) is another instance of this sort of device. For this reason it is appropriate to say that this aggregation rule itself has no concern for distribution.

Simple maximization can also be applied to the monetary values of goods (as in the maximization of National Income), to life years, to disability-free life years, or to QALYs, but the same measurement properties are required in each case for this to make sense. In the latter case, the QALY must be measured on an interval scale with a unique zero and must be interpersonally comparable (i.e. a QALY must have the same social value no matter who is enjoying it). Interpersonal comparability requires some postulate to be made about what is assumed to be of equal social value across all

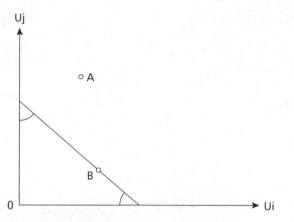

Fig. 2.3 Simple sum of individual utilities

individuals (Williams 1996). In the case of QALYs this is typically that being dead is to be regarded as of equal value (zero) for everybody, and that healthy (equal to 1) is to be regarded as of equal value to everybody. Note 'is to be regarded as' is not the same as 'is'. This is a matter of what the underlying assumptions are, not of the facts of the situation. The question to be asked is not 'is this assumption true?' but 'is this assumption appropriate in the particular policy context?'. Yet again there is no explicit concern with distributional issues here.

2.3.2 The no-loser constraint

The no-loser constraint, which is the distinctive feature of Paretian Welfare Economics, means that none of the individuals within the group should become worse off under the alternative scenario compared to the baseline. Any measure that will enable a judgement to be made at individual level about whether that individual regards him/herself as better or worse off can be subjected to this rule. In order to determine whether or not the alternative outcome is better than the baseline, this constraint itself does not require either cardinality or interpersonal comparability of individual utilities. However, if the extent to which one outcome is better than the other is also required, then sum ranking becomes necessary. Figure 2.4 illustrates the no-loser constraint by using broken lines. Unlike usual indifference curves, where points on the line represent alternatives which are neither better nor worse than the baseline, the broken lines here are better than the baseline, because along these lines, the utility of one individual is improved without decreasing the utility of the other individual. In order to satisfy the constraint, point A now has to lie either to the north-but-not-west, or to the east-but-not-south, of point B. At a practical level, this means that if any party expresses dissatisfaction with the alternative scenario, then it cannot be unambiguously an improvement in social welfare. Since the implication of this is that the baseline scenario will be maintained unless there is unanimous agreement for change, the no-loser constraint is a very conservative rule.

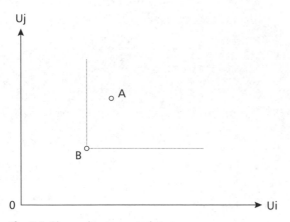

Fig. 2.4 The no-loser constraint

Since everybody, including the worst off, is guaranteed that they will not be made worse off, it may be said that there is some concern for distribution. However, given that the rule will approve of a change that benefited only the best off, this concern for distribution is severely limited.

2.3.3 The no-loser constraint with hypothetical compensation in terms of goods (the theory of CBA)

The no-loser constraint denies the relevance of the relative amount of benefit enjoyed by the gainers and losers, so an alternative situation which, compared with the baseline, would yield enormous benefits to most individuals in the society but which imposes very small losses on a few, will be ruled out of consideration. This made the no-loser constraint *with hypothetical compensation* rather more attractive for policy purposes, since it allows the evaluation of alternatives such as the one just described. This corresponds to the Kaldor–Hicks criterion, and to some extent constitutes the theoretical foundation for cost-benefit analysis (CBA).

If the alternative scenario will make some individuals better off and other individuals worse off, it stipulates that what we need to test is whether, by rearranging the distribution of the targeted item from the potential winners to the potential losers, it would be possible for all parties to be at least as well off as under the baseline outcome. (Note the closeness of this thought experiment to compensating variation.) Figure 2.5 shows a community indifference curve, which is defined as a locus of those points that offer enough goods so that, with appropriate redistribution (i.e. with the winners compensating to the losers) both parties could remain exactly as well off as at the baseline distribution.[7] The axes now represent goods, 1 and 2, and no longer individual

---

[7] A community indifference curve is defined for a given *distribution* of output mix *B* between individuals *i* and *j*, indicated by point D_b, and not simply for output mix *B*. The curve is formed by combining the individual indifference curves I_i and I_j. For details, see Boadway and Bruce (1984).

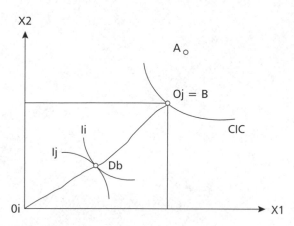

Fig. 2.5 The Kaldor criterion

utility. If point *A* lies to the north-east of the community indifference curve, it satisfies the 'no-losers with hypothetical compensation' constraint. Now, if this redistribution were in fact to take place, then the alternative scenario will satisfy both of the earlier rules above: there will be a net increase in the sum of individual utilities, and there will be no losers. However, since the criterion does not require that the redistribution actually takes place, not only is the second rule not satisfied, but neither is the first. There are several things to note. First, the focus of this criterion is on the total level of goods or output that, with some appropriate redistribution amongst the parties, has the potential to satisfy the no-loser constraint. In other words, the criterion is not concerned about actual individual utility, or its sum. Second, as is mentioned above, when there are more than two goods, total output cannot be represented by a simple addition of the natural units, and so a community indifference curve has to be adduced. It is important to keep in mind that this curve is based on the marginal rate of substitution of individual indifference curves, and therefore is usually expected to be convex to the origin. Third, since the central concern of the criterion is total goods, regardless of whose hands they are in or how individuals fare in terms of utility, there is no concern for the distribution of utility.

2.3.4 The no-loser constraint with hypothetical compensation in terms of money (Practical CBA)

The rule just discussed in Section 2.3.3 operates in an abstract world, and has severe practical limitations in the real world, because testing whether or not the alternative scenario lies to the north-east of the community indifference curve for the baseline scenario is quite impractical. The solution to the problem within actual CBAs is to refer to the sign of the simple sum of individual compensating variations as a test for the satisfaction of the Kaldor criterion. In other words, the (hypothetical) redistribution of goods is here replaced with (hypothetical) compensation in money. If an individual is a winner (loser) then his/her compensating variation is positive (negative), and thus if the sum of all individual compensating variations is positive, then the

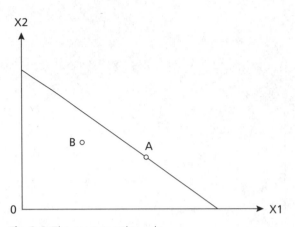

Fig. 2.6 The compensation rule

money value of the gains exceeds the *money value* of the losses, and there must therefore be a net benefit of some kind at the societal level.

However, it is known that, strictly speaking, passing this test does not necessarily guarantee the satisfaction of the criterion, unless stringent and unrealistic conditions regarding individual value functions are met.[8] An intuitive illustration is given in Figure 2.6. (For a more technical argument, see Boadway 1974; Foster 1976; Boadway and Bruce 1984). The gradient of the straight line represents the exchange rate between goods 1 and 2 under the alternative outcome. This gradient, in the case leading from Figure 2.1 above, represents the marginal rate of substitution between the two goods, which is shared across all individuals. In the case leading from Figure 2.2, the gradient is the average marginal rate of substitution across all affected individuals.[9] Now, the requirement that the sum of individual compensating variations be positive is equivalent to requiring that point *B* lies to the south-west of this straight line. This is because goods under point *A* can (hypothetically) be converted to a larger sum of money than those under point *B*, and therefore an appropriate redistribution of the yield of the alternative outcome must make all parties at least as well off as under the baseline scenario. However, whereas the satisfaction of the Kaldor–Hicks criteria shown in Figure 2.5 adopted as the border between good and bad changes a convex curve in the goods space, this test adopts as the border between good and bad changes a straight line in the same space, and therefore they cannot be equivalent. This arises because in the earlier case we were measuring individual compensating variation under a given distribution of goods, whereas now we are measuring individual

---

[8] The same applies to the relationship between the sum of individual equivalent variations and the satisfaction of the Hicks criterion.

[9] If Figure 2.2 is operationalized in the context of some *unit* of health (or year of life), and not in the actual degree of improvement each individual will get, and if the change in health under the alternative scenario is to differ across recipients, then a weighted average reflecting this variation is necessary. A necessary assumption is that compensating variation is constant over different degrees of health improvement.

compensation under all distributions of goods, and diminishing marginal rates of substitution at individual level are left out.

An alternative to this is to re-interpret aggregated compensating variations in light of maximizing aggregated individual utility, and not the Kaldor criterion. In this case, a functional relationship from individual income to individual utility, and another from individual utility to social welfare needs to be specified. The implied assumption of equating the simple sum of individual compensating variation with social welfare is that marginal social welfare of individual income $(\partial W / \partial y_i)$ is equal across all individuals.[10] While there are some theoretical efforts to account for variation in this in terms of weights that correct for income distribution (Little and Mirrlees 1974; Ray 1984; Layard and Walters 1994), such attempts are limited in the empirical literature.

CBA conducted by simply aggregating individual compensating variation exhibits no concern with distributional issues, unless appropriate distributional weights are applied.

2.3.5 Cost-per-QALY analysis

We will now move into an explicitly non-welfarist framework, i.e. one in which consequences of alternative policies are not necessarily valued in the way that each affected individual would value them. In the health care field, these consequences are typically health gains within a community. These health gains do not have to be conceived of in QALY terms, but since the QALY is the distinctive contribution of contemporary health economics, it is the use of the QALY that we will concentrate on here. In the non-welfarist framework, the 'quality-adjustment' in the QALY will be standardized, and applied uniformly to all affected people, no matter what their own individual valuations might be.

So far we have presented CBA as an analysis of individual compensating variations, in which all matters relevant to the comparison between the baseline and alternative scenarios have to be evaluated in monetary terms by the affected individuals. However, there is a variant of CBA that defers the introduction of monetary values until the final phase of the process. One central outcome measure, in this case the number of QALYs gained, will be left in non-monetary units while all of the other inputs and outputs are valued and aggregated in money terms. The decision rule then becomes: choose that option which produces QALYs at least cost (the latter expressed in money terms). This is equivalent to maximizing QALYs subject to a resource constraint, as with simple maximization in Section 2.3.1 above. Instead of generating and using an explicit money value for a QALY, an implicit value emerges only when the decision-maker decides whether or not the cost of the extra QALY can be afforded. If it can, we know the minimum value of a QALY from the decision-maker's standpoint, and if it can't we know the maximum value.

One reason for not adopting a money valuation from the outset is typically that many people are very uneasy about setting explicit money values on life and suffering,

---

[10] The terminology often used in the literature is 'marginal social utility of income' and 'social marginal utility of income'.

even though such decisions have to be made, and the monetary valuation of goods such as preserving human life and limb cannot be avoided altogether.

But can the measurement properties of the QALY sustain this treatment? As noted earlier the aggregation of QALYs across individuals requires some special assumptions to be made about what is to be regarded as of equal social value between individuals (namely being dead and being healthy). In this version of CBA matters are typically carried one stage further, and a common set of values is attached to each and every health state, usually based on the mean or median values assigned to that state either by patients or by the general population. In either case the values of the particular individuals who are gaining or losing QALYs are not the key feature. The argument for using population values (in a public policy context) is that they are the people who both meet the costs (through taxation) and are the potential beneficiaries (in a state system with universal coverage). But the important matter to note here is that we have moved away from the welfarist position that claims the welfare of individuals as judged by themselves is the only legitimate consideration to take into account when making judgements about changes in the welfare of a group. Here we are maximizing the health of a community in terms of QALYs that reflect some kind of societal valuations. Depending on how these valuations are elicited, they may or may not have the required interval properties, but they are always treated as if they do have them.

Cost-per-QALY analysis using a standardized set of values for everybody shows some concern for distributional equity in the sense that a unit of health is valued equally across the population.

2.3.6 Introducing explicit equity weights

It has been noted *en passant* that occasionally an attempt has been made to accommodate various distributional concerns through special devices (such as assuming diminishing marginal utility of goods or of income, or introducing 'caring externalities', or having a 'no losers' constraint). The one specific distributional issue that has always interested economists is the reduction of inequalities, usually in income and wealth. But in the context of health economics it is inequalities in health that have been the central concern (and they seem to be closely related empirically to inequalities in income and wealth). Much effort has been devoted to finding appropriate ways of measuring the extent of such inequalities, all of which implicitly entail attaching some weight to an individual according to where he/she is located in frequency distribution of the target variable, be it income, or wealth, or health. (For a review of these measures, see Cowell 1995.) These weights then function as a kind of 'equity weight' if these summary measures are used as the basis for social judgements about how good or bad one distribution is compared with another.

Although the reduction of inequalities in health has frequently been displaced as the focus of policy interest by reducing inequalities (after controlling for health) in health care resources, in access, or in utilization (Culyer and Wagstaff 1993; Wagstaff and van Doorslaer 2000), recently there has been an upsurge of interest in the direct elicitation of such weights from individuals in the relevant population (Neuberger *et al.* 1998; Ubel *et al.* 1999; Ratcliffe 2000).

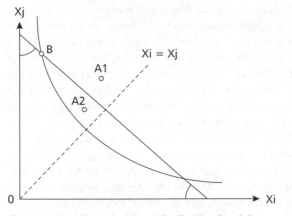

Fig. 2.7 CBA with and without distributional weights

Figure 2.7 is an illustration of how such weights would be incorporated in a cost-per-QALY analysis. (Ignore the curve for the time being.) On the two axes are the amount of the health (measured as quality-adjusted life expectancy) on offer to individuals i and j. If the analysis were to be neutral to distribution, the critical locus is a straight line through point B with gradient of -1. If point A lies to the north-east of this line, (e.g. at A_1) the alternative outcome is preferable to the baseline outcome. There are two ways in which to introduce concern for distribution and equity into the analysis. One is by looking at the distribution of the outcome measure across individuals (i.e. the consequences), and the other is by looking at individual choice and liability (i.e. the process).

In the first of these strategies we would introduce a social welfare contour through point B (the existing distribution of health) which is convex to the origin and thus reflects an aversion to health inequalities in that society. The stronger this aversion, the greater the curvature of the contour (i.e. the more different it is from the straight line through B, which reflected no aversion to inequality). In this new situation a point such as A_2 will be preferable to B, even though it lies to the south-west of the straight line. What this says is that the people in that community would be prepared to lower the average level of health in the community as a whole in order to reduce inequalities in its distribution. Since a move from point B to point A_2 implies a loss for individual j, the no loser constraint is violated.

Let us suppose that this social welfare contour came from a social welfare function with constant elasticity of substitution, that is:

$$W = (\alpha h_i^{-r} + \beta h_j^{-r})^{-1/r}, \quad h_i, h_j \geqslant 0, \alpha + \beta = 1, r \neq 0,$$

where W stands for (health related) social welfare, h_i represents the level of health of individual i, α and β are scale parameters, and r is for the degree of aversion to inequality. (For a similar approach, see for example Little and Mirrlees 1974; Layard and Walters 1994; Wagstaff 1994.) Here, it is assumed that $\alpha = \beta$. The curve pictured in the figure is an iso-welfare curve of such a social welfare function, where $r > -1$. (cf.

the straight line in the same figure corresponds to the case where $r = -1$.) The implication of such a social welfare function is that gains to the better off are less socially valuable than gains to the worse off. The 'equity weight' which reflects this would be derived from the marginal rate of substitution along the iso-welfare curve (i.e. the tangent at whatever point we happen to be). For examples that explore the application of such weights see Little and Mirrlees (1974) or Ray (1984), who use them to adjust for income distribution in a full-scale CBA, and Williams (1997), who uses them to adjust for variation in expected lifetime QALYs, in a non-welfarist context.

But this same social welfare function can also be interpreted in another way that is relevant to equity weights. Instead of assuming that $\alpha = \beta$, we could give more weight to the one than to the other. This offers a way to reflect different moral claims that individuals may have on social resources designed to improve their health which may depend on whether the individual is regarded as responsible, to some extent at least, for the bad situation they are in. In the field of health care this issue is hotly debated concerning smokers versus non-smokers, but it can be extended to cover any action which might be held to indicate that the individual has knowingly placed his/her own health in jeopardy. The issue then is whether this was in a 'good cause' (e.g. rescuing someone from a fire) or whether it was purely for enjoyment (e.g. sporting injuries), since the moral claim on other people's resources might depend on such judgements. For a much fuller analysis of the various ways in which concerns about distributive justice can be incorporated into welfare economics, see Williams and Cookson (2000).

2.4 Concluding remarks

The key concepts that appear in the foregoing sections are summarized in Tables 2.1 and 2.2. Table 2.1 is for the outcome measures at the individual level explored in Section 2.2, and represents how the kinds of outputs and the categories of their measurement relate to each other. Table 2.2 lists the six criteria discussed in Section 2.3, and gives brief notes regarding their implied maximand and their concern for distribution.

Our main purpose in this chapter has been to identify the methodological differences that exist between economic evaluations conducted according to welfarist principles, and economic evaluations that have stepped outside that framework in various

Table 2.1 The outcome measure at the individual level

Types			
Category	Goods	Life years	Health
Natural units	Amount of the good	Life expectancy Mortality rates	Diseases (?) Morbidities (?)
Subjective values	Ordinal utility Cardinal utility	(Utility of life years)	Utility of health QALYs
Monetary values	Compensating variation Equivalent variation	Of statistical life Of a life year	Of health Of QALYs

Table 2.2 The criterion for aggregation at the social level

	Implied social maximand	**Concern for distribution**
Simple maximization	Natural units Subjective values Monetary values	None
The no-loser constraint	Natural units Subjective values Monetary values	Nobody should be worse off than in the initial situation
The no-loser constraint with hypothetical compensation in terms of goods	Natural units	None
The no-loser constraint with hypothetical compensation in terms of money	Monetary values	None
Cost-per-QALY analyses	Health	All QALYs are equal
Explicit equity weights	Health, traded off with equity	By outcome levels By individual liability

ways. To the latter we have applied the term 'non-welfarist', to indicate that the only thing they have in common is that they are *not welfarist*. By 'welfarist' we mean postu-lating that the only arguments that are permitted to enter a social welfare function are those encapsulating measures of individual utility as assessed by each individual at the relevant moment. Non-welfarist approaches may differ markedly one from another, so there is no single paradigm which encompasses them all. For this reason we have eschewed the use of the term 'extra-welfarist', because some people seem to think that this is a particular methodological position which goes beyond welfarism.

When appraising alternative methodological approaches it is essential to have conceptual clarity about the respects in which they differ. It is also advantageous to have terminological clarity, though this is not absolutely essential. The great danger with terminological ambiguity is that people do not realize that the same term is being used by different people to mean different things. As an example of this we may take the rival positions taken by different people about terms such as cost-effectiveness analysis, cost-utility analysis, and cost-benefit analysis. According to one school of thought, if both inputs and outputs are expressed in money terms, then the analysis is a cost-benefit analysis; but if the inputs are in money terms and the primary outcome is in a preference-based non-monetary unit such as the QALY, then the analysis is a cost-utility analysis; and finally, if the inputs are in money terms and the central output is in a non-preference-based non-monetary 'natural' unit, then the analysis is a cost-effectiveness analysis. This is the position taken for example by Johannesson (1996); Drummond *et al.* (1997). Another set of terminology, advocated by, amongst many others, Gold *et al.* (1996), holds that cost-utility analysis (as defined above) is a subset of cost-effectiveness analysis, but from the societal perspective. Nord (1999) deals with the matter by calling them 'cost-value' analyses if they purport to value outcomes at all. Yet another approach refers to analyses that concern allocative efficiency as cost-benefit analyses, and those that address technical efficiency as cost-effectiveness analyses, which is the view of Donaldson (1998) and Currie *et al.* (2000). We have tried to avoid the issue as to whether 'cost-utility analysis' is a subset of CBA or a subset of CEA by simply calling it 'Cost-per-QALY analysis', which, after all, is what most such studies actually are. This leaves open the issue of how the 'quality adjustment' in the QALY is carried out, which could range from the average monetary value assigned by a group of individuals to some idiosyncratically defined health state, to the median value assigned by that same population to a generic health state when asked to say how that state should be regarded as a matter of public policy. So cost-per-QALY analysis could range over a very broad range of alternative methodological positions concerning whose values count and how they are to count. The important general message, however, is that it is essential to be clear about what the underlying conceptual differences are between the different approaches to economic evaluation, and to be aware that these broad classificatory terms are not always used in precisely the same way by all writers.

There is a growing body of research investigating the conditions under which what we are here calling 'cost-per-QALY analysis' will be equivalent to full-scale CBA (see for example Phelps and Mushlin 1991; Johannesson 1995; Garber and Phelps 1997; Donaldson 1998; Dolan and Edlin 2000). These studies demonstrate that some very restrictive conditions need to be placed on individual utility functions regarding QALYs if this equivalence is to be established. How is this to be interpreted? If the objective is to work within a welfarist framework, then this is bad news. It implies that it is not easy to justify the belated introduction of a unique monetary value for a QALY. However, for non-welfarists, whose objective is *not* to reproduce the results of standard welfarist full-scale CBA, this demonstration of non-equivalence is a great relief!

The choice between whether to work within a welfarist or a non-welfarist framework when conducting a piece of policy analysis is not a simple one, and there are circumstances when doing both might be appropriate. When assessing a health care technology, those with a commercial interest in it might well be primarily interested in knowing what the beneficiaries would be prepared to pay for it, and what it will cost the private producers to provide it. If discriminatory pricing were possible, this would bring the economic appraisal very close to a financial appraisal. But as well as marketing the technology directly to 'consumers', a major potential purchaser might be a health provider who wishes to know whether the technology is cost-effective rather than profitable. This will point to the use of a non-welfarist framework in which a wider range of service costs (and perhaps also costs borne by others) has to be taken into account, and in which health gains are measured not by what the beneficiaries are willing to pay for them, but by what the funders (e.g. taxpayers or policy-holders) are willing to pay for them. Even the commercial producers of the technology will need to know this if they are to be able to provide the evidence to get the technology accepted by the providing agency. Conversely, when provider agencies are trying to persuade their funders that their policies are justified, they may well find it useful to have data on what different groups of individuals would be willing to pay for the benefits of rival technologies. So there is no simple rule to apply, such as that the private sector will be interested in a welfarist approach and the public sector in a non-welfarist approach.

Finally, it is not helpful to approach these issues looking for the 'theoretically correct' approach which is then to be regarded as 'the gold standard' by which to judge the inadequacies of the other approaches. Economic evaluations are conducted to help people make specific decisions, and each such decision is set in a particular policy context. It is this policy context which is important in determining what is the *appropriate* methodology to use. If it is the case that policy is to be based only on the effects of each alternative on the welfare of each individual in some specified group, as judged by each of them for themselves, and any policy option which leaves any individual in that group worse off is to be rejected, then that makes one of the methodological stances sketched out above the appropriate one to use. But if it is the case that policy is to be based primarily upon its capacity to reduce inequalities in the distribution of socially-valued health between the individuals in the relevant group, then quite a different methodological stance, also discussed above, will be the appropriate one to adopt. You cannot get the methodological stance right until you have got the decision context right!

Acknowledgements

At the time of writing, Aki Tsuchiya was an Overseas Post-Doctoral Research Fellow of the Japan Society for the Promotion of Science and a Visiting Research Fellow of the Centre for Health Economics, University of York. Alan Williams is grateful to his colleagues in the Centre for Health Economics at the University of York for keeping him going despite his being well past his sell-by-date! Richard Cookson, Mike Drummond, Hugh Gravelle, Katharina Hauck, Atsuo Kishimoto and Ali McGuire have given helpful comments. The usual disclaimer applies.

References

Boadway, R. (1974). The welfare economic foundations of cost-benefit analysis. *Economic Journal*, 84, 926–39.

Boadway, R. and Bruce, N. (1984). *Welfare economics*. Basil Blackwell, Oxford.

Broome, J. (1978). Trying to value a life. *Journal of Public Economics*, 9, 91–100.

Broome, J. (1993), Qalys. *Journal of Public Economics*, 50, 149–67.

Brouwer, W. and Koopmanschap, M. (2000). On the economic foundations of CEA: Ladies and gentlemen, take your positions! *Journal of Health Economics*, 19, 439–59.

Cowell, F. A. (1995). *Measuring inequality*. (2nd ed.). Prentice Hall, Englewood Cliffs, NJ.

Culyer, A. J. and Wagstaff, A. (1993). Equity and equality in health and health care. *Journal of Health Economics*, 12, 431–57.

Currie, G. R., Donaldson, C. and McIntosh, E. (2000). *'Cost-effectiveness' analysis and the 'societal approach': should the twain ever meet?* Paper presented at the HESG meeting, Newcastle.

Dolan, P., Edlin, R. (2000). *Is it really possible to build a bridge between cost-benefit analysis and cost-effectiveness analysis?* Paper presented at the HESG meeting, Newcastle.

Donaldson, C. (1998). The (near) equivalence of cost-effectiveness and cost-benefit analyses. *Pharmacoeconomics*, 13(4), 389–96.

Drummond, M. F., O'Brien, B., Stoddart, G. L. *et al.* (1997). *Methods for the economic evaluation of health care programmes*. (2nd edn). Oxford University Press, Oxford.

Foster, E. (1976). The welfare foundations of cost-benefit analysis – A comment. *Economic Journal*, 86, 353–8.

Garber, A. M. and Phelps, C. E. (1997). Economic foundations of cost-effectiveness analysis. *Journal of Health Economics*, 16, 1–31.

Gold, R. M., Siegel, J. E., Russell, L. B. *et al.* (eds). (1996). *Cost-effectiveness in health and medicine*. Oxford University Press, Oxford.

Johannesson, M. (1995). The relationship between cost-effectiveness analysis and cost-benefit analysis. *Social Science and Medicine*, 41(4), 483–9.

Johannesson, M. (1996). *Theory and methods of economic evaluation of health care*. Kluwer Academic Publishers, Dordrecht.

Johansson, P. O. (1991). *An introduction to modern welfare economics*. Cambridge University Press, Cambridge.

Jones-Lee, M. W. (1989). *The economics of safety and physical risk*. Basil Blackwell, Oxford.

Layard, R. and Walters, A. A. (1994). Allowing for income distribution. In R. Layard and S. Glasiter (eds). *Cost-benefit analysis* (2nd edn). Cambridge University Press, Cambridge (reprinted from R. Laylard and A. A. Walters (1978). *Microeconomic Theory*. McGraw-Hill).

Little, I. M. D. and Mirrlees, J. A. (1974). *Project Appraisal and Planning for Developing Countries*. Basic Books, New York.

Neuberger, J., Adams, D., Maidment, A. *et al.* (1998). Assessing priorities for allocation of donor liver grafts: Survey of the public and clinicians. *British Medical Journal*, 317, 172–5.

Ng, Y.-K. (1983). *Welfare economics: introduction and development on basic concepts*. (Revised Edition). Macmillan, London.

Nord, E. (1999). *Cost-value analysis in healthcare: making sense out of QALYs*. Cambridge University Press, Cambridge.

Phelps, C. E. and Mushlin, A. I. (1991). On the (near) equivalence of CE and CB Analyses. *International Journal of Technology Assessment in Health Care*, 7(1), 12–21.

Ratcliffe, J. (2000). Public preferences for the allocation of donor liver grafts for transplantation. *Health Economics*, 9(2), 137–48.

Ray, A. (1984). *Cost-benefit analysis: issues and methodologies*. World Bank/Johns Hopkins, Baltimore.

Ubel, P., Baron, J. and Asch, D. A. (1999). Social responsibility, personal responsibility, and prognosis in public judgements about transplant allocation. *Bioethics*, 13(1), 57–68.

Wagstaff, A. and van Doorslaer, E. (2000). Equity in health care finance and delivery. In: A. J. Culyer and J. P. Newhouse (eds). *Handbook of Health Economics* (Vol. 1B). Elsevier Science, Amsterdam.

Wagstaff, A. (1994). QALYs and the equity-efficiency trade-off. In: A. Laylard and S. Glaister (eds). *Cost-benefit analysis* (2 edn). Cambridge University Press, Cambridge (reprinted from *Journal of Health Economics*, 10, 21–41, 1991).

Williams, A. (1977). Income distribution and public expenditure decisions. In: M. Posner (ed.). *Public expenditure: allocation between competing ends*. Cambridge University Press, Cambridge.

Williams, A. (1996). *Interpersonal comparisons of welfare.* Discussion Paper 151, Centre for Health Economics, University of York.

Williams, A. (1997). Intergenerational equity: An exploration of the 'fair innings' argument. *Health Economics,* 6. 117–32.

Williams, A. and Cookson, R. (2000). Equity in health. In: A. J. Culyer and J. P. Newhouse (eds). *Handbook of Health Economics* (Vol. 1B). Elsevier Science, Amsterdam.

Chapter 3

Output measures and valuation in health

Paul Dolan

3.1 Introduction

In all countries throughout the world, there is a considerable degree of government involvement in the market for health care. If governments are going to deploy the resources at their disposal where they will be of greatest benefit, then information on the benefits associated with alternative allocations is required. This raises questions about how benefit is to be defined and measured and how it is to be allocated amongst the population. This chapter addresses these questions from a normative perspective. That is, it is concerned with how health outcomes *ought* to be measured and with how benefits *ought* to be weighted according to who receives them.

The measurement of outcomes, not only in health but elsewhere, is central to economics. The discipline is premised on the notion that every decision made by a consumer, producer, bureaucrat or politician involves some kind of trade-off between the different bundles of attributes that make up each choice. *Implicit* trade-offs can be revealed from decisions made by policy-makers in the public sector, e.g. how the benefits from additional expenditure on education are weighed against the benefits from using those resources to reduce the risk of death or serious injury. By studying such choices, it is possible to infer the implied value of different goods (for example, the value of a statistical life).

Since all resource allocation decisions, then, imply some marginal rate of substitution between different attributes, economists typically argue that consistent decision-making requires for all implicit trade-offs to be made *explicit*. This is premised on the notion that the benefits from all allocation decisions are ultimately commensurable with one another, otherwise it would be impossible to estimate a marginal rate of substitution between attributes. This in turn means that it must be possible to quantify the value of different attributes with some degree of precision. When all of these conditions are satisfied, policy-makers are able to apply a consistent set of weights which allow for *generalizability* across a wide range of different decision contexts. This means that any health outcome measure must allow for comparisons between different health care programmes which may impact upon different aspects of health in different ways.

Traditionally the impact of health care has been measured in terms of its effects on mortality but, since health is much more than merely being alive, its effects on morbidity are increasingly being taken into account. However, mortality and morbidity data say nothing about what the priority weights given to one condition relative to another ought to be. Therefore, it is necessary to not only say what conditions people are suffering from but also to say something about the impact that these conditions have on their lives. The measurement of health-related quality-of-life (HRQoL), as distinct from more clinically focused measures, aims to achieve this.

To capture the health effects of policies and programmes, then, it is necessary to say something about their effects on life expectancy and HRQoL. There now exist a number of approaches which try to combine these two attributes into a composite measure of health. One of the most widely used is the Quality-Adjusted Life Year (QALY) approach which assigns to each period of time a value corresponding to the HRQoL during that period (see Weinstein and Stason 1977). The value typically lies on a scale between 0 (to represent death) and 1 (to represent full health), although negative values for states rated as worse than dead are possible. The number of QALYs relating to a health outcome are then expressed as the value given to a particular health state multiplied by the length of time spent in that state.

The QALY has been the subject of much criticism. Many economists hold the view that the approach is too narrow in that it does not incorporate society's preferences for a fair distribution of health (see Nord 1995), or that it does not pick up a whole range of wider non-health benefits (see Mooney 1994). The responses to such criticisms from proponents of the QALY has been varied, but one common theme emerges; that is, every utility affecting characteristic and any equity preference could in principle be built into the QALY as weights. Thus, it is argued, all the arguments within the health-related social welfare function (HRSWF) can be captured within a 'super-QALY' (see Dolan and Olsen 2000a).

Other economists have rejected the QALY approach and have instead drawn on methods used in other areas of economics in an attempt to capture a wider range of benefits than those in the QALY model. For example, the contingent valuation (CV) method, which uses answers to survey questions to estimate an individual's willingness-to-pay (WTP) for a particular commodity, has been developed from its original use in estimating the value of environmental changes to value health programmes and health improvements (see Olsen and Donaldson 1998). For any health care programme, as for an environmental good, respondents can be asked for its *use* value (i.e. its value to current patients), for its *option* value (arising from its availability should care be needed in the future), and for its *existence* value (to represent the value of any concern that people may have for the programme being available to others).

More recently, conjoint analysis (CA), which uses ranking, rating or pairwise comparisons exercises to estimate the relative weights that people attach to different attributes of a commodity, has been developed from its original uses in transport economics and market research to value different treatment attributes (see Ryan and

Hughes 1997). CA can be used to: (i) calculate the QALY gains from different interventions when the various dimensions of health are used as attributes; (ii) calculate the implied WTP for those interventions when money is included as an attribute; (iii) express the value of different attributes in terms of one another (see Ryan 1998).

3.2 Theoretical questions

3.2.1 What role should health outcomes play?

Although economists agree that it is important to measure health outcomes so as to inform (and hopefully improve) decision-making, they are more divided about the precise role that health outcomes *per se* should play in determining priorities.

Broadly speaking, there are the 'welfarists' who believe that the output of health care should be judged according to the extent to which it contributes to overall welfare, as determined by individual preferences over health relative to other arguments in the utility function. Welfarists often stress the importance of equality of access to effective health care, so that, whilst individuals face the same opportunities to use health care, the exercising of individual choice is a legitimate reason for differences in health (Herrero 1996).

Then there are the 'extra-welfarists' who define the output of health care according to its contribution to health itself. This school of economists will typically focus attention on equality of health, whereby it is justifiable, at the margin, to override individual preferences in the interests of improvements in the overall level or distribution of health. This is justified on the grounds that health is fundamental to an individual's capacity to 'flourish' as a human being (Culyer and Wagstaff 1993). However, and crucial in the context of this chapter, what constitutes a health improvement is *to some extent* defined according to individual preferences by welfarists and extra-welfarists alike.

3.2.2 How should health outcomes be evaluated?

There is considerable debate amongst health economists about how health outcomes should be evaluated when comparing alternative allocations. Specifically, it is about whether or not the same health state should be given the same value across all individuals. On this issue, it is again possible to distinguish between welfarists and extra-welfarists. Because they are committed to respecting individual preferences, welfarists will take each individual to be the source of their own value. However, this may be damaging in the context of interpersonal comparisons since we might choose to return to full health a less seriously ill person over a more seriously ill person on the grounds that the former perceives the utility loss from her condition to be greater.

To avoid such problems, extra-welfarists assume that a particular health state has the same effect on all individuals. But this raises interpersonal comparability problems of its own. For example, paraplegia is likely to have much more of an effect on a builder's life than on an academic's life yet assigning the same value to the condition would imply that the utility loss was the same for both people. There is no simple solution to this problem and it remains a normative judgement about which approach to adopt. Much, of course, will turn on the extent to which any *non*-health benefits an Iindividual receives from health care are considered to be relevant.

3.2.3 How should health outcomes be distributed?

Economists typically aggregate benefits according to sum-ranking which could be justified on the grounds that it is morally preferable to confer greater benefit than less. However, in choosing how to prioritize between patients, the size of the benefit may not be the only consideration. Wagstaff (1991) proposed that an HRSWF could be used to determine the optimal distribution of the gains from health care across the population. In his analysis, the individuals start with identical endowments. However, Nord (1995) suggests that the no-treatment health profile is important in its own right and, in developing the 'fair innings' argument, Williams (1997) suggests that a person's stock of health up to the decision point should also be taken into account. Dolan and Olsen (2000b) suggest that it may also be useful to distinguish between health obtained thus far as a result of past health care and health obtained otherwise 'free'. This suggests that there may be a range of endogenously determined 'lifestyle'characteristics by which the gains received by one person might be weighte differently to those received by someone else (see Le Grand 1991).

In addition, there are a range of other potentially important personal characteristics that health gains might be weighted by. For example, those who have family who are dependent upon them might be given priority over those who do not, or those with rare skills might be given priority over those without those skills (although strictly speaking such considerations are broadening out the definition of efficiency to include the benefits received by others). A consideration motivated more by concerns for equity is that priority might be given to those who are deemed to have a greater claim, either through having previously been deprived (i.e. to compensate them) or as a result of having previously contributed a lot to society (i.e. to reward them). There are then six main equity considerations: (1) the distribution of benefits; (2) the no-treatment profile; (3) the previous health profile; (4) endogenously-determined lifestyle; (5) the impact on others; and (6) claims based on compensation or reward.

3.2.4 What is to be valued?

With regards only to health benefits that accrue to an individual recipient, the answer to this question is a simple one: it is the alternative states of health that an individual might experience over the course of her lifetime, combined with the different lengths of time that she might be in each state for. One approach, then, would be to construct profiles for all possible life paths and then to elicit individual preferences over them.

The valuation of profiles is the key feature of the healthy-years equivalent (HYE) approach which asks individuals to state the number of years in perfect health that are considered equivalent to a particular profile (see Mehrez and Gafni 1989). This approach has the advantage that it places very few restrictions on individual preferences. Specifically, in order for the number of HYEs to be a valid representation of an individual's preferences over different profiles, it is only necessary to assume that she is risk neutral with respect to (discounted or undiscounted) years in full health.

The problem with the HYE approach is that in most contexts there will be a large number of possible health profiles, each of which would require preference measment. To allow greater generalizability, an alternative approach would be to elicit preferences for one health state (of a specified duration) at a time. The value of any given profile of health could then be estimated by taking the (discounted or undiscounted) weighted average of the value for each of the health states in that profile multiplied by the time spent in each state. This is the approach adopted in the calculation of QALYs. Of course, this places greater restrictions on individual preferences since a number of assumptions have to be made when calculating this weighted average.

Bleichrodt *et al.* (1997) have established the least restrictive conditions under which the QALY model will represent individual preferences over a health profile of constant quality. In essence, they show the model will hold if an individual is risk neutral with respect to gambles over life years for *all* health states. Whilst attitudes towards time are often (and mistakenly) subsumed within attitudes towards risk, the standard QALY model assumes risk neutrality over *discounted* life years. In addition, for profiles in which health changes over time, each individual's utility function is required to b strongly separable on the time dimension; that is, the utility derived from a profile of health is equal to the sum of the utility derived from each state in that profile. Therefore, for the QALY model to fully represent individual preferences over health *outcomes*, two main assumptions are required: (i) risk neutrality over discounted life years; and (ii) additive separability.

Mooney and others have suggested that the utility associated with the treatment *process* should also be taken into account when making resource allocation decisions. Whilst it would seem that some of the examples of 'process utility' that are given, such as the fear of dentists (see Mooney 1994, p. 74), are better defined as the outcome utility associated with treatment, other examples, such as autonomy in the decision-making process (see Mooney 1994, p. 19), might represent genuine *process utility* and would be much more difficult to capture within the QALY approach. If these and other possible non-health benefits are considered to be relevant arguments in the HRSWF (and much will of course depend upon whether a welfarist or extra-welfarist approach is adopted), they could be better captured by using the CV method or CA, neither of which require the benefits of health care to be expressed solely in terms of quality and length of life. The choice of approach to valuation, then, will be largely determined by a normative judgement about the extent to which health outcomes fully capture the benefits from health care.

Those studies that have used Qualy-type apperoach, the CV method, or CA, have usually attempted to measure the (health or non-health) benefits derived from health care by an *individual* patient. However, the results are often treated as a mesure of *social* value in which they represent society's preferences over different interventions. To interpret the results in this way, it must be assumed that social preferences over different allocations of the health care budget can be represented by an HRSWF which is simply the sum of individual benefits. But it is widely acknowledged that people are also concerned with the distribution as well as the size of the benefits generated. A number of authors have proposed ways of measuring this efficiency-equity trade-off (see Wagstaff 1991, Olsen 1997, Dolan 1998). An alternative approach, discussed more fully below, has been suggested by Nord (1995), who argues that the social value of health benefits should reflect responses to person trade-off (PTO) questions asked in a social decision-making context.

3.2.5 How is it to be valued?

There are a number of different ways in which the benefits from health care can be quantified. If values are to be placed on changes in HRQoL, first a decision about the way in which health is to be described has to be made. In the context of informing resource allocation decisions across a wide range of conditions, it is necessary to measure health status across a range of different dimensions and also to combine the relative value of the different dimensions, and levels within dimensions, so as to form an overall single index. There are a number of measures which appear to fulfil these criteria, although it has been argued that, of these, the McMaster Health Utility Index (see Feeny *et al.* 1995) and the EQ-5D (see Brooks 1996) are to be preferred (see Brazier *et al.* 1999).

Once a health state descriptive system has been developed, it is necessary to determine the values to attach to the states so described, and this raises the question of which method(s) should be used. An important consideration here is the level of measurement that is required. It is now well established that different social welfare functions require different types of comparability (see Sen 1977). For example, adoption of a Rawlsian-type criterion of maximizing the welfare of the worst-off individual requires only that we know whether one person is better or worse off than another. This is referred to as level comparability and requires only that health states are expressed on an ordinal scale with no indication of how much more severe one state is compared to another. Maximizing the sum of individual utilities requires that differences in utilities can be compared; that is, unit comparability is required.

For most purposes, including those relating to the various types of economic evaluation, full comparability, which subsumes both level and unit comparability, is required. In going beyond individual orderings, full comparability means that problems associated with Arrow's General Possibility Theorem (Arrow 1951) can be avoided. For full comparability, a valuation method must produce a set of values which lie on an interval or a ratio scale. An interval scale provides information on how far apart those states are in terms of severity but it does not indicate the absolute magnitude of severity. A ratio scale is achieved when the distance from zero is known for at least one state, and thus the absolute severity can be determined for all states.

Valuations that lie on an interval scale are sufficient for the purposes of economic evaluation (see Lipscomb 1982).

The three most widely used methods that in principle generate valuations that lie on an interval scale are the visual analogue scale (VAS), the standard gamble (SG) and the time trade-off (TTO). The VAS requires respondents to rate health states on a scale, usually with endpoints represented by 0 and 100. The SG asks respondents to choose between the certainty of an intermediate health state and the uncertainty of a treatment with two possible outcomes, one of which is better than the certain outcome and one of which is worse. The object is to find the probability at which the respondent is indifferent between the certain and the uncertain alternatives. The TTO asks respondents to choose between living for a given time in a poor health state and living for a shorter time in full health. The time in full health is varied until the respondent is indifferent between the two alternatives. For more detailed descriptions of these methods, see Torrance (1986).

Because valuations from the VAS are elicited in a choice*less* context, and thus do not require people to make trade-offs between different arguments in their utility function, the method is commonly regarded by economists as theoretically inferior to the choice-based SG and TTO methods. Based on two assumptions about individual preferences, it might be expected that SG values will be higher than TTO ones. The first is that people are risk averse, implying that they will be reluctant to accept the gamble outcomes in the SG. The second is that people have a positive rate of time preference, implying that they will be more willing to give up years of life at the end of a profile, as in the TTO. Therefore, the choice of method might have important implications and, as a result, there has been considerable debate about the theoretical merits of SG and TTO.

In developing Expected Utility Theory (EUT), von Neumann and Morgenstern (1953) showed that if a cardinal utility could be expressed as equivalent to a gamble, under certain assumptions (including transitivity and independence), it would be a linear function of the risk involved in the gamble. This has led many to regard the SG as the 'gold standard' for health status measurement (see Gafni 1994). However, considerable doubt has been cast on EUT both as a positive and as a normative theory (see Camerer 1993; Richardson 1994). The SG is also advocated on the grounds that almost all decisions about health care are made under conditions of uncertainty (see Mehrez and Gafni 1991). However, the appropriateness of a valuation method is determined by its ability to act as a proxy for utility and not by its capacity to model the situation being valued (see Buckingham and Drummond 1993). In this respect, the TTO may be considered to be more appropriate since it collapses the relationship between the health profile (or state), its duration and its value into one single measure (see Richardson 1994).

However, Dolan and Jones-Lee (1997) have shown that for a response to a TTO question to provide a direct and unbiased estimate of health state value, it is necessary that: (i) there is no re-allocation of lifetime consumption; and (ii) there is no discounting of future utilities. It turns out that the effect of lifetime re-allocation is likely to be very small but that discounting can produce significantly biased estimates. Of course, time preference will play a part in *all* valuation methods since all profiles and health states are for a specified duration. But if utility independence holds, SG values will not be affected by discounting since the time spent in full health and the health state being valued is the same (Johannesson *et al.* 1994). And since time is used as the means of valuation itself in the TTO, attitudes towards time will be a more important determinant of value using this method.

It is difficult, then, to choose between SG and TTO on theoretical grounds since valuations from neither method can automatically be assumed to map directly on to utility. This is an important point since it implies rejecting the idea that the SG should be regarded as the 'gold standard' for measuring health state values. As well as the on-going debate about the relative merits of the SG and TTO, in recent years there has been a controversy of a different kind. In proposing the HYE, Mehrez and Gafni (1989) suggest how the number of healthy-years considered equivalent to a given profile should be calculated. However, the 'two-stage SG procedure' that they propose, which requires the indifference probability from a conventional SG question to be used in a second gamble over life years, has been shown to be formally equivalent to a TTO question (see Loomes 1995). Therefore, it is difficult to see what advantages there are from using a much more complicated and burdensome technique.

Besides risk and time, another important argument in an individual's utility function is wealth and in principle it would be possible to measure the extent to which an individual is willing to sacrifice wealth in order to experience one health profile or health state relative to another. Using the CV method to value HRQoL has the advantage that it allows preferences for health to be considered alongside other non-health attributes that the individual values. In contrast, for the SG and TTO methods to fully represent utility, the individual benefit from health care must be a function only of the size of the health improvement. In addition, the ability of an individual to enjoy income cannot be affected by illness. The latter of these conditions is central to a number of theoretical models (see Johannesson and Meltzer 1998) but it is not supported by empirical evidence (see Evans and Viscusi 1993 and Sloan *et al.* 1998).

However, in valuing a health state, the extent to which a respondent will consider the consequent non-health effects is likely to be limited. Moreover, it is not clear whether it is appropriate to take account of non-health preferences when valuing health outcomes. If a welfarist approach is adopted then no greater weight is given to one kind of preference over another. Therefore, if basing allocation decisions on responses to SG or TTO questions means that relevant information relating to such factors as income is ignored, then this will be seen by welfarists to be a serious weakness of the methods. However, if an extra-welfarist approach is adopted and if only health-related preferences are considered to be relevant, then the fact that the SG and TTO methods might abstract respondents away from non-health considerations will be seen as an advantage of these methods.

Rather than being used to value changes in HRQoL, the CV method is typically used to value the overall benefits of health interventions (see Olsen and Smith 2001). Respondents could be given information regarding a range of (process and outcome) attributes associated with different treatments and then asked for their maximum WTP for each treatment, thus allowing the relative value of the different attributes to be calculated. Alternatively, entire health care programmes could be described to respondents who would then be asked for their maximum WTP for each programme, perhaps through increased taxation in the context of a publicly-funded health care system. In addition, and as noted above, CA is also now being used to estimate the relative weights attached to the different attributes of different interventions. Although it is possible to infer these weights from responses to ranking and rating exercises, the majority of CA studies conducted in health care have presented respondents with a series of pairwise choices (see Ryan 1998).

In addition to the measurement of individual utility (in a much wider welfarist sense than the QALY model allows), the CV method and CA can both be used to elicit preferences over distributional concerns, or over any other factors that contribute towards the social value of health interventions. However, people's preferences over the distribution of health benefits (typically in the narrow extra-welfarist sense) have most often been elicited using the PTO method. The method was originally developed by Patrick *et al.* (1973) who called it the equivalence of numbers procedure but Nord's terminology is now widely adopted (see Nord 1993). The approach involves asking respondents how many outcomes of one kind they consider equivalent in terms of social value to a different number of outcomes of another kind. It is Nord's contention that PTO responses, unlike those to methods based on the measurement of individual utility, capture concerns that are relevant to social decision-making, such as consider-ations about the initial severity of illness (see Nord 1995).

3.2.6 Who is to value it and from which perspective?

The debate about whose values to elicit has been most prominent in the literature on valuing HRQoL although the issues raised are also relevant to the valuation of non-health benefits using the CV method and CA. Preferences can be elicited from a number of population sub-groups; from health care professionals, from patients, from those with some experience of the condition or health state, and from samples of the general public. Whilst few people recommend that HRQoL should be valued according to the preferences of health care professionals, many consider that it is most appropriate to elicit valuations from those people who are currently experiencing the health states for which values are sought (see Nord *et al.* 1999). The argument is that these are the only people who know what it is really like to be in those states and therefore the only ones capable of expressing a 'true' preference over different states of health.

However, the received wisdom is increasingly that the preferences of the general public should be used. A consensus panel convened by the United States Public Health Service recommended that the source of values should be a representative sample of the general population (see Gold *et al.* 1996). The Panel's principal reason for this was that, since the public bears the costs associated with health care decisions, they ought also to have some say in the determination of the benefits. Public preferences are also considered the most appropriate by those who advocate the 'insurance principle', the logic of which is that the preferences used to determine coverage patterns under health insurance plans should be those of the beneficiaries, as determined empirically prior to any need for specific treatments (see Hadorn 1991). In addition, if one of the purposes of the health care system is to give reassurance to the public, then resources should in part be allocated so as to reassure the public that treatment is available to alleviate the health states they fear the most (see Edgar *et al.* 1998).

In reality, of course, the distinction between patients and the public is blurred. Even in supposedly 'healthy' general populations, there is a substantial degree of ill health. Also, many people have experienced ill health at some time in their lives and many have relatives or close friends who are currently experiencing ill health (see Dolan 1999). Since there is a well-established direct positive link between the time spent in ill health and adaptation to that ill health (see Cassileth *et al.* 1984), the real question is whether or not such adaptation should be accounted for in HRQoL values. If the extent to which people are able to cope with different conditions *is* considered relevant then, since adaptation is a gradual and continuous process, there is still the question of *when* to ask patients for their preferences. Therefore, if patient preferences are to be given any weight, the question is not *whether* adaptation to illness is considered relevant (since it is) but rather *the extent* to which it is considered relevant. The literature has been almost silent on this issue.

In addition to the question of whose values should be used, there is the question of which perspective these values should be elicited from; that is, in *whose shoes* should a respondent be placed. There are essentially three types of preferences that an individual can be asked for: (i) her personal preferences regarding her own treatment independent of the treatment of anyone else; (ii) her interpersonal preferences regarding her own treatment *vis-à-vis* the treatment of other people; and (iii) her social preferences regarding the treatment of others. Many economists are critical of the social decision-maker perspective on the grounds that the respondent is not motivated by self-interest (see Johannesson 1999) but if an ethically defensible set of preferences can be derived from moral intuition or forms of ethical reasoning which are separate from self-interest, then the social perspective may be a legitimate one (see Menzel 1999). The literature has been quieter still on this issue.

3.3 Empirical evidence

3.3.1 Valuing HRQoL

The validity of the assumptions of the QALY model

With regard to the first assumption, risk neutrality, the evidence overall is of moderate risk aversion (see McNeil *et al.* 1978; Stiggelbout *et al.* 1994; Verhoef *et al.* 1994). With regard to the second assumption, additive separability, there is some evidence that the value of a health profile depends upon whether health is improving or deteriorating during that profile: if it is improving, then the profile value is higher than the value that would be implied by combining the scores for discrete states, and vice versa if health is deteriorating (see Richardson *et al.* 1996; Kupperman *et al.* 1997). Specifically, the results suggest that people focus more on the change in health in the final period. Such results cast doubt on the validity of the QALY model. However, in a different test of additive separability, Krabbe and Bonsel (1998) found that the majority of respondents were indifferent to the sequencing of health states, thus lending support to the QALY model. Therefore, the evidence relating to the assumptions of the QALY model is mixed.

Differences in SG and TTO values

There is clear evidence that the SG and TTO methods yield different valuations from the same respondents for identical descriptions of health. In accordance with *a priori* expectations, most studies have found SG values to be higher than TTO ones (see Torrance 1976; Wolfson *et al.* 1982; Read *et al.* 1984; Bleichrodt and Johannesson 1997a; Lenert *et al.* 1998) although there is some evidence for the opposite relationship (see Hornberger *et al.* 1992; Dolan *et al.* 1996). Even if differences do exist between the methods, it might be that a systematic relationship exists between them. Of particular interest is the possibility of converting values from the simple VAS method into theoretically superior SG and/or TTO ones. In a comparison of mean VAS and TTO values, Torrance (1976) suggested that the two sets of values are related to one another by a power function. Since then, a number of authors have used this function to estimate SG and TTO values from VAS ones (see Loomes 1993; van Busschbach 1994; Stiggelbout *et al.* 1996).

However, there are a number of reasons to be cautious about such findings. First, the power coefficients differ across studies (for example, a VAS score of 0.10 would convert into a TTO score of 0.23 in the Stiggelbout *et al.* study and 0.34 in the van Busschbach study). Second, the analyses were performed on aggregate- rather than individual-level data, thus making the choice between competing models more difficult as well as making inefficient use of the data. Third, the models presented by Torrance did not hold at the individual level (this is confirmed in studies reported in Dolan and Sutton (1997) and Bleichrodt and Johannesson (1997b). Fourth, van Busschbach (1994) found that the power model offered no improvement over a linear one (in a comparison of a number of different models, Dolan and Sutton (1997) conclude that linear ones perform best). It would seem, then, that VAS valuations cannot be converted into SG or TTO ones with any degree of confidence.

The relative merits of SG and TTO

Empirical assessment of the relative merits of the SG and TTO methods involves considerations of feasibility, reliability and validity. Feasibility means that the method must be acceptable to respondents. It would appear that both methods are feasible in that most studies have reported high response and completion rates (see Froberg and Kane 1989). However, in a comparison of the SG and TTO in a sample of the UK general population, Dolan *et al.* (1996) found that a variant of the TTO which used a specially designed board produced fewer missing values than the analogous version of the SG and fewer missing values than variants of the methods which used a self-completion booklet. Reliability refers to the stability of responses when all pertinent conditions remain unchanged, and is usually assessed in terms of the stability of values over short periods of time. Most studies have found little to choose between the two methods on these grounds (see Churchill *et al.* 1984; O'Connor *et al.* 1985) although Dolan *et al.* (1996) found that the 'board-based' variant of the TTO performed best.

Essentially a method is valid if it accurately reflects the concept it claims to measure. The most rigorous way to establish validity is to test construct validity. A construct is a theoretically derived notion of what an instrument is intended to measure. For example, it might be expected that the rankings of health profiles implied by calculating QALYs from SG and TTO valuations would be the same as the direct rankings of the same profiles from the same respondent. In a test of this, Bleichrodt and Johannesson (1997a) found that the correlation between the two rankings was significantly higher for TTO than for SG. Overall, then, there would appear to be little compelling evidence to favour one method over the other, although the 'benefit of the doubt' might be given to the TTO.

Differences in values according to respondent characteristics and perspective

In the first empirical study on this issue, Sackett and Torrance (1978) reported that home dialysis patients assigned higher values to health states associated with kidney dialysis than did the general public. Similarly, Boyd *et al.* (1990) found that colostomy patients valued various states of health related to their condition higher than did a healthy population, and Hurst *et al.* (1994) found that patients with rheumatoid arthritis gave higher scores to these states than did a general population sample. However, Balaban *et al.* (1986) reported no differences between valuations elicited from rheumatoid arthritis patients and those elicited from a general population sample, and Jenkinson *et al.* (1997) found no differences between how BHP patients valued their health and how the general public valued the same health states. Therefore, the evidence on this subject is not unambiguous. The results from some studies suggest that patients have higher valuations than the public; the results from others suggest that there is no difference between the preferences of the two groups.

These studies have all sought to elicit *personal* preferences from the perspective of an actual or hypothetical patient. There have been very few studies which have elicited *interpersonal* preferences, although there is currently some interest in the 'veil of ignorance' approach, behind which people do not know their precise position in society (see Richardson and Nord 1997). There are more studies relating to the elicitation of *social* preferences, most of which have asked people for their responses to PTO questions (see Nord 1995). However, it is difficult at this stage to tell how people's preferences are affected by the shoes they are placed in.

3.3.2 Valuing health outcomes using the CV method

In addition to the benefits that an individual receives directly from health care, the CV method in principle can capture both the option value and existence value of health programmes. However, this has certainly not been the case in practice. In a review of 54 CV studies from 1985 to 1998, Olsen and Smith (2001) found that 41 studies were concerned with use value only (of the remaining 13, five elicited option value, one elicited existence value, and seven studies elicited information regarding both option and existence values). Another advantage of the CV method is that it can be used to value the utility associated with the process of treatment as well as with the treatment outcomes. In this regard, the empirical evidence is more plentiful. Olsen and Smith's (2001) impression is that 'for the majority of studies there has been a WTP for a health care *product* rather than the *health produced* by the product'. In this way, the CV method is attractive to those adopting a welfarist viewpoint.

However, it is very difficult to draw general conclusions about the monetary value attached to various health and non-health outcomes from the CV studies to date. Unlike the QALY approach, which is designed to allow for comparability across health care programmes, the CV method has primarily been used to value all the attributes associated with specific programmes. This means that the aggregated WTP values from one study cannot be meaningfully compared to the aggregated WTP values from another study which valued a different programme with a different set of characteristics. Against this background, Olsen and Smith (2000) could not find any study which suggested that the WTP figures could be transferred to the valuation of another programme.

3.3.3 Valuing health outcomes using CA

CA can be used to establish the weights given to different attributes of health within the QALY model. For example, the approach has been used to estimate health state values for alternative types of treatment for breast cancer patients (see Verhoef *et al.* 1994). If price (or cost) is an attribute to be traded-off against other process and/or outcome attributes, then CA can also be used to estimate the WTP for different treatments. For example, Propper (1995) used CA to estimate the WTP to reduce NHS waiting lists and Ryan (1997) used it to look at women's WTP for assisted reproductive techniques.

However, since a large part of the motivation behind using CA in health care was to measure the importance of non-health outcomes and process attributes (see Ryan 1998), it has largely been used in the context of measuring the trade-offs that people make between the process of treatment and its consequent outcomes. From samples of patients, or respondents asked to imagine themselves in the role of patients, a number of studies have shown that people are seemingly willing to trade-off quite substantial expected gains in health (for example, in the probability of having a child in the case of fertility treatment) for better care during the process of treatment (for example, a good relationship with doctors and nurses) (see Ryan 1997). Of course, the weight that is given to information of this kind will again turn on which of the welfarist or extra-welfarist viewpoints is adopted.

3.3.4 Valuing distributional considerations

There is an ever-increasing body of evidence relating to the extent to which people are willing to trade-off the maximization of health for each of the six equity considerations highlighted above. With regard to the *distribution of benefits*, there is evidence that people are unwilling to discriminate between patients on the grounds of the size of the QALY benefit they could receive (see Nord 1993; Cookson and Dolan 1999). Other studies have shown that when asked to choose among patients with the same illness, respondents will often distribute resources in ways that will equalize outcomes (see Ubel and Loewenstein 1995, 1996). There is evidence of similar trade-offs between efficiency and equity in the context of preventative programmes (see Ubel *et al.* 1996; Lindholm *et al.* 1997). Also, people are not indifferent to the distribution of the same total gain over populations of different sizes. Specifically, it seems that there is a threshold level of benefits to the larger group above which people prefer to distribute gains to as many people as possible (see Choudhry *et al.* 1997; Olsen 2000).

With regards to the *no-treatment profile*, Nord (1993) observed that respondents often prefer to treat more severely ill patients, even if that does not bring as much benefit as treating less severely ill patients. Dolan (1998) found that the social value given to health gain was higher at lower levels of health. In contrast, Dolan and Green found that many subjects favoured treating those patients with most to gain, seemingly on the grounds that the health state the worse off would be in *after* treatment was not sufficiently good enough to warrant giving them priority. So far as the *previous health profile* is concerned, there is strong evidence to suggest that health benefits to younger people are valued more highly than similar benefits to older people (see Williams 1988; Lewis and Charny 1989; Bowling 1996).

There is now evidence to suggest that many people wish to give less priority to those whose illness is considered to be the result of an *endogenously-determined lifestyle*, such as through smoking or heavy drinking (see Williams 1988; Charny *et al.* 1989; Bowling 1996; Dolan *et al.* 1999). However, the issue of whether or not to discriminate against certain lifestyles is a hotly contested one (see Dolan and Cookson 2000). With regard to the *impact on others*, there is also evidence that people wish to discriminate in favour of those with dependants (see Williams 1988; Charny *et al.* 1989; Dolan *et al.* 1999). There is much less evidence relating to the extent to which *claims based on compensation or reward* are concerned to be relevant equity criteria, although Charny *et al.* (1989) claim that some of those who chose to give higher priority to elderly people did so because they believed that a significant purpose of the NHS was to compensate for inequalities elsewhere in society.

3.4 Discussion

This chapter has raised a number of important questions which need to be addressed by future theoretical and empirical research. One of the most important of these is the question of which perspective people should be asked to adopt in valuations studies. Whilst there has been some debate in the literature about whose values ought to be used to inform resource allocation decisions, there has been almost no discussion of what the most appropriate perspective is. It is important that a discussion of this issue takes place since there might be expected to be important differences, particularly in a publicly-funded health care system. For example, it has been observed that, from the perspective of a patient, an individual will place a relatively high value on those attributes of his health care which do not directly contribute towards his health, such as process attributes associated with the treatment itself (see Ryan 1997). This may be because he feels he has already contributed towards them through taxation or because someone else is subsidizing his treatment at the point of use.

However, from the perspective of a potential patient who does not have the 'luxury' of such cross-subsidization and who might be faced with higher taxes or higher insurance premiums, the individual might be expected to focus more on the health-related attributes of treatment and less on the process attributes. From the perspective of a citizen being asked to contribute towards the treatment of others, health-related attributes are much more likely to be seen as the public good aspect of health care than process-related attributes and hence the focus on health outcomes is likely to be even greater. Empirical evidence, which is lacking at present, would shed light on the extent to which perspective matters and this would help to focus the theoretical debate.

Whilst the perspective of a patient has typically been the one adopted, studies that have attempted to value HRQoL have used many different descriptive systems and valuation methods, thus making comparisons across studies almost impossible. Against this background, a US panel on cost-effectiveness in health and medicine (Gold *et al.* 1996) recommended a 'reference case' for use in cost-effectiveness analyses. Amongst other things, they suggested that the health state descriptive system should be generic and that the valuation method should be preference-based. Whilst these recommendations have attracted few dissenting voices amongst health economists, a review by Neumann *et al.* (1997) highlights how much of the current practice has to change to meet the recommendations. To facilitate comparability between studies, all future studies should use the Gold *et al.* 'reference-case'.

As noted above, most studies that have used the CV method have been concerned with eliciting the WTP for a particular programme or intervention. Similarly, studies which have used CA have tended to focus on the specific attributes of a particular intervention. Consequently, it is not possible to transfer from the results from existing CV or CA studies to other contexts. Whilst each programme is likely to have its own set of characteristics which will require separate and independent valuation, it would be desirable if future CV and CA studies valued a core set of health-related attributes which would then allow for some cross-study comparisons. It might even be possible to establish a 'reference-case' for such studies analogous to the Washington Panel recommendations. Not only would generalizability be enhanced as a result, but it would also be possible to undertake more rigorous tests of construct validity if a core set of results were directly comparable across studies.

Much of the empirical research that has been undertaken into establishing the validity of measures designed to value health outcomes has been conducted within the psychometric tradition, largely in terms of construct validity. Economists, on the other hand, are more concerned that hypothetical decisions are validated against actual decisions. This has attracted a great deal of attention in the literature on the use of the CV method in valuing environmental goods, where the question is whether an individual really would be willing to pay her stated WTP (Mitchell and Carson 1989). It is important that wherever possible similar tests of validity are undertaken in the area of assigning monetary values to health outcomes. Such tests could also be performed in health state valuation or CA studies. For example, it should be possible to compare the choices implied by QALY calculations with decisions made in direct choices between the same alternatives (see Loomes and McKenzie 1989).

Of course, all of this implies that people's stated and/or revealed preferences can be interpreted in some meaningful way. It is striking, however, that so few empirical studies have considered the nature of these preferences. The received wisdom amongst mainstream economists is that individuals behave as if they had clear, well-defined preferences over all the possible decision options they might face (see Williams 1995). Economists involved in eliciting *stated* preferences have largely accepted the received wisdom, arguing that well-defined preference functions can be 'tapped into' by appropriate questions (see Fischhoff 1991). Therefore, economists tend to focus on ensuring that preference elicitation questions are formulated and understood as intended, arguing that any 'slip' could invoke a precise, thoughtful answer to a 'wrong' question. However, the idea that people read their preferences off of some in-built master utility function is called into question by psychologists and by the many studies which have shown that seemingly subtle changes in question framing or problem structure can change the stated preferences of respondents.

These findings could be accounted for by a number of alternative views about the nature of individual preferences. A view that is the extreme opposite to that put forward by mainstream economists is that behaviour is hardly ever motivated by preferences which would satisfy even the weakest of consistency conditions (see Slovic 1995). Adopting this viewpoint would mean that responses in preference elicitation studies are merely constructed 'on the spot' by people. Equally though, there are many studies which suggest that the most general representation of preferences lies somewhere in between the two extremes (see Jones-Lee and Loomes 1995; Cookson and Dolan 1999). Of course, the spectrum of possibilities that this viewpoint covers is very wide, and where a particular person's preferences lie on this spectrum will be largely determined by the extent to which she is familiar with the choices she faces. In very general terms, though, most people's preferences are unlikely to be very clearly defined over most of the issues they are presented with in studies designed to elicit values for different health outcomes.

This suggests that: (1) elicitation procedures can help to shape preferences; and (2) it might be possible to find 'true' preferences but only after deliberation and reflection that improves the understanding of the decision and its implications. Many economists appear to be increasingly aware of the first point and are attempting to gain a better understanding of the cognitive processes that people use in order to arrive at their responses. But most are yet to grasp the fact that studies which do not provide people with sufficient time to carefully consider their responses, as well as the opportunity to provide the reasons underlying them, will not provide the type of preference data that is appropriate for informing resource allocation decisions (see Dolan and Cookson 2000).

The amount of time and opportunity that people should be given to think about a response to a particular question, and precisely how this is achieved, will depend on where their preferences are assumed to be located on the spectrum between being well-defined and constructed on the spot. But whatever the precise details of future studies, the collection and analysis of qualitative data is crucial if economists are to get a better understanding of individual preferences. This may not conform to the standard welfare economics framework but there is more to economics than this particular framework. For example, there are many economists who would deny that actual preferences represent underlying true preferences, pointing out that people sometimes prefer things that make them worse off, possibly as a result of incomplete information or bounded rationality (see Broome 1991). Seen this way, to recommend that economists should aim to 'get behind the numbers', is merely to suggest that they find out which preferences are the ones that are most likely to be make people better off.

3.5 Concluding remarks

It should be clear that many of the issues discussed in this chapter are inextricably linked to a debate about the appropriateness of welfarism. This probably stems from the fact that health has certain characteristics which make it unlike most other commodities and which challenge many of the assumptions of standard welfare economics. By focusing attention on health outcomes, this chapter has served to show where future theoretical and empirical research might be conducted into such issues as the role that individual preferences should play in determining priorities and whether there is more to health care than health. Rather than attempting to find ways in which to reconcile the different approaches to valuation, health economists engaged in outcome measurement should focus their attention on the relative merits of welfarist and non-welfarist philosophies in the context of allocation decisions in health care.

References

Arrow, K.J. (1951). *Social choice and individual values.* Wiley, New York.

Balaban, D. J., Sagi, P. C., Goldfarb, N. I. *et al.* (1986). Weights for scoring the quality of well-being instrument among rheumatoid arthritics: a comparison to general population weights. *Medical Care*, 24, 973–80.

Bleichrodt, H. and Johannesson, M. (1997a). Standard gamble, time trade-off and rating scale: experimental results on the ranking properties of QALYs. *Journal of Health Economics,* 16, 155–75.

Bleichrodt, H. and Johannesson, M. (1997b). An experimental test of a theoretical foundation for rating scale valuations. *Medical Decision-Making*, 17, 208–16.

Bleichrodt, H. Wakker, P. and Johannesson, M. (1997). Characterizing QALYs by risk neutrality. *Journal of Risk and Uncertainty*, 15, 107–14.

Bowling, A. (1996). Health care rationing: the public's debate. *British Medical Journal*, 312, 670–3.

Boyd, N. F., Sutherland, H. J., Heasman, Z. K., Trichler, D. L. and Cummings, B. J. (1990). Whose utilities for decision analysis? *Medical Decision-Making*, 10, 58–67.

Brazier, J.E., Deverill, M. and Green, C. (1999). A review of the use of health status measures in economic evaluation. *Journal of Health Services Research and Policy*, 4, 174–84.

Brooks, R. (1996). EuroQol: the current state of play. *Health Policy*, 37, 53–72.

Broome, J. (1991). *Weighing Goods*. Basil Blackwell, Oxford.

Buckingham, K. and Drummond, M. (1993). *A theoretical and empirical classification of health valuation techniques*. HESG Conference, Strathclyde.

van Busschbach, J. (1994). *The validity of QALYs*. PhD Thesis, Erasmus University, Rotterdam.

Camerer, C. (1993). Individual decision-making. In: J. Kagel and A. Roth, *Handbook of Experimental Economics*. Princeton University Press, NJ.

Cassileth, B. R., Lusk, E. J., Strouse, T. B. *et al.* (1984). Psychosocial status in chronic illness: a comparative analysis of six diagnostic groups. *New England Journal of Medicine*, 311, 506–11.

Charny, M. C., Lewis, P. A. and Farrow, S. C. (1989). Choosing who shall not be treated in the NHS. *Social Science and Medicine*, 28, 1331–8.

Choudhry, N., Slaughter, P., Sykora, K. *et al.* (1997). Distributional dilemmas in health policy: large benefits for a few or smaller benefits for many? *Journal of Health Service Research and Policy*, 2, 212–16.

Churchill, D. N., Morgan, J. and Torrance, G. W. (1984). Quality-of-life in end-stage renal disease. *Peritoneal Dialysis Bulletin*, 4, 20–3.

Cookson, R. and Dolan, P. (1999). Public views on health care rationing: a group discussion study. *Health Policy*, 49, 63–74.

Culyer, A.J. and Wagstaff, A. (1993). Equity and equality in health and health care. *Journal of Health Economics*, 12, 431–57.

Dolan, P. (1998). The measurement of individual utility and social welfare. *Journal of Health Economics*, 17, 39–52.

Dolan, P. (1999). Whose preferences count? *Medical Decision-Making*, 19, 482–6.

Dolan, P. and Cookson, R. (2000). A qualitative study into the extent to which health gain matters. *Health Policy*, 51, 19–30.

Dolan, P., Cookson, R. and Ferguson, B. (1999). Effect of discussion and deliberation on the public's views of priority setting in health care: focus group study. *British Medical Journal*, 318, 916–19.

Dolan, P. and Green, C. (1998). Using the person trade-off approach to examine differences between individual and social values. *Health Economics*, 7, 307–12.

Dolan, P., Gudex, C., Kind, P. *et al.* (1996). Valuing health states: a comparison of methods. *Journal of Health Economics*, 15, 209–31.

Dolan, P. and Jones-Lee, M. (1997). The time trade-off: a note on the effect of lifetime re-allocation of consumption and discounting. *Journal of Health Economics*, 16, 731–9.

Dolan, P. and Olsen, J. A. (2000a). Desperately seeking numbers: The not-so-holy grail of the super-QALY. *Mimeo*, University of Sheffield.

Dolan, P. and Olsen, J. A. (2000b). The equity-efficiency trade-off across different streams of health. *Mimeo*. University of Sheffield.

Dolan, P. and Sutton, M. (1997). Mapping visual analogue scale scores onto time trade-off and standard gamble utilities. *Social Science and Medicine*, 44(10), 1519–30.

Edgar, A., Salek, S., Shickle, D. *et al.* (1998). *The ethical QALY: Ethical issues in healthcare resource allocations.* Euromed Communications.

Evans, W. N. and Viscusi, W. K. (1993). Income effects and the value of health. *Journal of Human Resources,* 28, 497–518.

Feeny, D., Furlong, W., Boyle, M. *et al.* (1995). Multi-attribute health status classification systems: health utilities index. *PharmacoEconomics,* 7, 490–502.

Fischoff, B. (1991). Value elicitation: is there anything there? *American Psychologist,* 46, 835–47.

Froberg, D. G. and Kane, R. L. (1989). Methodology for measuring health state preferences II: scaling methods. *Journal of Clinical Epidemiology,* 42(5), 459–471.

Gafni, A. (1994). The standard gamble method: what is being measured and how is it interpreted? *Health Services Research,* 29(2), 207–24.

Gold, M., Siegal, J. E., Russell, L. B. *et al.* (1996). *Cost-effectiveness in health and medicine.* Oxford University Press, Oxford.

Hadorn, D. (1991). Setting health care priorities in Oregon: cost-effectiveness meets the rule of rescue. *Journal of the American Medical Association,* 265.

Herrero, C. (1996). Capabilities and utilities. *Economic Design,* 2, 69–88.

Hornberger, J. C., Redelmeier, D. A. and Petersen, J. (1992). Variability among methods to assess patients well-being and consequent effect on a cost-effectiveness analysis. *Journal of Clinical Epidemiology,* 45(5), 505–12.

Hurst, N. P., Jobanputra, P., Hunter, M. *et al.* (1994). Validity of EuroQol – a generic health status instrument – in patients with rheumatoid arthritis. *British Journal of Rheumatology,* 33, 655–62.

Jenkinson, C., Gray, A., Doll, H. *et al.* (1997). Evaluation of index and profile measures of health status in a randomized controlled trial: comparison of the Medical Outcomes Study 36-item short form health survey, EuroQol and disease specific measures. *Medical Care,* 35, 1109–18.

Johannesson, M. (1999). On aggregating QALYs, a comment on Dolan. *Journal of Health Economics,* 18, 381–6

Johannesson, M. and Meltzer, D. (1998). Some reflections on cost-effectiveness analysis. *Health Economics,* 7, 1–7.

Johannesson, M., Pliskin, J. S. and Weinstein, M. C. (1994). A note on QALYs, time trade-off and discounting. *Medical Decision-Making,* 14, 142–9.

Jones-Lee, M. W. and Loomes, G. (1995). Scale and context effects in the valuation of transport safety. *Journal of Risk and Uncertainty,* 11, 183–203.

Krabbe, P. and Bonsel, G. (1998). Sequence effects, health profiles, and the QALY model. *Medical Decision-Making,* 18, 178–86.

Kupperman, M., Shiboski, S., Feeny, D. *et al.* (1997). Can preference scores for discrete states be used to derive preference scores for an entire path of events? *Medical Decision-Making,* 17, 42–55.

Le Grand, J. (1991). *Equity and Choice.* London, Harper Collins.

Lenert, L. A., Cher, D. J., Goldstein, M. K. *et al.* (1998). The effect of search procedures on utility elicitations. *Medical Decision-Making,* 18, 76–83.

Lewis, P. A. and Charny, M. (1989). Which of two individuals do you want to treat when only their ages are different and you can't treat both? *Journal of Medical Ethics,* 15, 28–32.

Lindholm, L., Rosen, M. and Emmelin, M. (1997). Health maximization rejected: the view of Swedish politicians. *European Journal of Public Health Policy,* 7, 405–10.

Lipscomb, J. (1982). Value preferences for health: meaning measurement and use in program evaluation. In: R. L. Kane, and R. A. Kane, *Values and long term care*. Lexington Books Mass.

Loomes, G. (1993). Disparities between health state measures: is there a rational explanation? In: W. Gerrard, *The economics of rationality*. Routledge, London.

Loomes, G. (1995). The myth of the HYE. *Journal of Health Economics*, 14, 1–7.

Loomes, G. and McKenzie, L. (1989). The scope and limitations of QALY measures. *Social Science and Medicine*, 28, 299–308.

McNeil, B. J., Weichselbaum, R. and Pauker, S. G. (1978). Fallacy of the five-year survival in lung cancer. *New England Journal of Medicine*, 299, 1397–401.

Mehrez, A. and Gafni, A. (1989). Quality-adjusted life years, utility theory, and health-years equivalents. *Medical Decision-Making*, 9, 142–9.

Mehrez, A. and Gafni, A. (1991). The health-years equivalents: how to measure them using the standard gamble approach. *Medical Decision-Making*, 11, 140–6.

Menzel, P. (1999). How should what economists call 'social values' be measured? *The Journal of Ethics*, 3, 249–73.

Mitchell, R. C. and Carson, R. T. (1989). *Using surveys to value public goods: the contingent valuation method, Resources for the future*. Washington.

Mooney, G. (1994). *Key issues in health economics*. Harvester Wheatsheaf, London.

von Neumann, J. and Morgenstern, O. (1953). *Theory of games and economic behaviour*. Wiley, New York.

Neumann, P. J., Zinner, D. E. and Wright, J. C. (1997). Are methods for estimating QALYs in cost-effectiveness analyses improving? *Medical Decision-Making*, 17, 402–8.

Nord, E. (1993). The trade-off between the severity of illness and treatment effect in cost-value analysis of health care. *Health Policy*, 24, 227–38.

Nord, E. (1995). The person trade-off approach to valuing health care programs. *Medical Decision-Making*, 15, 201–8.

Nord, E., Pinto, J. L., Richardson, J. *et al.* (1999). Incorporating societal concerns for fairness in numerical valuations of health programs. *Health Economics*, 8, 25–39.

O'Connor, A. M., Boyd, N. F. and Till, J. E. (1985). *Influence of elicitation technique, position order and test-retest error on preferences for alternative cancer drug therapy*. Paper to 10th National Nursing Conference, University of Toronto.

Olsen, J. A. (1997). Theories of justice and their implications for priority setting in health care. *Journal of Health Economics*, 16, 625–40.

Olsen, J. A. (2000). Eliciting distributive preferences for health: some problems and a few lessons. *Journal of Health Economics*, 19, 541–50.

Olsen, J. A. and Donaldson, C., (1998). Helicopters, hearts and hips: using willingness to pay to set priorities for public sector health care programmes. *Social Science and Medicine*, 46, 1–12.

Olsen, J. A. and Smith, R. (2001). Who have been asked to value what? A review of 54 WTP-based surveys on health and health care. *Health Economics*. 10, 39–52.

Patrick, D. L., Bush, J. W. and Chen, M. M. (1973). Methods for measuring levels of well-being for a health status index. *Health Services Research*, 8, 228–45.

Propper, C. (1995). The disutility of time spent on the United Kingdom's National Health Service waiting list. *The Journal of Human Resources*, 30, 677–700.

Read, J. L., Quinn, R. J., Berrick, D. M. *et al.* (1984). Preferences for Health Outcomes: Comparison of Assessment Methods. *Medical Decision-Making*, 4(3), 315–29.

Richardson, J. (1994). Cost-utility analysis: what should be measured? *Social Science and Medicine*, 39(1), 7–21.

Richardson, J., Hall, J. and Salkfeld, G. (1996). The measurement of utility in multiphase health states. *International Journal of Technology Assessment in Health Care*, 12, 151–62.

Richardson, J. and Nord, E. (1997). The importance of perspective in the measurement of quality-adjusted life years. *Medical Decision-Making*, 17, 33–41.

Ryan, M. (1997). *Assessing the benefits of health interventions: a role for conjoint analysis?* Paper presented for the Labelle Lectureship in Health Services Research, McMaster University, Hamilton, Canada.

Ryan, M. (1998). *Conjoint – what's the point?* Paper presented to the HESG Conference, Galway.

Ryan, M. and Hughes J. (1997). Using conjoint analysis to value surgical versus medical management of miscarriage. *Health Economics*, 6, 261–73.

Sackett, D. L. and Torrance, G. W. (1978). The utility of different health states as perceived by the general public. *Journal of Chronic Diseases*, 31, 697–704.

Sen, A. (1977). On weights and measures: informational constraints in social welfare analysis. Econometrica 45, reprinted in Sen, A (1982) *Choice, welfare and measurement*. (Blackwell, Oxford and MIT Press, Cambridge, Mass).

Sloan, F. A., Viscusi, W. K., Chesson, H. W. *et al.* (1998). Alternative approaches to valuing intangible health losses: the evidence for multiple sclerosis. *Journal of Health Economics*, 17(4), 475–97.

Slovic, P. (1995). The construction of preferences. *American Psychologist*, 50(5), 364–71.

Stiggelbout, A. M., Eijkemans, M. J. C., Kiebert, G. M. *et al.* (1996). The 'utility' of the visual analog scale in medical decision-making and technology assessment: is it an alternative to the time trade-off? *International Journal of Technology Assessment in Health Care*, 2, 291–8.

Stiggelbout, A. M., Kiebert, G. M., Kievit, J. *et al.* (1994). Utility assessments in cancer patients: adjustment of time trade-off scores for the utility of life years and comparison with standard gamble scores. *Medical Decision-Making*, 14, 82–90.

Torrance, G. W. (1976). Social preferences for health states: an empirical evaluation of three measurement techniques. *Socio-economic Planning Sciences*, 10, 129–36.

Torrance, G. W. (1986). Measurement of health state utilities for economic appraisal. *Journal of Health Economics*, 5, 1–30.

Ubel, P. and Loewenstein, G. (1995). The efficacy and equity of retransplantation: an experimental survey of public attitudes. *Health Policy*, 34, 145–51.

Ubel, P. and Loewenstein, G. (1996). Public perceptions of the importance of prognosis in allocating transplantable livers to children. *Medical Decision-Making*, 16, 234–41.

Ubel, P. M. D., Baron, J. and Asch, D. (1996). Cost-effectiveness analysis in a setting of budget constraints. *The New England Journal of Medicine*, 334, 1174–7.

Verhoef, L. C. G., Maas, A., Stalpers, L. *et al.* (1994). The feasibility of additive conjoint measurement in measuring utilities in breast cancer patients. *Health Policy*, 17, 39–50.

Verhoef, L. C. G., de Haan, A. F. J. and van Daal, W. A. J. (1994). Risk attitude in gambles with years of life: empirical support for prospect theory. *Medical Decision-Making*, 14, 194–200.

Wagstaff, A. (1991). QALYs and the equity-efficiency trade-off. *Journal of Health Economics*, 10, 21–41.

Weinstein, M. C. and Stason, W. B. (1977). Foundations of cost-effectiveness analysis for health and medical practices. *New England Journal of Medicine*, 296, 716.

Williams, A. (1988). *Economics and the rational use of medical technology*. In: F. F. H. Rutten and S. J. Reiser (eds), *The economics of medical technology*. Springer, Berlin.

Williams, A. (1997). Rationing health care by age: the case for. *British Medical Journal*, 314, 820–2.

Willliams, M. (1995). *The Philosophy of economics: a critical survey*. Department of Economics Discussion Paper No. 95–02, De Monfort University, Leicester.

Wolfson, A. D., Sinclair, A. J., Bombardier, C. *et al.* (1982). Preference measurements for functional status in stroke patients: interrater and intertechnique comparisons. In: R. L. Kane and R. A. Kane (eds), *Values and long term care*. Lexicon Books, MA.

Chapter 4

Costing in economic evaluations

Werner Brouwer, Frans Rutten and
Marc Koopmanschap

4.1 Introduction

In this chapter the methods related to costing in economic evaluation are discussed. Costing involves identifying, measuring and valuing all resource changes that occur as a certain health care intervention is carried out. The aim is to value the use of scarce resources (materials, drugs, time of physicians, time of patients etc.) that is needed to produce a certain health effect – the outcome of the intervention. Then, we may be able to weigh the sacrifices against the gains of the intervention and thus determine the relative desirability of such an intervention. In Figure 4.1 we indicate which resource uses may in general be distinguished and need to be identified, estimated in quantitative terms and valued monetarily.

Considering Figure 4.1 it becomes clear that relevant resource changes occur both within (boxes A and E) and outside of the health care sector (boxes B, C and D), now and in the future, making the identification and measurement of such changes in resource use more difficult. A problem in determining the values of the cost-items is that for many of them there is no straightforward method of valuation. For instance patient time, sacrificed for instance to seek and undergo treatment, is difficult to value. But also the real societal costs of traded services, like physician's time or care in a nursing home, are not always clear, as for instance tariffs for these services may be only a poor approximation. This also relates to the fact that the health care sector is far from being a perfectly competitive, transparent market. Only in such markets are prices proper indicators of the opportunity costs of the medical services. As prices in the health care market cannot be considered to reflect opportunity costs, costs should be estimated in other ways, for example using specific cost calculations or shadow prices.

Looking at Figure 4.1 one may also wonder whether costs outside the health care sector are relevant for economic evaluations of *health care* interventions. The answer to that question lies in the adaptation of the societal perspective, which is discussed in more detail in Section 4.2. The main message is, that in order to make a good assessment of an intervention, we need to examine all costs (and consequences) regardless of who bears the burden or where they occur in society.

The level of detail in the costing method used can be varied with the purpose of a study. If the aim of a study is to give a global impression of total costs, 'gross-costing' may be appropriate. In this case a global cost-indicator (e.g. an existing tariff for an

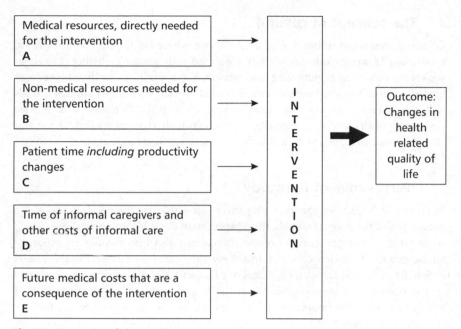

Fig. 4.1 Categories of changes in resource use

intermediate product or a 'diagnosis related group') is used to determine the total costs of a cluster of activities (e.g. a patient day in a general hospital or even the treatment of a specific disease case). 'Gross-costing' has the advantage of consuming less resources and providing better opportunity for generalization, but at the expense of the level of precision. On the other hand, one could opt for 'micro-costing' which entails detailed inventory, measurement and valuation of all separate cost-items involved. This method is much more laborious, but provides the researcher with more specific insight in the relationships between characteristics of activities and their costs, the economies of scale of a production process, and the relative importance of sepa- rate activities. The choice of which costing method to adopt depends on the level of precision required, the desired scope for generalization and the feasibility and costs of adopting either method (Gold *et al.* 1996). This is further discussed in Section 4.4.

The outline of this chapter is as follows. First, in Section 4.2, the concept of costing is further addressed. Then, in Section 4.3 we will explore the identification and measurement of resource use. In Section 4.4 we will discuss how the value of the resource use may be determined, addressing subjects like costs versus tariffs, shadow prices and so on. After having discussed the three main steps of costing (identification, measurement and valuation), we deal with two specific cost-items: informal care (Section 4.5) and related and unrelated costs in normal and added life- years (Section 4.6). Finally, Section 4.7 will conclude this chapter.

4.2 **The concept of costing**

Economic evaluation of health care interventions is based in the tradition of welfare economics. This economic discipline is concerned with assessing whether changes in society can be viewed as enhancing total welfare. Two key notions for this chapter may be derived from this simple statement. First of all, welfare economics ultimately deals with the welfare of society as a whole. Second, economists try to assess the relative desirability of changes relevant to that society, which are changes in resource use and changes in outcome. Below we will address these key notions further.

4.2.1 **Perspective of the study**

In economic evaluations the focus on society as a whole is translated in terms of the perspective of the study. Normally, the perspective of the study is a societal one, which means that all changes in resource use should be taken into account regardless of whose budget is affected or where in society they occur and that all health effects should be taken into account, regardless of who gains. This broad perspective ensures that all resource changes and outcomes are taken into account in the determination of whether or not a programme should be implemented as a consequence of a positive or negative change in total welfare. Taking other perspectives, like the health care budget perspective, is therefore to be discouraged as being narrow and not recognizing that budgets are arbitrary divisions in how resources are organized (compare Chapter 3). For example, although from a health care budget perspective waiting lists may be defendable, the high burden imposed on the rest of society due to production losses and quality-of-life losses, of waiting employees, should encourage the further reduction of waiting times because of welfare losses. It should be noted that taking a societal perspective has consequences for all three steps of costing procedure: identifying, measuring and valuing the resource use.

4.2.2 **Relation to production function**

Economic evaluation deals with the assessment of changes in society. An intervention under study requires certain resources to be sacrificed producing a certain outcome. In some way the outcomes need to be compared with these sacrifices in order to make a judgement about whether or not the outcomes outweigh the total costs. To study the changes in resource use one may consider the different input factors required to produce a good or service in the health care sector. In that way, one may determine a so-called *production function* that gives the relationship between the different inputs (labour, capital and so on) and the outcomes of the intervention. For micro-costing this entails the full determination of the production function, with all the different arguments of the function to be identified, measured and valued, while for gross-costing the production function is estimated on more general cost-items, such as hospital days or doctors' visits. By subsequently determining the valuation of the different cost-items in the production function and incorporating them in that function, we derive a *cost-function* that provides the relationship between costs and outcomes. This cost-function ultimately describes what needs to be sacrificed in monetary terms in order to gain certain outcomes. This information may help a decision-maker to decide whether or not a programme should be implemented and/or reimbursed.

4.2.3 Opportunity costs

In general, the resources used should be valued at their opportunity costs, the value of their best alternative use. These opportunity costs should reflect true societal valuations of the sacrificed resources. As suggested above, in a competitive market opportunity costs are reflected in the market prices. However, in health care markets prices are often not adequate as indicators of opportunity costs or simply not present (like the 'prices' for patient time). Therefore, analysts need to be cautious in using tariffs and other prices in the health care sector as they may not reflect real opportunity costs.

4.2.4 Average versus marginal costs

One of the problems is whether to use average or marginal costs in an economic evaluation. Average prices include fixed costs, such as costs of hospital buildings and costs of overheads, as well as variable costs. Marginal costs only cover the costs of producing one additional unit of outcome of the intervention. Thus, fixed costs are left out of the calculation. Which one to choose depends on the specific research question and the policy-context of the evaluation. For instance, when it is likely that expansion of infrastructure is necessary in order to implement the intervention under study nation wide, marginal costs derived in a setting with an existing infrastructure will clearly underestimate true societal costs of such an implementation. When the evaluation entails the comparison of two programmes that require a different type of health care infrastructure or when a generalization of cost consequences to a national level is necessary, the use of average or integral costs is recommended. Also when longer-term cost consequences are calculated, average costs may be more appropriate, because many cost-items that are fixed in the short term, may become variable in the long term.

4.2.5 Relation to time

The influence of time should be well noted. Not only may some cost-items occur after a longer period, but also the degree of variability of cost-items changes over time as noted above. Furthermore, time may have an influence on the magnitude of certain cost-parameters (e.g. Aletras 1999). For instance, through learning effects future costs of interventions may decrease. This may occur through learning and better performing techniques (like cardiovascular surgery) or through learning about better organizing interventions. This is further discussed in Section 4.4.

Choosing an appropriate time horizon for the evaluation is important, since shifting the time horizon of the evaluation may have a substantial impact on the results of the study. Ideally, the time horizon should be chosen in such a way that all cost consequences of the intervention under study can be taken into account in the analysis. Basing longer-term costs on real measurement data is preferred. Often, however, measurement of resource changes is limited to the length of the clinical trial to which the economic evaluation is attached. Still, costs that occur beyond this period need to be taken into account, e.g. in follow-up measurements added to the initial (clinical) study-design or through modelling longer-term cost consequences using other data (e.g. literature, registries). Such longer-term consequences may also entail above mentioned learning effects that may be projected in the analysis.

4.3 Identifying and measuring resource use

Costing involves three distinct phases: identifying the relevant cost-items, measuring the use of the identified cost-items (quantity) and placing a value on these cost-items (e.g. Gold *et al.* 1996; Drummond *et al.* 1997). In this section, we will discuss the first two steps.

4.3.1 The identification of resource-items

As already mentioned above, the process of identifying resource items can be seen as a study of the *production function* of the health care programme under study. All relevant resource items, both outside and inside the health care sector should be identified and quantified. Amongst other things, this requires both knowledge about the resources needed to perform the intervention, as well as epidemiological knowledge (the disease process before, during and after treatment and what resources will then be consumed) and knowledge about the duration of changes (how long will persons have to be monitored, etc.). Also, issues like productivity changes in the patient group and side-effects of the treatment that may require other treatment (leading to additional costs) need to be identified. To build a detailed decision tree specifying all possible courses of the disease and treatment options is a useful step in this phase.

When the analyst has a broad idea of which resource-items will be relevant in the programme under study, he may decide that some resource changes are expected to be too small to incorporate in the analysis (and to measure and value). Although there may be a sound reason to leave out a resource item from further analysis, it is important to indicate its existence in the identification phase. As Gold *et al.* (1996) note, ease of measurement should not be the initial criterion for identification.

It should be noted that the choice for gross-costing or micro-costing also has consequences for the identification phase. Generally, in gross-costing the intervention is broken down into large components (intermediate products) and these larger components have to be identified. In micro-costing the intervention is broken down further to the extent that all underlying activities and resource-inputs, which together form the intervention, are identified. For example, one may use the inpatient day as a separate cost-item or one can break this hospital day down into smaller components (care, food, tests, cleaning, housing, medication, overheads etc.) that together constitute a patient day, but may differ between patient groups.

4.3.2 Measuring resource use

When measuring resource use, the level of detail required in the study is also crucial. When a study is performed using micro-costing, information on resource use on a very detailed level is required. The individual resource components of the intervention under study (e.g. each diagnostic test) need to be indentified and measured. For gross-costing, the intervention is broken down into larger intermediate products (e.g. hospitalizations) for which resource use is determined. As the choice for gross-costing or micro-costing has implications for valuing resource use as well we consider this choice in more detail in Section 4.4.

Prospective studies generally provide more opportunity for detailed measurement than retrospective studies. Some issues regarding the analysis of resource use data are considered here. First, the analysis should be based on 'intention to treat', where it does not suffice, as in clinical studies, to consider drop-outs simply as failures. Rather a precise estimate of resource use of these cases is necessary as they may drive the cost difference between the arms of a prospective trial. Another issue is the extra-polation of costs beyond the observation period of a prospective study. van Hout *et al.* (1993) showed for heart-transplant patients, that different estimation methods of future hospital consumption based on a mean (after transplant) observation period of about one year yield a twofold difference in total patient-days. They suggested that the best strategy may be to estimate average costs per period in a particular treatment stage as the average costs across all patients for whom data for that period are available. By summing up these chronological estimates of costs per period a cumulative cost curve is determined where systematic increases in costs (e.g. due to annual follow-up) can be identified and no assumptions have to be made on the relation between costs and duration in a treatment phase. Finally, there is often discussion on whether one should test for significant differences between arms considering separate resource items or perform a test on an aggregate indicator of resource use (e.g. total costs). If there is information about different items being complementary or substitutes this may help to direct the answer to this question. Often power is lacking to show significant differences for resource items which are relatively rare.

4.3.3 Collection of resource use data

Whether one may collect data prospectively or not and the level of precision required in the study have clear consequences for the methods used in data collection of resource use. In the case of a prospective study the method of collection of data on resource use should be selected well in advance of the start of the study. The specific method for determining unit prices may be decided on at a later stage as the availability of unit prices is required only in the phase of final analysis. The choice of method for data collection depends furthermore on a number of other characteristics of a study, such as the perspective of the study, the requirements for representativeness and generalizability, the (expected) impact of the specific resource item on total or incremental costs, and the availability of existing data and the effort needed to collect additional data.

Regarding perspective, a societal viewpoint is assumed as indicated above. For data collection this means that one should critically assess whether existing data from registries or accounting systems cover all relevant resource items. In a cost benefit analysis from the perspective of a hospital manager, data from the hospital accounting system may incorporate all relevant resource changes, but from a societal perspective other resource components such as patient travel costs may be important as well. Furthermore, relying on the hospital accounting system may lead to missing certain activities which use up resources but are not billed and therefore not registered.

Regarding representativeness and generalizability, it is important to consider the objective of the study, which may be targeted to support a decision in a specific setting or to inform national policy. In the first case using data from the specific setting is more appropriate whilst in the latter case the use of data from national registries may be the preferred option. Such data may represent the average picture as drawn from multiple settings and provide better opportunity for being representative for a country.

Third, the estimated impact of a specific resource item on the final result determines the precision, with which that resource item should be measured. *A priori* determination of the desired precision can be done by performing a sensitivity analysis up front using best guesses for the different relevant parameters (in terms of resource use and costs). In this way information is offered as to which resource items and relating cost items are crucial.

Finally, given the previous criteria, the availability of data from existing registries may allow shortcuts to be made in the calculation of costs. The effort to be put in the calculation of a specific cost-item is dependent on the required precision but also on the resources required for the different alternative options for data collection.

When considering existing data one may distinguish national registries and accounting systems of relevant health care organizations. In most countries there are national registries for resource use in several sub-sectors in health care, which may be operated by a specific health statistics organization or by a research institute. These registries are often used for national surveys of health care costs and may be used for cost of illness studies (top down type see Section 4.4) and for economic evaluation, especially when national representativeness is important. At a level of a health care institution, cost accounting systems may be used but it should be acknowledged that the objective of such systems is to provide the information for billing purposes or for internal management rather than producing detailed data as required for economic evaluation.

Where an economic evaluation is conducted alongside a clinical trial, data on the resource quantities can be collected on the case report forms. The preferred option is to incorporate such items in the same case report form, which is used for collecting the medical/clinical information. Often the medical case report form already contains some quite useful information for the calculation of resource use and, subsequently, costs. In other cases the medical records of patients in the GP practice or in the hospital can inform about resource use of relevant patients. Some resource use like domiciliary nursing visits may only be collected through the patient himself, for instance through a patient survey or patient diary. Standardization in the collection of resource use data and cost data for economic evaluation is lacking, one of the few examples being the labour and health status questionnaire of van Roijen *et al.* (1996).

4.4 **Estimating the value of resources**

In this section we will further discuss the third step of the three-fold identifying, measuring and valuing resources: placing a value on resources used. As indicated above, the aim of an evaluation from a societal perspective is to provide a decision-maker with cost-information – the opportunity costs of the resources used – in order to decide on whether or not a certain programme is relatively worthwhile to implement or reimburse. After the identification and measurement of the resource changes in society, the analyst faces the difficult task of valuing them. This valuation is hampered by the fact that many of the resources used are not priced in a transparent and competitive market. Tariffs or prices in the health care sector therefore often do not represent a fair reward for a well-defined product, but are mere components in mechanisms to compensate health care providers for their resource input. Therefore the analyst often has to determine the true societal opportunity costs through a separate cost analysis. In this section we will discuss some common ways to do so and related problems.

4.4.1 **Gross versus micro-costing and level of refinement**

As already mentioned, the level of precision required in the analysis broadly determines all three phases of the costing process. The level of precision of cost estimates can vary substantially and depends on the specific research question. A very precise estimate of the savings in health care costs arising from primary prevention of cardiovascular disease may not be required as the impact of these savings on the resulting cost-effectiveness ratio is low because of discounting. On the other hand, if in a cost-effectiveness analysis of breast cancer screening there is the choice between a fixed or a mobile screening unit, the costs attached to either option should be calculated precisely in order to support such a choice. The level of precision required is an important determinant for the costing methods used. Far ends of the total spectrum of precision, gross-costing and micro-costing can be distinguished. Note that in practice most economic evaluations use a combination of these methods for different parts of a study. In gross-costing often composite intermediate products have to be valued that are not broken down further into their underlying components. Thus the valued components are relatively large in relation to the total value of resources needed for the intervention under study. For this type of analysis it is important that the valuation of the large components of the intervention is close to the true societal opportunity costs. Prices and tariffs need to be critically reviewed on whether they reflect these opportunity costs or whether they are merely financial parameters with no relation to actual costs. For micro-costing, the calculation of opportunity costs of separate resource items is necessary and may be quite tedious. Therefore, the analyst will have to determine for which resource items it is feasible and worthwhile to perform detailed cost-studies.

The general approach in a costing study is that for a specific health care service one determines the necessary amount of each input: personnel, equipment, material, floor surface, etc. and the costs per unit of each input. Aggregating the product of costs per unit and the number of units of each input gives the costs of the health care service ('bottom up cost calculation'). However, this procedure can be carried out on several levels of refinement and depends on the setting in which a service is being produced. A hospital ward may have a relatively homogeneous production, e.g. inpatient days, allowing a broad calculation of costs per unit of output using the total costs of the department, divided by the total number of inpatient days. On the other hand, a radiology department produces many services (X-rays, CT-scans, ultra-sounds, MRI-scans), using multiple equipment. Hence the calculation of the cost of a CT-scan requires data on personnel, equipment, occupancy rate, depreciation, maintenance etc., on a very detailed level, in order to assign a specific part of the cost of a hospital department to a specific medical service.

To illustrate the degrees of refinement let us consider the cost per hospital day for a stroke patient on the neurology department, which can be determined in several ways:

1. If one assumes that the costs of nursing and physician input are the same as for the average patient in the department, one could estimate the total costs of the department by summing all department costs for personnel, equipment, material, medication and accounting for the costs of catering, cleaning, location costs and overhead costs by assigning a proportional part of hospital costs for these categories. Total costs divided by the number of inpatient days gives the hospital costs per day.

2. If one suspects the stroke patients to be more care-intensive than the average neurology patient with respect to the costs of nursing, one could correct the costs of nursing personnel using patient classification data. With patient classification data, such as the San Joaquin classification (for normal inpatient wards, see Bergman *et al.* 1995) or the TISS-score (for intensive care units, see de Keizer *et al.* 1998), one can estimate nursing costs for individual patients or groups of patients. Using classification data requires knowledge on the exact relation between specific classes of nursing intensity and nursing time (costs).

3. If it is very important to have a reliable detailed estimate of the cost of a hospital day for a specific patient group and if data as mentioned under (2) are not available, one may consider setting up a multi-moment measurement study. In such a study the time spent by nurses and physicians and the medication and material used for each patient are measured in a standardized way, using multiple observations. This procedure can produce very refined cost estimates which can be linked to patient characteristics and data on patient classification (de Keizer *et al.* 1998.)

4.4.2 Handling of overhead costs

One of the problems in costing an activity or product is how to deal with those resources that serve various production units (e.g. administration, cleaning, power, etc.). Drummond *et al.* (1997) give ample advice on different methods of allocating the costs of such resources to final products or services. Direct allocation of overhead costs to final products seems to be the preferred approach, as more sophisticated methods require detailed data that most health care organizations cannot produce from their accounting systems. In this method of direct allocation first, overhead costs for the various overhead departments are allocated to a final production centre using an appropriate allocation-key (e.g. square metres for allocating the costs of cleaning services). Note that cleaning services are also done for other overhead departments so that allocation may take place in two steps: allocating a proportional part of the costs of cleaning to an overhead department (e.g. central administration), which costs are then allocated to a final production centre using yet another allocation-key (e.g. personnel in full time equivalents). Second, one should establish what proportion of the capacity of this final production centre is used for the product or programme under consideration. The same proportion of overhead costs is then allocated to this product or programme.

There are various ways to avoid performing a detailed cost study and instead use existing prices or other information. We will discuss using market prices or tariffs and adjusting market prices or using shadow prices in the next two paragraphs.

4.4.3 Costs versus tariffs

In economic evaluation studies cost estimates should generally reflect opportunity costs and not costs in a strict financial sense. For example if hospital buildings are fully depreciated the financial costs may be zero, but the opportunity costs are positive, since alternative use of the buildings could generate revenue. It is important to note this discrepancy between financial costs and economic or opportunity costs. This difference is especially important when the analyst considers using tariffs as an approximation of opportunity costs. In health care tariffs charged are generally not suitable for this purpose for several reasons:

• tariffs may not cover full costs, if in addition lump sum financing exists or if investment costs are financed separately;

• tariffs associated with products (e.g. patient days) are often merely vehicles for allocating resources to health care providers (e.g. hospitals) without having any relationship with the real costs of these products (for some countries like the Netherlands and Belgium the tariff per hospital day is larger than the actual cost of a hospital day, whereas the outpatient tariff is lower than the actual cost).

The general advice is to use tariffs only if there is a clear indication that a tariff for a service represents a reasonable approximation of the actual costs and if the service makes up only a small part of total cost. In all other cases costs per unit should be analysed in detail. At the start of a study, it may not be clear which cost categories are substantial for the particular patient group studied. Interviews with medical experts may offer some information on what type of medical services are the most important and the most likely to be influenced by the intervention studied. If the latter is not sufficient, analysing the medical consumption of a small sample of patients, e.g. by studying patient records, may be very useful to select the medical services for which detailed cost studies are required.

For hospital services such as inpatient days and outpatient visits, using tariffs is to be discouraged because hospitals are multi-product and multi-department organizations with many possibilities for cross-subsidies. For simpler, labour intensive services such as those of general practitioners and physical therapists, using tariffs has fewer complications, because the more homogeneous production leaves little room for cross subsidization. However, if capitation payment prevails, one needs an additional step in order to calculate the costs per unit of service. Through available data on the average workload for each practitioner one may calculate an imputed fee for service that may be used in cost calculations.

Sometimes economic evaluations are supplemented by an analysis of the financial costs for third party payers. In that case the tariffs charged should be the basis for the cost estimates. In addition, comparing tariffs and reimbursement schedules with opportunity costs can be useful to highlight adverse incentives in the reimbursement system, which may inhibit the introduction of cost-effective health care services. For example, in the Netherlands the cure and care sector have different financing regimens, which clearly hampers the introduction of transmural stroke services that may improve the quality and continuity of care for these patients in a cost-effective way. If such a financial analysis is being performed, the viewpoint should be clearly stated in order to avoid confusion.

4.4.4 Adjusting market prices and using shadow prices

Another disturbing factor in using prices of some products is that these may incorporate a relatively large component of profit. When this profit rate is above a fair return on investment and risk compensation, these prices cannot be seen as reflecting the opportunity costs for society. A solution to this problem, mainly adopted in the USA, is to adjust the prices for the excess profit component using so-called cost-to-charge ratios. These ratios indicate how the price could be deflated in order to better reflect real opportunity costs. Naturally, when using such ratios, the analyst needs to ensure that the cost-to-charge ratios are applicable in the specific context of the intervention under study (Gold *et al.* 1996).

In other cases there may not exist a market price or tariff for the activity to be costed, but there may be a comparable activity for which such a price does exist. The latter may be used as a shadow price with or without some adjustments. This method is rarely used for activities within the health care sector, but more often for activities outside health care (e.g. using the wage rate of a professional housekeeper for the valuation of an informal caregiver, see Section 4.5).

4.4.5 Recommended prices

In order to get more uniform methodology in cost calculation, several countries such as Canada, Australia and The Netherlands have included costing appendices in their guidelines for economic evaluation of pharmaceutical products (CCOHTA 1997; Commonwealth Department of Human Services and Health 1995; Oostenbrink *et al.* 2000). In these guidelines, sometimes recommended prices for use in evaluation studies are also indicated for several types of care. In the Australian Manual of Resource Items and their Associated Costs, 'costs per episode' and 'costs per bed day' are quoted for the Australian national diagnosis related groups. For the Dutch case several unit prices per day for different types of hospitals and nursing homes are recommended. In that way analysts may benefit from earlier research and more uniform cost-figures will be used in different studies, enhancing comparability of results.

4.4.6 Costing in relation to context

It is quite difficult to provide reliable estimates of the additional costs or savings of implementing a specific health programme. The approach to be taken depends largely on the specific circumstances under which the intervention will be implemented. The simplest situation seems to be if the health care programme is carried out in a new stand-alone organization, allowing a simple assignment of the total cost of the organization to the services provided. However, the introduction of many programmes can be seen as the extension or reduction of the production of an existing health care organization. The extra costs of such an extension depend on the type of cost categories affected. If a programme only produces some extra hospital days on a previously not fully occupied ward, only variable patient related costs such as the costs of medication, material and catering will change. If the number of extra inpatient days is not negligible, personnel costs may increase as well. Extending a hospital ward also yields extra costs for location, cleaning, equipment and other facilities, whereas setting up an entire new ward will have large implications for fixed costs and may also affect overhead costs for the rest of the hospital.

Personnel cost is a special cost category: these costs may be quite fixed in the case of long-term contracts for specialized personnel. On the other hand less specialized (nursing) personnel can often be redeployed swiftly within other parts of an organization. In the latter situation, personnel costs are a much more variable cost component. As discussed above, the analyst will have to determine and specify the assumptions underlying his cost-calculations, especially when dealing with longer-term consequences. A sensitivity analysis may demonstrate the robustness of results and the influence of such assumptions.

The above examples highlight that it is crucial to have insight in the scale of health care programmes and how they affect existing infrastructure in order to derive sound cost estimates. In addition the time frame is important. As noted above, in the short run only some cost categories may be variable, in the long run organizations have much more discretion to change the production process and overhead, turning most costs into variable costs. Most economic analysts view health care programmes as structural long-term additions to existing health care and therefore calculate full (average) costs. The latter also has the advantage of generalizability, facilitating the extrapolation of costs to other settings and from local to regional or national scales.

4.4.7 Monitoring costs and learning curves

In order to get a better impression of the additional cost of an operational health care programme, one should monitor the costs after implementation, perhaps for several years. Unfortunately the literature does not provide many examples of systematically monitoring costs. An example from the Netherlands shows that during the first years of setting up the national breast cancer screening programme for women of age 50–70, the regional variation in costs was considerable. Later on, the cost differences decreased considerably, which may be due to some kind of learning effect. However, when the screening was extended to age 75, organizations had to adapt to this change and regional variation in costs became larger again (LETB 1999).

Examples of learning curves are numerous. The most frequently mentioned example is the shortening of time for surgical techniques as surgeons become experienced. Hui *et al.* (2000) for instance report the learning effects of an inexperienced group of surgeons and indicate how the learning effect ends at a certain level of achievement. This may be expected to exist in many different procedures and techniques. Learning effects may also occur because of a very cautious attitude of physicians at the start of experimental programmes. For example, in the first year of the Dutch lung transplantation programme, patients on the waiting list were often admitted to the hospital to monitor their fitness before the transplantation (van Enckevort *et al.* 1997). Later on this turned out to be a superfluous precaution for many patients. The same phenomenon occurred for patients during the follow up after the lung transplantation. In both instances the most recent admittance pattern was used in the cost estimates of the economic evaluation of the lung transplantation programme (Al *et al.* 1998). A similar learning effect was observed for liver transplants in patients with chronic liver failure. van Agthoven (1998) reports a strong decrease in the number of days that these patients were screened in order to assess their eligibility for transplantation. Over time the knowledge about which patients were eligible for the transplant was gathered more quickly than before, shortening the screening period. Also, the number of re-admissions after transplantation decreased over time, due to the fact that the surgeons learned to pick the best moment for transplantation. Table 4.1 indicates the decrease in screening days and re-admissions over a four-year period.

4.4.8 Should transfer costs be included?

An issue that needs some attention here is whether transfer payments need to be taken into account when prices can be used as cost-estimates. First of all, it is important to note that within the context of this chapter, we mainly refer to transfer costs as meaning social transfers like income-taxes, VATs and social premiums. It is possible to

Table 4.1 Learning effects in liver transplantation: screening days and re-admission in four years

Year	Screening days	Re-admissions
1993	37	30
1994	24	17
1995	26	12
1996	22	10

Source: Van Agthoven (1998)

view these transfer costs as not being real economic costs, since they represent simple transfers from one party in society to another, without real resource use. On the other hand, however, one may argue that in deciding on the deployment of capital or labour inputs, decision-makers will consider the full costs of labour and capital (including VAT, social premiums and so on). In that sense, the full cost to the health care organization is reflected in the full price paid by the organization, including all transfer payments. It is recommended here to adopt the latter approach in the analysis of medical costs in order to stay close to the practical decision-making level. Note that the use of transfer payments (like social benefits to the disabled) are not to be used as proxies for productivity losses due to illness, disability or premature death.

4.4.9 Problems in analysis of cost data

When the resource use is measured in different centres (throughout a country or in different countries) issues arise in analysing such data. Raikou *et al.* (2000) indicate two possible ways of transforming the multi-centre trial data into an average cost per unit. First of all, it is possible to calculate average treatment costs by applying unit costs averaged across treatment centres to centre-specific volumes of resource use. Thus, only the volume component is effectively allowed to differ between the different centres. A second option is to use centre-specific information for both the unit costs and the resource volumes, and then averages across centres. Both prices and quantities are thus varied over different centres. Raikou and colleagues show that these two methods lead to differences in average treatment cost estimates. An important lesson that they draw from this result is that caution is warranted in the collection, calculation and interpretation of treatment costs in multi-centre studies. It is recommended here that differences between centres in a trial, both in terms quantities and in terms of prices are shown clearly in the presentation of results. Also, the method of calculating overall findings from the different centre-specific results should be made clear. Raikou and colleagues conclude:

> These findings highlight the need for more caution in calculating treatment costs in multi-centre studies. They also emphasize the need for more and better information on the production process in the health care sector. Little is known about the degree of factor substitution in this sector. What is known is that there is considerable variation in treatment patterns across centres. Even when this is regulated through clinical trial procedures, caution is required in assuming that an average cost is a true average cost.

When the centres included in the evaluation are situated in different countries, difficulties may exist in arriving at overall conclusions as well as at conclusions for a specific country. Different resource uses may be found in such a trial in the included countries, for instance due to differences in health care culture. Also, the costs of different resource items may differ substantially between countries and regions. Often, the subsample of patients within a national context is not large enough to draw firm conclusions, and conclusions for all patients are subsequently hampered by the large differences between subgroups. Willke *et al.* (1998) discuss these problems extensively and demonstrate the problem with actual data from a multinational clinical trial.

Their findings suggest that a simple generalization of trial-wide cost-estimates to specific countries can be (and in their example is) inappropriate. They present a model which may assist analysts in making results more applicable at the level of individual countries. Again, in a context of a multinational trial the calculation methods used in the analysis should be made clear and differences in resource use and costs between the countries and centres should be made clear. This subject is discussed in detail in Chapter 11.

As indicated in Chapter 9 the amount and costs of medical consumption across patients is mostly right-skewed, has a large variance and may contain many observations with zero medical consumption. This pattern holds for the number of units of service consumed. The variation in the unit cost across organizations is less known, but may be substantial. If one needs a national or regional average for the cost per unit of a service it is not easy to give a simple rule of thumb on the number of observations (c.q. sites) needed in order to get a robust estimate. What can be said is that the cost per unit differs between specific settings such as teaching, specialized and general hospitals, between health care services in big cities and the countryside (wage levels). The best provisional advice may be to use at least three to five observations for each specific organizational setting and to make overall estimates as a weighted average using the prevalence of the specific settings as weights.

Cost functions may be estimated by means of regression analysis, where a measure of total costs is related to different explanatory variables representing various units of output and where the regression parameters may be interpreted as indicators for marginal cost and average cost per unit. This is an elegant option if one has enough observations for a meaningful analysis. Still one should be cautious, because of the non-experimental nature of the data: health care organizations are influenced by markets, government regulation, bureaucracy, mergers, interaction of management and professionals etc. This contextual influence may be very different for specific health care providers. The *ceteris paribus* clause necessary to interpret the regression parameters properly as attributes of a robust cost function may often not apply (Spanos 1995).

4.5 Costing informal care

Apart from professionals who may provide all sorts of care for a patient, in some instances this care can be provided by so-called informal caregivers. These non-professional informal caregivers are defined here as family, friends, acquaintances or neighbours of a patient, who provide care for which they do not have to be financially compensated (e.g. Wright 1987; Smith and Wright 1994). Costing informal care can be important when dealing with the economic evaluation of interventions aimed at patient groups who typically need and often get a large amount of informal care, such as schizophrenia and Alzheimer's disease (van Busschbach *et al.* 1998).

Besides several types of costs that are incurred to facilitate informal care such as costs related to home adaptation and consumer durables (e.g. special beds), the time invested in the care for a patient by informal caregivers is difficult to value and opinions on how to value this time vary considerably. The main problem in costing the time invested by informal caregivers is probably that the full impact of this time use should be expressed in monetary terms, in order to be able to capture informal care fully on the cost-side of the C/E ratio in a cost-effectiveness analysis. However, while providing informal care entails giving up leisure time, investing energy and making fewer social contacts, it proves difficult to capture the impact of informal care fully in terms of costs. That may be one of the reasons that influential guidelines and textbooks on economic evaluation of health care often provide analysts with little guidance on this subject (e.g. Gold *et al.* 1996; Drummond *et al.* 1997).

4.5.1 Should informal care be valued?

A first question one has to ask is whether informal care should be valued in an economic evaluation. One can easily argue that this type of care does not constitute a cost for the insurer or the government, since the informal caregiver engages in informal care freely and uncompensated. Naturally, such a line of thinking cannot be supported merely from the fact that an economic evaluation should be conducted from a societal perspective. This also holds for the time input of volunteers. Caring for specific patient groups can only be performed by not caring for other patient groups or by giving up paid or unpaid work, constituting in opportunity costs. So, although the costs borne by the informal caregiver, for instance due to investing time, may not be experienced by others in society, these costs may have to be taken into account. Interestingly, if providing informal care yields certain intangible effects (e.g. fatigue, social isolation, sacrificing leisure time or sleep), these effects should be taken into account as well in an economic evaluation from a societal perspective, but rather in terms of quality-of-life than as costs. Note, that this introduces an outcome measure in addition to patient health-related quality-of-life, that is relevant in decision-making but cannot simply be summed with patient quality-of-life, because it is care-related rather than health-related.

4.5.2 Valuing the time input of informal caregivers

In this section we will focus on the time input of informal caregivers in the intervention. Since informal caregivers give up on normal time uses in order to provide informal care, opportunity costs are incurred. The costs related to this time input in the treatment of the patient may be valued in several ways (e.g. Smith and Wright 1994; Gold *et al.* 1996; Posnett and Jan 1996; Drummond *et al.* 1997). Here, we will discuss the market price method, the reservation wage method and an alternative valuation method which was presented by Brouwer *et al.* (1999).

Before valuing the time spent on informal care, it is important to recognize that both the amount of time and the valuation of time are important. It may prove difficult to determine the amount of time effectively spent on informal care. For instance, in the case of surveillance (e.g. in the case of caring for a demented patient) informal caregivers may provide informal care 24 hours a day. However, taking this amount as input in the analysis would ignore the fact that during surveillance one can probably perform many of one's normal tasks (joint production). Also, it may turn out to be difficult to separate caregiving from normal activities. For instance cooking a meal by a housewife for her sick husband may be a normal use of her time, but helping him to eat not. Structured interviews or detailed diaries may be useful in determining the exact loss of time spent on normal time uses (van Busschbach *et al.* 1998). Validation and standardization of methods used are encouraged to enhance the comparability of results between different studies.

A first method of valuing the time input of informal caregivers is by attaching a value to the output of the informal care process (Posnett and Jan 1996). This may be done by valuing the activities performed by an informal caregiver at the market price that one would otherwise have had to pay if formal caregivers would have provided these tasks. Two ways of operationalizing such a method are possible. First, one may attach the hourly wage-rate of a professional who otherwise would have performed these tasks to the hours spent on the tasks by the informal caregiver (using a shadow price). In principle one could even use different hourly wage-rates for different care-tasks, e.g. a lower one for simple tasks like cleaning and a higher one for more advanced caregiving activities. A problem with this method is that if informal care-givers are less efficient in performing these tasks, they may use more time than a professional would have, overestimating the real value of their performance. Therefore, a second way may be preferred, in which the market price of performing a certain task is set equal to the amount of time that a professional would have spent on that task and multiplying this amount of time by the wage-rate of that professional. A general problem with this method is that its result does not necessarily reflect the opportunity costs of the time that is invested by the informal caregiver.

A second method is therefore to attach a value to the time equal to the wage-rate the informal caregiver earns or would have earned if he or she would have worked for pay (Gold *et al.* 1996). In agreement with Posnett and Jan (1996), this method may be considered a valuation of input rather than output and therefore appears to be more closely related to the opportunity costs principle. In general, a wage-rate that the informal caregiver earns when working for pay is attached to all time effectively invested in informal care. If the informal caregiver does not work for pay, a wage-rate of someone with similar characteristics who does work for pay may be used as a proxy for his or her opportunity costs of time. Note that this wage-rate is subsequently attached to all time and normal activities sacrificed (e.g. paid work, unpaid work and leisure). However, wage-rates may be inadequate to reflect the full opportunity costs of time, because quality-of-life aspects are left out and some time uses can best be valued in terms of quality-of-life in full, like leisure time (Brouwer *et al.* 1999).

An alternative approach suggested by Brouwer *et al.* (1999) is to use different valu-ation techniques depending on what time is sacrificed and using a combination of costing principles and quality-of-life measurement. This valuation method is closely related to the valuation methods sometimes used to estimate the value of time of patients and productivity costs with (see Chapter 4 for further discussion on produc-tivity costs). Time is separated in sacrificed time otherwise spent on paid work, unpaid work and leisure. Here we will briefly discuss the valuation of that time for these different cases.

- Paid work: If informal caregivers have to give up (a part of) paid work, temporarily or permanently, this time may be valued with a method like the friction cost method (e.g. Koopmanschap *et al.* 1995; Koopmanschap and Rutten 1996). Lost utility because of lost role functioning in a paid job may additionally be captured in terms of the informal caregiver's quality-of-life.[1]

- Unpaid work: Unpaid work is viewed as yielding both process and product utility. The latter originates from the endproduct itself. These endproducts may also be produced by someone else (e.g. a professional housekeeper). Lost production in terms of endproducts could be valued by estimating the time that a professional housekeeper would need to produce these products and subsequently multiplying such time period with the wage-rate of professional housekeepers. Process utility is gained by performing activities (e.g. raising children) yourself, which may be interpreted as home role functioning and be captured in terms of the informal caregiver's quality-of-life. Therefore, only the cost of lost production itself is valued in monetary terms.

- Leisure time: When leisure time is sacrificed in order to provide informal care it may best be treated as time in which one can do the things that make life valuable: sporting, hobbies, socializing and so on. As for patients, the loss of leisure time can most meaningfully be captured in terms of quality-of-life, instead of a monetary valuation (Johannesson 1997; Brouwer *et al.* 1998).

Note that the aspects proposed to be captured in terms of quality-of-life are already incorporated in questions of quality-of-life questionnaires for patients, such as the EQ-5D and the SF-36. However, this valuation method invokes the problem that, while the patient's quality-of-life is clearly health-related, the caregiver's quality-of-life change is care-related, making a comparison between the two difficult. A provisional solution is to mention the influence of caregiving on the quality-of-life of caregivers as a separate item, not entering the cost-utility ratio.

Explicit attention for caregiver quality-of-life makes it possible to give an appropriate weight to changes in caregiver quality-of-life.[2] This also seems to be dictated by taking a societal perspective, since these quality-of-life changes are relevant effects that occur in society. Parker (1990) states:

> I have tried to raise in the readers' minds some doubts about the advisability of measuring the quality-of-life of any single individual, without also taking into account the quality-of-life of those who support and care for him or her. (page 127)

Gold *et al.* (1996) encourage analysts to think broadly about the incorporation of quality-of-life effects of 'significant others'. In that sense, it has to be noted that here we restrict the valuation of time and quality-of-life to those effects attributable to informal

---

[1] Lost income should not be captured in terms of quality of life, although some times proposed. For a discussion of this subject see Gold *et al.* (1996), Brouwer *et al.* (1997a), Weinstein *et al.* (1997) and Brouwer *et al.* (1997b). See also Chapter 5.

[2] Note that the quality of life of informal caregiver does indeed change when providing care as reported by Mohide *et al.* (1988) and Drummond *et al.* (1991)

care only. Naturally, the mere existence of illness in one's direct social environment will have effects on quality-of-life of persons as well. However, these 'family effects', although perhaps important, are not dealt with here. Also, in assessing quality-of-life changes due to caregiving, these family effects should be neutralized in order not to count them as effects due to the provision of informal care. Future research aimed at assessing these family effects of illness in one's social environment could provide valuable additional insight in the societal changes that occur due to the prevalence of certain illnesses (and may pinpoint the relative family burden of diseases).

Finally, the use of quality-of-life measurement also facilitates the valuation of 'intangible effects' of providing informal care like fatigue and disutility from having to perform unpleasant tasks. This makes a full indication of the quality-of-life change due to providing informal care possible. In that sense quality-of-life measurement may substitute or at least complement more sociological estimates of the burden of care-giving. The (further) development and validation of instruments and techniques to measure this impact is an important area for future research.

4.6 Incorporation of different cost-categories

An area of considerable debate is that of the costs in future life years and life years gained and whether or not these costs should be taken into account in an economic evaluation of a new treatment and to what extent. It is also useful to separate costs in life years that the patient would have lived without the new treatment from costs in gained life years and related medical consumption (i.e. medical consumption that is incurred due to health problems that are directly related to the intervention under study) from unrelated medical consumption.[3] Recommendations on inclusion of the different cost-categories are provided below.

4.6.1 Related medical and non-medical costs

Medical costs that are related to the intervention should always be included in a study (when significantly present), since they are a direct result of the intervention studied (Gold *et al.* 1996; Drummond *et al.* 1997). The related non-medical costs should also be a normal part of an economic evaluation from a societal perspective. This holds both for related medical and non-medical costs in years the patient would have lived anyway and in life years gained. Informal care, travelling expenditures, productivity changes and so on are normally captured in an economic evaluation, although the latter cost category is somewhat controversial. Although there are only few opponents of inclusion of these productivity costs, there does exist a discussion on how to include these costs. The debate mainly deals with the question whether to use the traditional human capital method, the more recent friction cost method (e.g. Koopmanschap *et al.* 1995) or quality-of-life measurement in order to estimate these costs (see Gold *et al.* 1996, and Chapter 5).

---

[3] Note that categorizing costs in this way is disputed and the lines between different categories are not always clear. Yet, as for the categorization of costs in general, an alternative is hard to find (at least a better one!).

4.6.2 Unrelated medical and non-medical costs in normal life years

It is normally argued that these costs can be omitted from the analysis as they occur similarly in the control group and the treatment group and therefore do not represent an incremental cost (Weinstein *et al.* 1996). If the costs are truly unrelated, differences in the two treatment arms can only occur by chance and thus, registration of unrelated costs should be discouraged, as it may lead to estimation errors.

4.6.3 Unrelated medical and non-medical costs in life years gained

The incorporation of unrelated costs in life years gained is most controversial and different recommendations may be found in the literature and in guidelines. One can argue that these costs should not be incorporated since they are irrelevant to the question whether the intervention under study is worthwhile (Russell 1986). On the other hand, the future unrelated costs can only occur due to the intervention under study and are in that sense a direct result from the intervention. This has been noted many times in the literature. Weinstein and Fineberg (1980) already state:

> Often ignored are the costs of medical care received during extended years of life. Credit given to control of blood pressure for reducing costs associated with treatment of strokes and myocardial infarctions must be balanced against the costs for other diseases incurred during the added years of life.

Recently, however, Garber and Phelps (1997) found that these costs do not have to be incorporated in an analysis. They conclude:

> We have shown that, within the framework of standard von Neumann–Morgenstern utility maximization, CE analysis can offer a valid criterion for choosing among health interventions. Surprisingly, the inclusion of unrelated future costs is without consequence so long as the practice is consistent.

Meltzer (1997), on the other hand, demonstrates that these costs should be taken into account in order to reach results consistent with lifetime utility maximization. He uses a more general formulation of lifetime expected utility maximization (with less restrictions on the substitution of income across time and potential outcomes) than Garber and Phelps and reaches the following conclusion:

> The theoretical section of this paper demonstrates that cost-effectiveness criteria for the allocation of medical expenditures are strictly consistent with a model of lifetime utility maximization only if they account for effects on future related and unrelated medical expenditures, as well as consumption and earnings. This is a potentially important finding since it is not common practice to include these costs in medical cost-effectiveness analysis and since there has been theoretical disagreement whether they should be included.

Weinstein and Manning (1997), in a reaction to both Garber and Phelps and Meltzer, indicate that it is important to understand that both their papers adhere to the economic welfare theory, that can lead to 'some conclusions that may be unsettling to many practitioners of CEA'. An alternative approach to CEA, most notably the extra-welfarist or decision-maker's approach may adhere less to strict welfare economic theory and may therefore have more degrees of freedom to deal with certain costs and characteristics of persons (e.g. the value of a QALY may not be directly dependent on income). By turning to the fundamentals underlying CEA, Weinstein and Manning leave open the room for alternative suggestions on methodology, including unrelated medical and non-medical costs in life years gained. Thus, the controversy seems to persist.

What needs to be noted here, is that although there exists controversy on the incorporation of unrelated medical costs in life years gained, the impact of these costs may be substantial. For example, when analysing treatment of sepsis, van Hout et al. (1993) found that when including unrelated medical costs the cost-effectiveness of medication in patients with gram-negative sepsis substantially differed between different disease categories (e.g. comparing acute trauma patients with terminal cancer patients). There may be a strong case in such circumstances to not leave out these indirect costs from the analysis.

In guidelines on how to conduct an economic evaluation the choice whether or not to include this controversial cost-category is generally left up to the analyst (Weinstein et al. 1996; Drummond et al. 1997). Indeed, one might conclude it to be best to leave the decision to include or exclude these costs to the analyst. He or she can determine whether or not these costs may be substantial and whether or not data on these costs for the specific population of the study is available. In a sensitivity analysis the influence of including or excluding these costs may then be demonstrated. In the light of the above debate, this 'soft' recommendation seems appropriate here.

If an analyst decides to incorporate non-related medical costs in added life years probably the most appropriate way to do so is to find age and gender specific data on average medical costs. One way of coming to such data is to use general cost-of-illness studies, as discussed in Section 4.4, and specifying the total costs to different patient-groups, selected on the base of age and gender. In the absence of reliable data, the analyst may only consider mentioning these costs as a possible additional cost-item, indicating what influence they could have on the results.

4.6.4 Expanding unrelated non-medical costs to basic needs

A final issue that we want to address here is whether non-related future costs in added life years should also entail costs for normal housing, food, clothes and so on, perhaps even weighed against the production value of the longer living individual. The analysis by Meltzer (1997) indicates that these costs ('earnings and consumption') should also be part of a study, as these costs are relevant for total welfare. Although we contend that this is the case, both in terms of an individual and of a society, we do not recommend the inclusion of these broader unrelated non-medical costs and gains here. The analyst may decide to present this cost-category when considered relevant for the final decision, but for reasons of feasibility a prescription to include these costs is not considered useful. Furthermore, discussion on where to draw the line in costs to consider in the analysis is encouraged here.

Table 4.2 Recommendations for incorporation of different cost-items

	Life-years normally lived	Gained life-years
Related medical and non-medical costs	Incorporate	Incorporate
Unrelated medical and non-medical costs	Leave out of the analysis	*May be incorporated at analyst's discretion in a sensitivity analysis

4.6.5 **Concluding**

In conclusion of this section, it has to be noted that the discussion on this subject is still continuing and that a final recommendation on whether and how to include all types of costs cannot be given. It is important to acknowledge that, next to welfare theoretical approaches to the problem, the societal decision-maker's view should also be considered (Brouwer and Koopmanschap 2000). As Hurley (1998) indicates, economic evaluation should reflect societal preferences and opinions. In that sense, some of the costs discussed above may be omitted from the analysis because the societal decision-maker does not want to consider them (e.g. the net production gain of saving the life of a productive person). Also, the incorporation of certain costs may make the task of the analyst extremely difficult, since these costs are difficult to assess. As a preliminary solution, Table 4.2 is presented with for each cost-category a recommendation on whether or not and how to include it in an economic evaluation (if they are at least significantly present).

4.7 **Conclusions**

This chapter has dealt with the cost-calculations in economic evaluation. Specifically, after an introduction and a discussion about the concept of costing, it has discussed the three steps of costing: identification of resources, measuring resource use and valuing the resource use. Some main points will be highlighted.

An economic evaluation should aim at presenting the opportunity costs of the intervention under study from a societal perspective. Taking this perspective has consequences for which costs to include in the analysis (in principle all) and also for the way in which they are measured and valued. In the identification phase all relevant cost-items need to be identified, regardless of their expected influence of the final outcome. The preferred methods for data collection need to be determined in relation to the study design and the context and aim of the study. In the phase of designing a study a choice between more precise micro-costing and more general gross-costing needs to be made. Subsequently, resource changes related to the intervention need to be measured, making it possible to specify a production function. As indicated in Section 4.3 several data collection methods exist and may be useful mostly depending on the aim and context of the evaluation. The third step entails costing the different resource items, which transforms the production function into a cost function.

In Section 4.4 several costing aspects were discussed. It is important to stress that the use of tariffs requires caution, as these may not reflect societal opportunity costs in many cases. Depending on the level of precision of cost estimates required and the availability of data, a choice must be made between different costing methods (gross or micro-costing). In many instances, a study will use a combination of these costing methods. The organizational setting, the scale of the intervention and the time span in which the intervention will be implemented and performed are important in cost calculations and need to be taken into account. Projections of learning curves may be used in order to get a tentative idea about the future development of costs. Systematically monitoring the costs of an implemented intervention may provide valuable insight in this respect. It is recommended here that in cost calculations all transfer costs are incorporated in the opportunity costs. Using gross-wages and prices including VAT, the cost parameters remain comprehensible for the decision-maker, who is indeed confronted with full prices. When using resource and cost data from a multi-centre or even a multi-national trial, it is important to carefully consider and specify the method for cost calculations.

Sections 4.5 and 4.6 dealt with specific cost categories, informal care and costs in life years gained. For recommendations on the latter, we refer to Table 4.2. For informal care, it is stressed that in an economic evaluation from a societal perspective, this cost item should not be left out of the analysis. The costing method should be made clear and, where relevant and possible, quality-of-life changes in informal caregivers should be measured and reported.

Finally, we want to stress that since costing is a complex process, clarity of the analysts about what cost-items were identified, how the resource use was measured and how this was subsequently valued is crucial. All choices, from study design to time horizon should be specified and explained. Also, all resource items should be listed, separating quantity from costs per item and total costs. In the end, although perhaps not perfect, economic evaluation in general, and costing specifically, should be a transparent tool in the complex environment of modern health care.

References

van Agthoven, M. (1998). *Costs of liver transplantation: a second opinion* (in Dutch). Department of Health Policy and Management, Erasmus University Rotterdam.

Al, M. J., Koopmanschap, M. A., van Enckevort, P. J., Geertsma, A. *et al.* (1998). Cost-effectiveness of lung transplantation in the Netherlands; a scenario-analysis. *Chest*, 113, 124–30.

Aletras, V. H. (1999). Comparison of hospital scale effects in short-run and long-run cost functions. *Health Economics*, 8, 521–30.

Bergman, L., van der Meulen, J. H. P., Limburg, M. *et al.* (1995). Costs of medical care after first-ever stroke in the Netherlands. *Stroke*, 26, 1830–6.

Brouwer, W. B. F., and Koopmanschap, M. A. (2000). On the economic foundations of CEA. Ladies and gentlemen, take your positions! *Journal of Health Economics*, 19, 439–59.

Brouwer, W. B. F., Koopmanschap, M. A. and Rutten, F. F. H. (1997a). Productivity costs measurement through quality-of-life? A response to the recommendations of the Washington Panel. *Health Economics*, 6, 253–9.

Brouwer, W. B. F., Koopmanschap, M. A. and Rutten, F. F. H. (1997b). Productivity costs in cost-effectiveness analysis: numerator or denominator: a further discussion. *Health Economics*, 6, 511–14.

Brouwer, W. B. F., Koopmanschap, M. A. and Rutten, F. F. H. (1998). Patient and informal caregiver time in cost-effectiveness analysis. A response to recommendations of the Washington Panel. *International Journal of Technology Assessment in Health Care*, 14, 505–13.

Brouwer, W. B. F., van Exel, N. J. A., Koopmanschap, M. A. *et al.* (1999). The valuation of informal care in economic appraisal: a consideration of individual choice and societal costs of time. *International Journal of Technology Assessment in Health Care*, 15, 147–60.

van Busschbach, J.J., Brouwer, W. B. F., van der Donk, A. *et al.* (1998). An outline of a cost-effectiveness analysis of a drug for patients with Alzheimer's Disease. *PharmacoEconomics*, 13, 21–34.

CCOHTA. (1997). *Guidelines for economic evaluation of pharmaceuticals.* (2nd edn). CCOHTA, Ottawa.

Commonwealth Department of Human Services and Health (1995). *Guidelines for the pharmaceutical industry on preparation of submissions to the pharmaceutical benefits advisory committee.* Australian Government Publishing Service, Canberra.

Drummond, M. F., O'Brien, B., Stoddard, G. L. *et al.* (1997). *Methods for the economic evaluation of health care programs.* (2nd edn). Oxford University Press, Oxford.

van Enckevort, P.J., Koopmanschap, M. A., TenVergert, E. M., *et al..* (1997). Lifetime costs of lung transplantation: estimation of incremental costs. *Health Economics*, 6, 479–89.

Garber, A. M. and Phelps, C. E. (1997). Economic foundations of cost-effectiveness analysis. *Journal of Health Economics*, 16, 1–32.

Gold, M. R., Siegel, J. E., Russell, L. B. and Weinstein, M.C. (1996). *Cost-effectiveness in health and medicine.* Oxford University Press, Oxford.

Groot, T. L. C. M., Evers, S. M. A. A. and Wenemoser, R. A. S. (1996). Management accounting praktijk in Nederlandse ziekenhuizen, *Tijdschrift voor bedrijfsadministratie*, 100, 1186.

van Hout, B., Bonsel, D., Habbema D., *et al.* (1993). Heart transplantation in the Netherlands; costs, effects and scenarios. *Journal of Health Economics*, 12, 1–124.

van Hout, B. A., Rutten, F. F. H. and Lorijn, R. H. W. (1993). Cost-effectiveness of the human monoclonal anti-body HA-1A in patients with sepsis (in Dutch). *Ned Tijdschr Geneesk*, 137, 360–4.

Hui, K. C., Zhang, F., Shaw, W. W. *et al.* (2000). Learning curve of microvascular venous anastomosis: a never ending struggle? *Microsurgery*, 20, 22–4.

Hurley, J. (1998). Welfarism, extra-welfarism and evaluative economic analysis in the health care sector. In: M. L. Barer, T. E. Getzen and G. L. Stoddard, (eds). *Health, health care and health economics: perspectives on distribution.* John Wiley & Sons Ltd, Chichester.

Johannesson, M. (1997). Avoiding double-counting in pharmacoeconomic studies. *Pharmacoeconomics*, 11, 385–8.

de Keizer, N. F., Bonsel, G.J., Al, M. J. *et al.* (1998). The relation between TISS and real paediatric ICU costs: a case study with generalizable methodology. *Intensive Care Medicine*, 24, 1062–69.

Koopmanschap, M. A. (1998). Cost of illness studies; useful for health policy? *Pharmacoeconomics*, 14, 143–148.

Koopmanschap, M. A. and Rutten, F. F. H. (1996). Indirect costs: the consequences of production loss or increased costs of production. *Medical Care*, 34, DS59-DS68.

Koopmanschap, M. A., van Roijen, L., Bonneux, L. *et al.* (1994). Costs of diseases in international perspective. *European Journal of Public Health*, 4, 258–64.

Koopmanschap, M. A., Rutten, F. F. H., van Ineveld, B. M., and van Roijen, L. (1995). The friction cost method for measuring indirect costs of disease. *Journal of Health Economics*, 14, 171–89.

LETB. (1999). *National evaluation of population screening for breast cancer in the Netherlands.* Report (in Dutch). Rotterdam.

Lindgren, B. (1990). The economic impact of illness. In : U. Abshagen and F. E. Munnich, (eds), *Cost of illness and benefits of drug treatment*, W. Zuchschwerat Verlag, Munich, pp. 12–20.

Meerding, W. J., Bonneux, L., Polder, J. J. *et al.* (1998). Demographic and epidemiological determinants of healthcare costs in Netherlands: cost of illness study. *British Medical Journal*, 317, 111–15.

Meltzer, D. (1997). Accounting for future costs in medical cost-effectiveness analysis. *Journal of Health Economics*, 16, 33–64.

Mohide, E. A., Torrance, G.W., Streiner, D. L. *et al.* (1988). Measuring the wellbeing of family caregivers using the time trade-off technique. *Journal of Clinical Epidemiology*, 41, 475–482.

Oostenbrink, J., Koopmanschap, M. A. and Rutten, F. F. H. (2000). *Costing manual for economic evaluation in health care* (in Dutch). Health Insurance Council, Amstelveen.

Parker, G. (1990). Spouse carers. Whose quality-of-life?. In: S. Baldwin, C. Godfrey, and C. Propper (eds). *The quality-of-life: perspectives and policies.* Routledge, London.

Posnett, J., and Jan, S. (1996). Indirect cost in economic evaluation: the opportunity cost of unpaid input. *Health Economics*, 5, 13–23.

Raikou, A., Briggs, A ., Gray, A. *et al.* (2000). Costing methodology centre-specific or average unit costs in multi-centre studies? some theory and simulation. *Health Economics*, 9, 191–8.

Rice, D. P., Hodgson, T. A. and Kopstein, A. N. (1985). The economic cost of illness: a replication and update. *Health Care Financial Review*, 7, 61–80.

van Roijen, L., Essink-Bot, M. L., Koopmanschap, M. A. *et al.* (1996). Labour and health status in economic evaluation of health care. *International Journal of Technology Assessment in Health Care,* 12, 405–15.

Russell, L. B. (1986). *Is prevention better than cure?* The Brookings Institution, Washington DC.

Smith, K. and Wright, K. (1994). Informal care and economic appraisal: A discussion of possible methodological approaches. *Health Economics*, 3, 137–48.

Spanos, A. (1995). On theory testing in econometrics modeling with nonexperimental data. *Journal of Econometrics*, 67, 189–226.

Weinstein, M. C., and Fineberg, H. V. (1980). *Clinical decision analysis.* W. B. Saunders, Philadelphia.

Weinstein, M. C., and Manning, W. G. Jr. (1997). Theoretical issues in cost-effectiveness analysis. *Journal of Health Economics,* 16, 121–8.

Weinstein, M. C., Siegel, J. E., Garber, A. M. *et al.* (1997). Productivity costs, time costs and health related quality-of-life: a response to the Erasmus Group. *Health Economics*, 6, 505–10.

Weinstein, M. C., Siegel, J. E., Gold, M. R. *et al.* (1996).Recommendations of the panel on cost-effectiveness in health and medicine. *Journal of the American Medical Association*, 276, 1253–8.

Willke, R. J., Glick, H. A., Polsky, D. *et al.* (1998). Costing methodology centre-specific or average unit costs in multi-centre studies? Some theory and simulation. *Health Economics*, 7, 481–93.

Wright. K. (1987). *The economics of informal care.* Centre for Health Economics, Discussion Paper 23, University of York, York.

Chapter 5

The role and estimation of productivity costs in economic evaluation

Mark Sculpher

5.1 Introduction

It has been recognized for some time that public sector investment decisions may have important implications for how individuals are able to allocate their time and, consequently, for the value of that time. Many cost-benefit studies have, therefore, sought to estimate how public sector projects might change how individuals spend their time, and to reflect the value of these changes within the calculus of the appraisal. Health care interventions and programmes influence the amount of time individuals are able to devote to the full range of leisure and working activities that are of value to them and to society more generally. As a branch of public sector appraisal, economic evaluation in health care has, therefore, attempted to reflect the value of changes in patterns of time allocation.

There is a general acceptance that individuals' time is a limited resource with opportunity costs. This is reflected in economic evaluation textbooks (Dranove 1995; Luce *et al.*. 1996; Drummond *et al.*. 1997). It is also shown in the current official guidelines for the economic appraisal of pharmaceuticals and other health technologies, usually for public funding, where a majority of statements explicitly (or by implication) support the incorporation of one or more aspects of time cost (Pritchard and Sculpher 2000).

Despite this general acceptance, the practical detail of how to incorporate time costs into economic evaluation has been controversial, and limited agreement exists regarding appropriate methods. Controversy has been most pronounced in the area of productivity costs, with disagreement about whether or not these costs should be included in economic evaluation and, if so, how they should be estimated. This methodological uncertainty is reflected in applied studies where, of 1039 cost-effectiveness studies on the Office for Health Economics' Health Economic Evaluation Database (HEED), only 10.4 per cent were found to have incorporated productivity costs (Pritchard and Sculpher 2000).

The objective of this chapter is to describe the methodological issues associated with the incorporation of productivity costs into economic evaluation in health care. Section 5.2 defines productivity costs and looks at the rationale for their inclusion in economic evaluation; Section 5.3 considers available approaches for the measurement of changes in time allocation which underlie productivity costs; Section 5.4 focuses on the alternative approaches that have been developed for the valuation of time to characterize productivity costs; and Section 5.5 offers some conclusions.

5.2 The rationale for including productivity costs in economic evaluation

5.2.1 Defining productivity costs

The term productivity costs has only recently become standard within economic evaluation to refer to the value of specific categories of individuals' time influenced by ill-health. Previously the term 'indirect costs' had been used, which caused some confusion given that this term is often used by cost accountants to mean something quite different. The US Panel on Cost-Effectiveness in Health and Medicine recommended the term 'productivity cost' to refer to 'the costs associated with lost or impaired ability to work or to engage in leisure activities due to morbidity and lost economic productivity due to death' (Luce *et al.* 1996, p. 181). Other time costs have previously been included under the heading of indirect costs, such as the value of the time patients allocate to receiving health care (e.g. visits to clinic for screening tests) and the value of the time individuals devote to the care of sick friends and relatives. The US Panel suggested that these latter components of time cost be included under the direct costs of care. Given some agreement with the Panel's suggestions regarding changes in terminology (Brouwer *et al.* 1997b), and an absence of clear disagreement, this is the working definition of productivity costs used in this chapter.

5.2.2 Societal perspective in economic evaluation

It is a widely understood principle of economic evaluation in health care that there should be a decision and a clear statement regarding the perspective from which costs and benefits are estimated within a study (Drummond *et al.* 1997). Although many studies adopt narrow perspectives, often that of the hospital or health service (payer), there are strong normative arguments that a societal perspective should be taken (Torrance *et al.* 1996b; Johannesson 1995). This argument relates to the principles of welfare economic theory which indicate that a given policy change may have a series of effects on different individuals and groups, and that an overall assessment of the efficiency of the policy needs to consider all of these implications.

The implication of this principle in health care is that taking a narrow perspective may lead to the adoption of inefficient changes in delivery. For example, if new interventions for dementia are evaluated from the perspective of the health care system, they may be rejected as inefficient in ignorance of the fact that their use can reduce the burden on resources outside the health care system in areas such as social services and the care provided by family members. In other words, any study taking a narrow perspective will only incorporate a partial view of the cost and benefit implications of changes in programmes.

5.2.3 **Inclusion of production costs: efficiency criteria**

If the principle of the societal perspective is accepted, then the impact of health care programmes on the time sick individuals are able to devote to working and leisure activities should be reflected in economic evaluation. This conclusion is widely accepted in the methods literature. Gerard and Mooney (1993) add an important caveat, however. They note that, as the dominant form of economic evaluation in health care, cost-effectiveness analysis (CEA) increasingly uses health outcomes as its measure of effect, typically in the form of life years or quality-adjusted life years (QALYs). They argue that the use of health-related outcomes to the exclusion of other non-resource effects removes the logic of including non-health care costs in the analysis. This is because, in terms of opportunity costs, the value of health care resources can only be measured in terms of forgone health. Non-health care resources (e.g. individuals' leisure and working time) have a range of alternative uses other than health producing activity, and this cannot adequately be reflected within CEA.

In response, it has been argued that the Gerard and Mooney argument does not recognize that budgets are arbitrary divisions in how resources are organized (Koopmanschap and Rutten 1996). This would be clear if the value of any savings in the use of resources outside the control of the health care sector (e.g. social services or productivity) as a result of using a specific intervention, were fed back into the health service budget.

This exchange raises a more general issue about the role of productivity costs in economic evaluation within an extra-welfarist paradigm, which focuses less on individual utility (as in conventional welfare economics) and more on the value of aggregate health gain (Culyer 1989; Hurley 2000). Rather than being viewed as true resource costs, productivity costs can be seen as non-health *effects* where individuals' loss of income through ill-health affects their wellbeing through its impact on their consumption rather than their health. Within the extra-welfarist approach, where a maximand of health gain operates, this view of productivity costs may be sufficient to rule it out of applied economic evaluation studies. Olsen (1994), however, develops a model which shows that, even with an objective function of maximizing the sum of utility from health, considering production gains may be warranted. Consistent with the argument of Koopmanschap and Rutten (1996) noted above, the analysis showed that giving priority to the productive – which is the ultimate implication of considering production costs in economic evaluation – could be justified to the extent that they could 'pay their way' by financing extra health care.

5.2.4 **Inclusion of production costs: equity criteria**

In contrast to the extra-welfarist position, several authors have sought to place societal CEA within a framework of conventional welfare economic theory (Johannesson 1995; Garber and Phelps 1997). An important feature of this work is the concept that a societal willingness to pay for a unit of health gain (which would be fixed between individuals) might provide a bridge between CEA, cost-benefit analysis (CBA) and hence applied welfare economics. In effect, this would offer an 'exchange rate' between the opportunity cost of resources in terms of health gain and non-health-affecting activities which, in principle, would overcome Gerard and Mooney's argument.

The consideration of productivity costs within a societal evaluation is prompted by efficiency arguments. Concerns have been raised regarding the equity implications of considering these costs (Williams 1992). These concerns reflect that the fact that, with the traditional methods of estimating productivity costs, the value of an individual's time is based on their level of productivity as reflected in their earnings from employment. Therefore, the logical conclusion of the inclusion of these costs is that interventions which are able to return more productive individuals to their usual activities will be deemed more cost-effective than other programmes. This may provoke concerns about the inclusion of productivity costs, particularly given that developments in economic evaluation in health have moved away from standard CBA where valuation of health benefit through stated or revealed valuation methods rests heavily on individuals' ability to pay. The egalitarian principle that exists in many countries in publicly-funded health care provision has led to an evaluative focus on CEA where health gain is valued equally regardless of who benefits, so the inclusion of productivity costs within the calculus may be considered inconsistent.

An analysis by Olsen and Richardson (1999) is one of the few to have addressed this broader perspective on productivity costs. Developing the themes raised by Olsen in his earlier paper referred to above (Olsen 1994), they argue that the methods literature on productivity costs has focused on the *positive* question of how to quantify the value of lost productivity due to illness, rather than the *normative* issue of which aspects of productivity cost should be included in social decision-making about health care resource allocation. On the basis of possible distribution principles relating to the health service, they seek to establish those components of productivity costs that should be relevant to resource allocation. They conclude that (a) production changes should only be considered in economic evaluation to the extent that they affect 'the rest of society' rather than the sick individual; (b) this 'external' effect could be through the effect of productivity gains on taxation levels and hence on additional health care expenditure and the funding of public goods – if it is considered that the only legitimate outcome of interest in economic evaluation is health effects, then only the implications for health care expenditure are relevant; (c) given that, even with this truncated perspective on relevant productivity costs, health gain for more productive individuals will be more highly valued than for others, there is a trade-off between the 'desirable' implications of productivity gains for health care funding and the 'undesirable' distributional effects – the optimal point on that trade-off will largely depend on a society's attitudes to inequality.

5.3 Measuring changes in productivity

Although Olsen and Richardson's analysis has raised normative questions about the *extent* to which productivity effects should be considered in economic evaluation in health care, it suggests that they are likely to play some role. Important questions, therefore, remain about the most appropriate methods for quantifying productivity effects.

It is important to make a distinction between the *measurement* of time affected by ill-health and the *valuation* of that time to estimate productivity costs. Whilst most literature has focused on issues associated with valuation, the measurement process has been under-researched. The increasing role of prospective data collection for economic evaluation – often alongside randomized controlled trials – has offered the opportunity of asking patients to record the amount of time they have missed from their usual activities as a result of illness. These developments have been supported by research showing high levels of correspondence between individuals' recall and administration records of days lost from work due to ill-health (Revicki *et al.* 1994).

Several questionnaires have been designed for this purpose. Reilly *et al.* (1993) developed a Work Productivity and Activity Impairment (WPAI) questionnaire to elicit the extent of lost time from work and loss in productivity whilst at work in patients with a specific health problem. Results were presented in percentages with an overall work productivity score calculated as the product of the proportion of scheduled work time spent working and the percentage productivity while at work. In addition, a set of items elicited individuals' ability to undertake everyday activities other than paid work and, again, results were presented as percentages. The authors showed the instrument correlated positively with established measures of perceived health and demonstrated adequate levels of reproducibility.

van Roijen *et al.* (1996) developed a similar instrument for individuals to self-complete – the Health and Labour Questionnaire (HLQ). The instrument had four modules: Module 1 focused on paid work and asked individuals, on a day-by-day basis, whether they had undertaken paid work, been unable to do so because of ill-health or been unable to do so because of other reasons. Module 2 related to loss of productivity while undertaking paid employment and asked respondents how many additional hours they would have had to work to compensate for lost productivity at work; additionally, a set of descriptive items sought information on aspects of work activity that were limited by illness. Module 3 considered unpaid production in four areas – household work, shopping, caring for children and odd jobs around the house. Respondents were asked to estimate the number of hours spent on each activity over a two week period; the effect of a specific health problem on this activity is established by comparing the results with data from a control group. Module 4 looked at impediments to paid and unpaid labour by asking respondents to indicate whether they had experienced any specific health impediments whilst undertaking paid or unpaid work.

In a representative sample of 995 individuals from the general population, the HLQ was tested for feasibility and validity by looking at response rates and comparison with other sources of data. The authors concluded that a 68 per cent usable response rate was acceptable for a postal questionnaire and that most measures of validity provided positive results. The main exception related to the measurement of productivity loss due to illness whilst at work where the HLQ measure showed poor correlation with two alternative measures.

Further research has been undertaken on the measurement of productivity loss whilst at work. Brouwer *et al.* (1999) compared the methods used for this purpose in the HLQ with two other approaches. The first of these is the Osterhaus method, which asks respondents the number of days over the past two weeks they went to work with health problems and the average efficiency of those days measured on a visual analogue scale (Osterhaus *et al.* 1992). The second comparator was the 'QQ' method which asks, on a daily basis using a visual analogue scale, the quantity of work they performed, compared with normal, and the quality of that work on a similar scale. The study considered the construct validity of the alternative measures, hypothesizing that the HLQ method would generate the lowest estimates because it focuses on production loss that is recoverable and is not yet made up for, the Osterhaus the highest because it concentrates in the work capacity of the individual and the QQ approach would lie somewhere in-between the extremes. In a survey of 216 workers in a Dutch trade firm, with a response rate of 50 per cent, the data were consistent with this hypothesis. The comparison also highlighted the large number of zero responses to the HLQ approach.

An aspect of the measurement task which has relevance to the valuation process is the extent to which lost productivity due to ill-health is compensated for, either by work colleagues or by the sick individual on return to work. If such compensating mechanisms are ignored, estimates of productivity costs may be overestimates of those that are actually incurred – Section 5.4.2 deals with this in more detail. Severens *et al.* (1998) explored this in the clinical area of dyspepsia. As part of two clinical studies including a total of 136 individuals with dyspepsia, questionnaires asked how many days were lost from work in the preceding four weeks due to dyspepsia or other health problems. Respondents were asked to indicate whether or not compensation mechanisms were available. The authors estimated that, if compensation mechanisms were allowed for, productivity costs for these patients would be only 25 per cent of the level that would result if such mechanisms were ignored.

5.4 Valuing productivity costs

The methods literature on productivity costs in health care evaluation has largely focused on how a value might be placed on measures of lost work and leisure time due to ill-health. It is possible to identify three distinct approaches to valuation, although these are not wholly mutually exclusive: the human capital approach, the friction cost approach and the US Panel approach.

5.4.1 The human capital approach

Valuing lost time from paid employment

Early examples of economic analysis of health care programmes were based largely on the principles of CBA where an important (often then only) component of benefit was taken as the gains in productivity resulting from getting sick individuals back into paid employment. In these early studies, productivity benefits were usually estimated on the basis of the present value of the additional stream of lifetime income for an individual as a result of a given health care programme – the human capital approach (Rice and Cooper 1967).

This approach was criticized for its tenuous link to welfare economic theory and its implicit assumption that the objective of health care was to maximize national productivity (Mishan 1971). Over the last 20 years CBA has played much less of a role in applied economic appraisal in health care, and CEA has become the predominant analytical approach where effects are typically represented by a measure of health such as life years or QALYs. Although 'health gain' has become a more widely used measure of benefit in economic evaluation, the need to reflect changes in productivity as a component of the time costs of interventions has resulted in the human capital approach retaining a role in CEA, albeit not as the main estimate of benefit.

As applied in health care evaluation, the human capital approach has largely been used to value changes in the amount of time individuals are able to allocate to paid work as a result of illness or programmes to alleviate ill-health. The principles of valuing this time rest firmly on neoclassical labour theory and theory of the firm. In particular, the theory that, assuming diminishing marginal productivity, a profit-maximizing firm would employ additional labour until the marginal revenue product of the last unit of employment equals the employment cost faced by the firm where the latter is the gross wage including additional costs of employment such as the employer's contribution to national insurance and superannuation.

According to the human capital approach, the gross wage thus becomes the unit of value for changes in paid working time resulting from health care programmes. In the case of a health care programme which can extend an individual's life (i.e. a reduc-tion in mortality risk), the change in productivity cost would be represented by the present value of the stream of additional days in paid work over the individual's life-time, with each day valued using the gross wage. In part, this value will be reflected in increased consumption (and utility) to the individual. However, 'external' effects will be experienced by others through, for example, increased tax revenue. The issue of external effects is considered further in Section 5.4.3. Similarly, changes in morbidity can be expected to result in additional working days and these too would be valued using the gross wage. In principle, reduction in productivity whilst at work as a result of illness could be valued in the same way, assuming such changes could be measured (see Section 5.3).

Valuing changes in leisure time

Leisure time forgone as a result of illness also has value to individuals. This is rarely considered as part of the human capital estimates of productivity change due to ill-health in applied studies, but the principles of the method indicate how such time could be valued. According to neoclassical theory, assuming diminishing marginal utility from leisure, an individual will devote time to paid work until the opportunity cost of that time equals the marginal benefit which is the wage-rate (net of taxes and other deductibles) received from employment. Assuming that an individual's time is allocated to either paid employment or leisure activities, the opportunity cost of working time is forgone leisure which, at the margin, can be valued as the net (take-home) wage.

There is another issue around the valuation of leisure time which has rarely been explicitly considered as part of the human capital approach. One of the implications of individuals having to take time off work as a result of illness is a corresponding increase in leisure. In principle, the value of this additional leisure time should offset the value of the loss in production through lost working time. In practice, it is usually assumed that the value of this increased leisure time is negligible given the patient's ill-health (Liljas 1998). Furthermore, within CEA, the valuation of changes in leisure time for the sick individual can be incorporated into some measures of health gain (see pp. 101–103).

Valuing changes in non-paid working time

Changes in days available for non-paid working time, such as housework or voluntary work outside the home, can also be valued using the principles of the human capital approach. Although examples of this are rare in the applied economic evaluation literature, economic theory would suggest that this time should be valued according to its opportunity cost which would probably be the value of forgone leisure time (Liljas 1998). As detailed above, labour theory would suggest that lost leisure time should be valued at the net wage that could be obtained by the individual if they were in paid employment – the reservation wage. A lower bound of this net wage can be inferred from that of individuals with similar characteristics, such as age and education level, who are in paid employment (Luce et al. 1996).

An alternative approach to valuing this time is to use the gross wage-rate of individuals in paid work which most closely matches that of the unpaid worker (Luce et al. 1996). In other words the cost of buying in this service if it was not being provided with no payment. For example, the time of an individual caring for a sick relative might be valued using the gross wage of a care assistant. In contrast to the valuation of this time using the reservation wage, this is likely to offer an upper bound of the value of non-paid work time because if the individual valued their leisure time to this extent, they would be expected actually to 'buy' the service rather than 'produce' it directly. The fact that an informal worker is likely to be less efficient at a service (e.g. through lack of training) again suggests this approach to valuing unpaid work will generate an upper band estimate. The methodological issues associated with costing non-paid working time were discussed in Chapter 4.

Human capital approach in cost-effectiveness analysis

The transplantation of the human capital approach from CBA to CEA has resulted in some complications. In particular, when the measure of effect in CEA is a generic measure of health, such as the QALY, which incorporates changes in both life expectancy and the health-related quality-of-life (HRQL), or even the simple life-year, there is a risk of double-counting when productivity costs are additionally valued in monetary terms (Johannesson 1997; Sculpher and O'Brien 2000). The clearest manifestation of this relates to the valuation of productivity changes due to mortality. Here, double-counting will exist – in part at least – if a monetary value is placed on lost productivity due to premature death, and additionally life years or QALYs are used as the measure of health. This double-counting exists as both are essentially valuing the same effect – the loss in healthy time. The use of life years or QALYs will not, however, reflect the value of lost production to individuals other than the deceased such as those who benefit from that individual's tax payments.

A second potential source of double-counting relates to the valuation of lost leisure time due to illness. When the QALY is used as the measure of effect, the value attached to leisure time can reasonably be expected to be included within the QALY as an important attribute of HRQL. Additionally to value this time in monetary terms using the human capital approach would be to double-count the effect.

A less obvious source of double-counting may exist in relation to the valuation of working time when a measure of health gain such as the QALY is used in CEA. The implications of health care programmes for HRQL are factored into the QALY by quality-weighting life expectancy according to the value individuals attach to a given level of HRQL or health state. These values, which are typically elicited on a 0 (equivalent to death) to 1 (equivalent to good health) scale, are often based on the preferences of a sample of the general public. This has been considered more appropriate than using a sample of patients or health professionals because the public are typically the payers for health care and potential beneficiaries (Gafni 1991). The extent of the risk of double-counting depends on what individuals consider when they value health states. It is possible that they may consider the effects of a given level of HRQL for their ability to perform paid work, and their value may then partly reflect the financial implications of lost work and hence the effects on their overall level of consumption and wellbeing. This 'income effects of lost health' is simply another way of valuing the productivity loss related to paid work resulting from ill-health (Weinstein *et al.* 1997).

Additionally to value time lost from paid employment in monetary terms within CEA would be to double-count that aspect of remuneration that an individual might consider in valuing a health state – namely the net (take-home) wage. The possible existence of this form of double-counting and ways to overcome it in CEA will be considered below under the third approach to valuing productivity costs (Section 5.4.3)

5.4.2 **Friction cost approach**

Limitations of the human capital approach

The friction cost approach was developed by a group of Dutch economists and focuses largely on the valuation of lost time from paid work as a result of illness (Koopmanschap and van Ineveld 1992; Koopmanschap and Rutten 1993; Koopmanschap *et al.* 1995). Hence the general issues considered above regarding the valuation of leisure time are largely unaffected by the friction cost approach. The method was developed as a result of the perceived crudeness of the human capital method and the unrealistic theories that underlie it. In particular, the neoclassical theory on which the human capital theory is based assumes flexibility in prices which, in turn, results in all markets clearing. This assumption is somewhat out of line with reality, particularly in relation to the labour market. If the labour market functioned as suggested by neoclassical theory, wage flexibility would ensure that the supply of labour was equal to its demand. This would result in the only unemployment being 'frictional' – that is, individuals only being out of work for a short time while they negotiated further employment. In reality, long periods of involuntary unemployment, often at quite high levels, in many parts of the world, suggest that labour markets do not operate according to neoclassical theory.

It can be argued that the existence of involuntary unemployment indicates that individuals (as paid labour) and firms do not make decisions at the margin in the way that is assumed as a basis of the human capital approach to valuing productivity. The most important implication of this is that, when an individual is not able to attend work due to ill-health, there is, in principle, a pool of unemployed people from whom the sick individual can be replaced. Although there will be costs associated with identifying and training the previously-unemployed individual who is replacing the sick worker and lost productivity during that 'friction' period, the value of lost production may be markedly less than under the assumption of the human capital method of zero involuntary unemployment. In other words, the human capital approach represents a measure of *potential* value of production loss due to illness rather than the actual loss.

The mortality case

The aim of the friction cost approach is to adjust the human capital estimates of productivity costs for the compensations that are likely to occur as a result of a labour market that does not adhere to neoclassical theory. In the case of the valuation of productivity changes associated with death, the friction cost approach simply values the loss in productivity during the friction period – that is, the time it takes to replace and to train a replacement worker. The friction period may be extended in the likely instance that a replacement chain ensues (Koopmanschap *et al.* 1997). Here a dead worker is replaced by someone already in employment who, in turn, requires replacement. Eventually, however, the replacement chain is assumed to terminate with the recruitment of an individual who was previously unemployed. Furthermore, the length of the friction period is likely to vary according to factors such as the relevant sector of the labour market. Therefore, in contrast to the human capital method, which uses the gross wage to value all working time lost due to premature death, the friction cost approach only considers productivity loss during the friction period.

According to the friction cost method, however, some additional costs should be included in estimates of the value of productivity change. The first is the resource cost associated with recruiting and training replacement workers – again, this can involve several levels within a replacement chain. The second additional cost to include with this method is the effect of a transitory change in productivity for labour productivity, per unit labour costs, international competitiveness and hence national income. This 'medium-term macroeconomic effect' requires estimation using a full econometric model of the macro economy but is the only cost that will remain after the friction period (Koopmanschap *et al.* 1995).

The morbidity case

Compensatory mechanisms play an important part in the friction cost approach to the valuation of changes in paid working time as a result of morbidity. In the case of long-term illness or disability where the worker is away from paid work longer than the friction period, the valuation of this time is the same as in the mortality case. In these circumstances, the bulk of the cost of lost productivity occurs during the friction period whilst a replacement worker is being identified and trained. After the friction period, the only productivity costs relate to any medium-term macroeconomic consequences.

In the case of short-term absences due to illness, the friction cost approach suggests there are two general implications for productivity. The first is that compensatory mechanisms result in no change in production or in the employment costs facing the firm. This would be the case if the sick individual made up the lost production on their return to work or if the firm held a permanent pool of 'reserve' labour which could be used as cover for sick colleagues. There would, however, still be medium term macro-economic consequences of these short-term absences.

However, other scenarios are considered which may result in short-term absences reducing productivity by a similar value as would be estimated with the human capital approach. One simple outcome would be for a once-and-for-all drop in production while the sick individual is away from work which is not compensated for. Another scenario is that the sick individual's lost production is compensated for in some way: overtime payments on their return to work, overtime to colleagues or the employment of temporary workers. Assuming that the sick individual's pay continues during the absence, this represents an increase in costs to the firm. A third scenario is some combination of the other two if the compensation mechanisms do not fully make up for the lost production despite employment costs increasing. As discussed in Section 5.3, an important issue is how to measure the extent to which compensation takes place.

Given the uncertainty in how a firm will choose and be able to react to short-term absence of a given worker, Koopmanschap *et al.* (1995) used aggregate Dutch data to estimate the elasticity of production with respect to changes in labour time. They found this to be 80 per cent – that is, every 1 per cent reduction in labour days would result on average in a 0.8 per cent reduction in production. The operationalization of the friction cost approach also requires country-specific estimates of a range of para-meters, which may also change over time, for example according to the business cycle. These parameters include the number and duration of the friction periods and the medium-term macroeconomic effects.

Comparing the human capital and friction cost methods

Some comparison has taken place of the alternative estimates of production costs generated by the human capital and friction cost approaches. In the context of a

Table 5.1 Productivity costs from illness in the Netherlands: a comparison of human capital and friction cost estimates (billions of Dutch guilders)[a]

Cost category	Friction costs 1988	Human capital costs 1988	Friction costs 1990
Absence from work	9.2	23.8	11.6
Disability	0.15	49.1	0.2
Mortality	0.15	8.0	0.2
Total (as a percentage of net national income)	9.5 (2.1%)	80.9 (18%)	12.0 (2.6%)

Note: [a] Medium-term macroeconomic consequences are not included

Source: Koopmanschap *et al.* (1995)

national cost-of-illness analysis for the Netherlands, Koopmanschap *et al.* (1995) found major differences between the two approaches, particularly in the valuation of productivity losses associated with disability (see Table 5.1). On the basis of 1988 data, the value of production losses due to ill-health according to the friction cost approach was only 12 per cent that of the human capital approach; that is, 2.1 per cent of net national income compared to 18 per cent.

Criticisms of the friction cost approach

The main source of criticism of the friction cost approach has been the implication of its rejection of key tenets of conventional microeconomic theory (Johannesson and Karlsson 1997; Liljas 1998). Perhaps the most important of these is the argument that, if the existence of involuntary unemployment effectively reduces the opportunity cost of labour to zero after the friction period, this has major implications for how direct labour inputs into health care (e.g. clinicians' time) should be valued in economic evaluation. In other words, if the value of production losses due to lost working time on the part of sick individuals is zero after replacement by and retraining of the previously unemployed, exactly the same situation applies to the valuation of the time of clinicians and other health service staff in applied studies. This has been refuted by the developers of the friction cost approach who argue that their focus is the aggregate effects of ill-health on production which, through macroeconomic effects, may extend past the friction period (Koopmanschap *et al.* 1997).

A further criticism levelled at the friction cost approach is that, although it can reasonably be argued that the neoclassical assumption that wage flexibility will generate zero involuntary unemployment is demonstrably wrong in practice in most developed economies, the assumption of the friction cost method that the value the unemployed put on their leisure time is effectively zero is also likely to be out of line with reality. If the opportunity cost of the leisure time of the unemployed were negligible, such individuals would be willing to offer their labour for any wage above unemployment benefit. If this is considered unrealistic, and the leisure time forgone on the part of a previously unemployed individual who is replacing a deceased or long-term disabled worker is taken as having value, part of the rationale for the friction cost approach disappears. The importance of this point has been emphasized in debate between the developers of the friction cost method and members of the US Panel (Brouwer *et al.* 1997a, b; Weinstein *et al.* 1997).

The friction cost approach to the valuation of short-term absences due to sickness is unlikely to generate markedly different estimates of production cost to the human capital approach. However, this aspect of the proposed method also rests on the abandonment of important elements of economic theory. The view that production loss might be limited if a sick worker can make up for production losses on return to work suggests that the worker is not normally generating output to the value of their gross wage or that they will have to work harder on their return to work thus forgoing leisure time which has value to them. The idea of compensation through internal labour reserves also suggests that firms are behaving in a manner which is inconsistent with maximizing profits. However, if the cost of recruiting and training new workers is high, for example when the labour market is 'tight', there may be good reason for a profit maximizing firm to retain labour reserves (Koopmanschap *et al.* 1995). Much depends, therefore, on how typical this type of behaviour is on the part of firms.

Much of the application of the friction cost approach has been in the context of cost-of-illness studies (Koopmanschap *et al.* 1995), rather than the CEA of alternative health care programmes from a societal perspective. Like the human capital approach, there are some aspects of the friction cost approach the use of which risks double-counting in CEA. The most important example of this is the valuation of productivity losses due to mortality. The full extent of this value would be appropriate to incorporate into a CEA where a measure of effect such as disability days avoided is used. Furthermore, a proportion of the value would be relevant to cover that element of production loss that affects individuals other than the deceased – for example, those benefiting from that part of the individual's output representing tax contributions. However, when the measure of effect within a CEA is QALYs or life years, the value of the change in life expectancy to the individuals to whom the interventions are targeted is fully represented in terms of the measure of health gain.

5.4.3 US Panel's proposals

In 1993, the US Public Health Service convened a multi-disciplinary panel to generate detailed guidelines for the cost-effectiveness analysis of health care interventions. The results of their research and deliberations were published in 1996 (Gold *et al.* 1996). Arguably, the panel's guidelines on the valuation of productivity costs have been its most controversial. The main source of the controversy was the view that an important element of the effect of disease on productivity could and should be valued

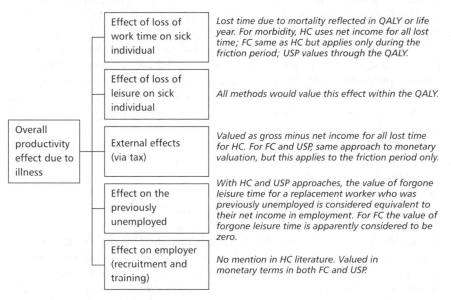

Fig. 5.1 The components of productivity cost and differences between the human capital (HC), friction cost (FC) and US Panel (USP) approaches to valuing each component

though a generic preference-based measure of health such as the QALY. Since the publication of the recommendations, key members of the team have further illuminated the Panel's views on productivity costs (Weinstein *et al.* 1997).

An important contribution of the US Panel was to delineate the various components of productivity cost. In particular, they emphasized that mortality or morbidity will result in a change in productivity that will be manifested in various areas of the economy and will affect a series of groups and individuals. Five possible productivity effects are considered in sections below and summarized in Figure 5.1, which also shows the differences and similarities between the three valuation approaches.

Effect on paid working time of the sick individual

The focus of the US Panel's recommendation was on appropriate methods for CEA and, in particular, for those studies where health is measured in terms of QALYs or a similar metric. This was, therefore, a more specific consideration of productivity costs than with the human capital and friction cost methods, and is partly responsible for the differences between the methods.

As discussed in Section 5.4.1, there has been concern that monetary valuation of changes in productivity will result in double-counting if the QALY is used as a measure of benefit. The clearest example of this is in the mortality case where premature death leads to a loss in time allocated to employment. Within a CEA, this lost time *to the deceased individual* is already given value in the non-monetarized benefit measure, if the latter takes the form of a QALY or life year. Additionally to value this effect in monetary terms as a 'cost' in a CEA would be a form of double-counting. The US Panel's argument that this element of the productivity effect should rightly be valued in non-monetary form does not seem to have been a source of controversy.

There is no such consensus regarding the Panel's recommendations on valuing the productivity effects of morbidity. When an individual is unable to work due to ill-health, they may lose financially which will have implications for a range of non-health-related aspects of their wellbeing (e.g. ability to partake in leisure activities). The US Panel accepted that this productivity effect on the sick individual could, as with the human capital and friction cost approaches, be valued in monetary terms in CEA. However, the Panel argued that the effect could also, logically, be valued within the QALY. This would be achieved by asking those individuals from whom health state values are elicited to consider the financial implications of health states and the effects of these on all areas of wellbeing, and to incorporate this 'income effect' into their values. The Panel emphasized that, unless the equivalence of the monetary and QALY-based approaches to the valuation of this aspect of the productivity effect was recognized, there was a risk of a further source of double-counting.

Although it emphasized the equivalence of these two approaches, the majority of US Panel members favoured the QALY-based approach to the valuation of the productivity effect on the sick individual. This preference was apparently due to the wish to retain the monetary valuation of all those effects of disease and interventions that were clearly on resources, from the valuation of effects that could be considered to be directly or indirectly associated with individuals' health. The Panel felt the latter category included effects on individuals' time and, given the rationale for CEA, these should be valued within the QALY.

The Panel's recommendation on the valuation of those productivity effects of morbidity experienced by the sick individual has been criticized (Brouwer *et al.* 1997b; Johannesson and Meltzer 1998). As mentioned in Section 5.2.3, it can be argued that, within an extra-welfarist paradigm where health gain is the maximand reflected in the QALY, it would be inappropriate to reflect non-health measures of wellbeing (i.e. consumption) in the measure of benefit. However, most criticism has not centred on the Panel's view that monetary and QALY-based valuation are conceptually equivalent, rather it has focused on the practicality of QALY-based valuation. First, it has been argued that the whole approach to health state preference elicitation would have to change. Instead of asking individuals to imagine experiencing the direct health effects in a health state, the Panel's suggested approach would require clear explanation that they were also to take into consideration, in turn, any effects the health state might have on their ability to work, the financial effects of any inability to work and the subsequent implications for other aspects of their life resulting from any loss of income. None of the existing multi-attribute valuation scales that are increasingly being used to categorize patients' health status in evaluation studies and to provide public values for health states ask the public to 'rule-in' these income effects when they value health states (Sculpher and O'Brien 2000). Indeed, one of the most widely used instruments, the Health Utility Index, actively asks individuals supplying health state values to 'rule-out' income effects (Torrance *et al.* 1996a).

Even if those multi-attribute valuation scales that are used to provide values for QALY estimation were actively to ask individuals to consider any income effects when they value health states, would this be a reliable way of valuing productivity effects? In many countries, the link between an inability to work and a loss of income is broken as a result of sickness insurance. In such instances, the individual valuing a health state will not necessarily associate poor health with income loss, so the resulting health state value will not incorporate a productivity element.

Furthermore, the generosity of sickness insurance schemes differ between countries. For example, in 1993 Canada devoted 0.1 per cent of gross domestic product to income maintenance during periods of sickness, compared to 2.6 per cent in the Netherlands and 2.1 per cent in Norway (Organisation for Economic Co-operation and Development (OECD) 1997). Therefore, when the individual is instructed to take income effects into consideration when providing preference data, a health state valuation exercise undertaken in a country with a generous welfare system may generate quite different values to a study based in a country with limited sickness insurance. These differences may have little to do with fundamental dissimilarities between how individuals perceive the direct health consequences of health states, and more to do with the differing extent to which poor health would be perceived to impact on them financially. If income effects generated variation in health state values between countries, there would be important implications for the generalizability and transportability of CEA across national boundaries.

Effect on the leisure time of the sick individual

The Panel identified the second distinct productivity effect of illness to be on the leisure time of the individual experiencing ill-health. Within CEA, the loss of leisure time associated with mortality would be valued within the non-monetarized benefit assuming, as in the case of the QALY and life-year, that life expectancy is an inherent element of that metric.

In the morbidity case, an effect of illness on the sick individual can be to increase leisure time (by virtue of being unable to undertake work), but to reduce the enjoyment of this time. The Panel recommend that the net effect of this productivity change is registered in CEA through the QALY (Weinstein *et al.* 1997), and this is also the position of the advocates of the friction cost approach (Brouwer *et al.* 1997a).

External effects

The US Panel very clearly distinguished two effects of ill-health on ability to undertake paid employment: first, the effect on the sick individual (see above, p. 107) and, secondly, the effect on others as a result of the loss of tax revenue. This distinction arises because, as noted in Section 5.4.1, the value of an individual's contribution to production is reflected in their *gross* income. A proportion of this income is received directly by the individual (net or disposable income), and the remainder is redistributed to others via taxation. In the situation when an individual is unable to work due to mortality or morbidity, those that benefit from tax-funded transfers will, in principle, experience a loss.

This 'external' productivity effect cannot be reflected in the benefit measure in CEA because, typically, the latter only relates to the health of the recipient of the heath care intervention. The US Panel, therefore, argued that it should be valued in monetary terms as a 'cost'. In the case of morbidity, this is consistent with the friction cost method, despite the fact that a clear distinction between a direct effect on the sick individual and an external effect was not necessary with the friction cost approach because the full productivity effect was valued in monetary terms. In the case of mortality, the loss of time to the deceased individual is valued explicitly within the QALY or life-year, and this does not seem to be a source of disagreement between the alternative valuation approaches. However, the external component of this effect can only be valued in monetary terms.

Effect on the employer

An important point of agreement between the US Panel and the advocates of the friction cost method was the need to consider the resource costs imposed on employers of individuals who are removed from their workforce as a result of mortality or long-term illness or disability. These costs are incurred as a result of the need to replace the worker and to train his/her replacement.

Effect on the previously unemployed

A second major area of disagreement between the US Panel and the friction cost method relates to the impact of illness on the previously unemployed worker. As described in Section 5.4.2, the fundamental rationale for the friction cost method is that the existence of involuntary unemployment means that productivity effects should only be valued during the friction period because the opportunity cost that an involuntarily unemployed individual attaches to their time is negligible. The US Panel reject this position and, instead, adhere to the conventional economic principle that, when an individual gains employment, the value of the their forgone leisure time is equal to the net income they receive.

The US Panel's position on this issue results in a major difference in their recommendations compared to those of the friction cost approach. Namely, that the productivity effect of mortality or morbidity on the individual experiencing the ill-health is not confined to the friction period. However, the *external* productivity effect on the recipients of tax-funded transfers only extends over the friction period. This is due to the fact that the replacement of the sick worker by someone who was previously unemployed results in a replenishment of tax revenues.

5.5 Conclusions

The incorporation of productivity costs into economic evaluation in health care is controversial at two levels. The first is the normative question of whether such costs *should* be reflected in such analyses. Although some have argued that, in health care systems based on non-market, egalitarian principles, productivity costs should have no role in resource allocation, most of the methods literature in this area has concluded that at least a proportion of productivity costs should be included in economic evaluation.

The other area of controversy has been the alternative methods that have been advocated for valuing productivity costs. Although the US Panel's deliberations have served to highlight some key issues and delineate the disparate effects of mortality and morbidity on production, the methods it advocated for valuation have been widely criticized for their impracticality. In identifying a preferred method between the human capital and friction cost approaches, much depends on a view being taken on the assumptions of neoclassical economics on how markets behave in practice.

Two aspects of the use of productivity costs in economic evaluation that have not been subject to much research are the measurement of lost time as a result of ill-health and the positive issue of the extent to which the presentation of productivity costs within studies actually influences decision makers.

References

Brouwer, W. B. F., Koopmanschap, M. A. and Rutten, F. F. H. (1997a). Productivity costs in cost-effectiveness analysis: numerator or denominator: a further discussion. *Health Economics*, 6, 511–14.

Brouwer, W. B. F., Koopmanschap, M. A. and Rutten, F. F. H. (1997b). Productivity costs measurement through quality-of-life? a response to the recommendation of the Washington panel. *Health Economics*, 6, 253–9.

Brouwer, W. B. F., Koopmanschap, M. A. and Rutten, F. F. H. (1999). Productivity losses without absence: measurement validation and empirical evidence. *Health Policy*, 48, 13–27.

Culyer, A. J. (1989). The normative economics of health care finance and provision. *Oxford Review of Economic Policy*, 5, 34–58.

Dranove, D. (1995). Measuring cost. In: F. A. Sloan, *Valuing health care: costs, benefits, and effectiveness of pharmaceuticals and other medical technologies*, Cambridge University Press, Cambridge.

Drummond, M. F., O'Brien, B. J., Stoddart, G. L. *et al.* (1997). *Methods for the Economic Evaluation of Health Care Programmes*. New York, Oxford University Press.

Gafni, A. (1991). Willingness to pay as a measure of benefits. *Medical Care*, 29, 1246–52.

Garber, A. M. and Phelps, C. E. (1997). Economic foundations of cost-effectiveness analysis. *Journal of Health Economics*, 16, 1–31.

Gerard, K. and Mooney, G. (1993). QALY league tables: handle with care. *Health Economics*, 2, 59–64.

Gold, M. R., Siegel, J. E., Russell, L. B. *et al.* (1996). *Cost-effectiveness analysis in health and medicine*. New York, Oxford University Press.

Hurley, J. (2000). An overview of the normative economics of the health sector. In: A. J. Culyer and J. P. Newhouse, *Handbook of health economics*. Amsterdam, Elsevier.

Johannesson, M. (1995). The relationship between cost-effectiveness analysis and cost-benefit analysis. *Social Science and Medicine*, 41, 483–9.

Johannesson, M. (1997). Avoiding double-counting in pharmacoeconomic studies. *Pharmacoeconomics*, 11, 385–8.

Johannesson, M. and Karlsson, G. (1997). The friction cost method: a comment. *Journal of Health Economics*, 16, 249–55.

Johannesson, M. and Meltzer, D. (1998). Some reflections on cost-effectiveness analysis. *Health Economics*, 7, 1–7.

Koopmanschap, M. A. and van Ineveld, B. M. (1992). Towards a new approach for estimating indirect costs of disease. *Social Science and Medicine*, 34, 1005–10.

Koopmanschap, M. A. and Rutten, F. H. H. (1993). Indirect costs in economic studies. *Pharmacoeconomics*, 4, 446–54.

Koopmanschap, M. A. and Rutten, F. F. H. (1996). The consequence of production loss or increased costs of production. *Medical Care*, 34, DS59–DS68.

Koopmanschap, M. A., Rutten, F. F. H., van Ineveld, B. M. *et al.* (1995). The friction cost method of measuring the indirect costs of disease. *Journal of Health Economics*, 14, 171–89.

Koopmanschap, M. A., Rutten, F. F. H., van Ineveld, B. M. and van Roijen, L. (1997). Reply to Johanneson's and Karlsson's comment. *Journal of Health Economics*, 16, 257–9.

Liljas, B. (1998). How to calculate indirect costs in economic evaluation. *Pharmacoeconomics*, 13, 1–7.

Luce, B. R., Manning, W. G., Siegel, J. E. *et al.* (1996). Estimating costs in cost-effectiveness analysis. In: M. R. Gold, J. E. Siegel, L. B. Russell and M. C. Weinstein. *Cost-effectiveness in health and medicine*. New York, Oxford University Press.

Mishan, E. J. (1971). Evaluation of life and limb: a theoretical approach. *Journal of Political Economy*, 79, 687–705.

Olsen, J. A. (1994). Production gains: should they count in health care evaluations? *Scottish Journal of Political Economy*, 41, 69–84.

Olsen, J. A. and Richardson, J. (1999). Production gains from health care: what should be included in cost-effectiveness analysis. *Social Science and Medicine*, 49, 17–26.

Organisation for Economic Co-operation and Development (OECD). (1997). *OECD health data 1997*. Paris, OECD.

Osterhaus, J. T., Gutterman, D. L. and Plachetka, J. R (1992). Health care resource and lost labour costs of migraine headache in the US. *PharmacoEconomics*, 2, 67–76.

Pritchard, C. and Sculpher, M. J. (forthcoming). *Productivity costs: principles and practice in economic evaluation*. London, Office of Health Economics.

Reilly, M.C., Zbrozek, A. S. and Dukes, E. M. (1993). The validity and reproducibility of a Work Productivity and Activity Impairment Instrument. *PharmacoEconomics*, 4, 353–65.

Revicki, D. A., Irwin, D., Reblando, J. and Simon, G. E. (1994). The accuracy of self-reported disability days. *Medical Care*, 32, 104–404.

Rice, D. P. and Cooper, B. S. (1967). The economic value of human life. *American Journal of Public Health*, 57, 1954–66.

van Roijen, L., Essink-Bot, M-L., Koopmanschap, M. A., *et al.* (1996). Labour and health status in economic evaluation of health care. *International Journal of Technology Assessment in Health Care*, 12, 405–415.

Sculpher, M. J. and O'Brien, B. J. (2000). Income effects of reduced health and health effects of reduced income: implications for health state valuation. *Medical Decision-Making*, 38, 460–8.

Severens, J. L., Laheij, R. J. F., Jansen, J. B. M. J. *et al.* (1998). Estimating the cost of lost productivity in dyspepsia. *Aliment Pharmacological Therapy*, 12, 919–23.

Torrance, G. W., Feeny, D. H., Furlong, W. J. *et al.* (1996a). Multiattribute utility function for a comprehensive health status classification system: Health Utilities Index Mark 2. *Medical Care*, 34, 702–22.

Torrance, G. W., Siegel, J. E. and Luce, B. R. (1996b). Framing and designing the cost-effectiveness analysis. In: M. R. Gold, J. E. Siegel, L. B. Russell and M. C. Weinstein. *Cost-Effectiveness in Health and Medicine*. New York, Oxford University Press.

Weinstein, M. C., Siegel, J. E. and Garber, A. M. (1997). Productivity costs, time costs and health-related quality-of-life: a response to the Erasmus group. *Health Economics*, 6, 505–10.

Williams, A. (1992). Cost-effectiveness analysis: is it ethical? *Journal of Medical Ethics*, 18, 7–11.

Chapter 6

Trial-based economic evaluations: an overview of design and analysis

Henry A. Glick, Daniel P. Polsky and
Kevin A. Schulman

In response to increasing health care costs, countries around the world have been exploring methods for their control. At the more macro level, responses have included greater risk sharing between payers, providers, and patients as well as a greater reliance on market-oriented incentives. At the more micro-level, government regulators, health care providers, members of managed care formulary committees, payers, and patients have begun to evaluate the value for the cost of individual medical therapies.

During the past ten years, one of the growing trends in this evaluation has been the incorporation of economic evaluations within randomized controlled trials of medical therapies. Most frequently these evaluations are incorporated into the drug development process (in phases II and III, during which a drug's safety and efficacy are evaluated prior to regulatory approval, as well as in phase IV, which occurs after the drug is marketed). To a lesser extent, they are conducted within trials of other medical therapies (e.g. surgical procedures, behavioural interventions, etc.). This approach to gathering economic data has been proposed by the US Food and Drug Administration (FDA) to pharmaceutical companies wishing to make economic claims about their products (FDA 1995).

Figure 6.1 indicates how the US pharmaceutical industry's interest in economic assessment has grown over time. In 1988, approximately 2.5 per cent of clinical studies incorporated health economic analyses, whereas by 1994, over 25 per cent of studies incorporated such analyses (Kim *et al.* 2000). Coincident with this increased attention has been a rapid development in the methodologies used to evaluate the value for the cost of new drugs. In 1988, the preponderance of these evaluations were developed using decision analyses, which, in some cases, derived only a single estimate (e.g. the clinical effectiveness of the new therapy) from a clinical trial. By 1994, many of these evaluations were based on the evaluation of patient-specific data on costs and outcomes of therapy measured directly within trials.

Table 6.1 reflects the growing interest in economic data within both the marketplace and the United States' regulatory community. Between 1995 and 1998 there has been a dramatic decline in the proportion of studies submitted to the US FDA that fail to

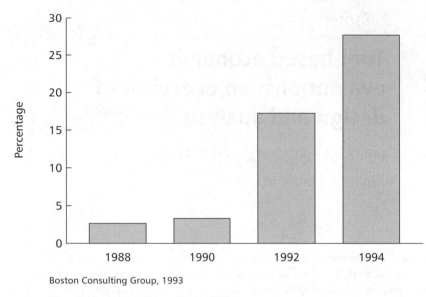

Boston Consulting Group, 1993

*Data for figure derived from Kim *et al.* (3)

Fig. 6.1 Percentage of clinical studies incorporating health economic analyses[a]
Note: Data for figure derived from Kim et al. (2000)
Source: Boston Consulting Group (1993)

Table 6.1 Use of Pharmacoeconomic Data by the US Food and Drug Administration (FDA)[a]

Variable	Submitted to FDA		Commented upon by FDA	
	1998	**1995**	**1998**	**1995**
Quality of life	50.0	39.1	57.7	31.6
Patient preferences	8.8	4.3	3.9	0.0
Resource use	23.5	13.0	19.2	10.5
Cost effectiveness	14.7	17.4	11.5	15.8
None	2.9	26.2	7.7	42.1

Note: [a] Data for table derived from Kim *et al.* (2001)

incorporate any economic outcomes. In addition, during this time period, there has been a dramatic increase in the proportion of economic claims upon which the US FDA has commented.

The information developed from economic evaluations is intended to inform decision-makers about the value for the cost of new drugs and technologies. This information will shed the most light on the question of value for the cost if the trial and the evaluation are appropriately designed, if appropriate data are collected and are correctly analysed, and if the many sources of uncertainty surrounding these evaluations are adequately addressed.

This chapter provides an introduction to issues in the design and analysis of economic assessments conducted as part of randomized trials. We first describe the gold standard economic evaluation and the tensions that exist in the design of such a study. Second, we discuss nine study design issues related to these evaluations. Finally, we describe issues in the analysis and reporting of the results of these evaluations.

6.1 **The gold standard**

The conduct of an economic evaluation as part of a randomized trial may be envisaged as six steps. In step 1, one quantifies the outcomes, while in step 2, one quantifies the costs. In step 3, one assesses whether and by how much mean costs and outcomes differ among the treatment groups (via the calculation of incremental costs and outcomes).

In step 4, one compares the magnitude of differences in incremental costs and outcomes and evaluates 'value for the cost', for example, by reporting a cost-effectiveness ratio or by reporting a therapy's net health benefits. A hypothesis that might be tested in such a study is that the ratio of the cost per quality-adjusted life year saved is significantly less than $60,000. This hypothesis might be confirmed by a finding of the upper confidence limit for the ratio that falls below $60,000 or by a finding of net health benefit – calculated using a ceiling ratio of $60,000 – that is significantly greater than 0.

In step 5, one evaluates the precision of these comparisons (e.g. by reporting a confidence interval for the cost-effectiveness ratio or for net health benefits). Finally, in step 6, one addresses other sources of uncertainty by performing other sensitivity analyses.

The gold standard economic evaluation within a clinical trial is conducted in naturalistic settings, and studies the therapy as it would be used in usual care. Such an evaluation is performed with adequate power to assess the homogeneity of results in the wide range of clinical settings and among the wide range of clinical indications in which the therapy will be used. It also is designed with an adequate length of follow-up to assess the full impact of the therapy. Fourth, it is conducted within a time frame that allows the resulting information to inform important decisions in the adoption and dissemination of the therapy.

Issues related to the type of analysis that will be conducted (e.g. cost-benefit, cost-effectiveness, or cost minimization analysis), the types of costs that will be included (e.g. direct medical, direct non-medical, productivity and intangible), and the perspective from which the study will be conducted apply equally to economic evaluations that are incorporated within clinical trials as they do to other economic evaluations. These issues have been well addressed in the literature (Eisenberg 1989; Detsky and Naglie 1990; Cost-Effectiveness in Health and Medicine 1996).

In gold standard evaluations, one measures all costs of all participants in the trial regardless of why the costs were incurred, starting prior to randomization and continuing for the duration of follow-up of the trial. Costs incurred after randomization constitute the cost outcome of interest in the trial (at least for the period of observation within the trial; in some cases, one may also want to project costs and outcomes beyond this period of observation). Costs incurred prior to randomization are a potential predictor of costs after randomization, and thus may explain variability in these costs.

Given that in the gold standard we measure all costs. We measure those future costs that are believed to be related to the disease and its treatment as well as those that might be expected to be unrelated. We do so because the gold standard evaluation is adequately powered; thus, rather than making judgements about the relationship between treatment and a particular element of resource use, we empirically determine the incremental costs that are related to the therapy. This measurement of all costs has implications for the debate about whether the analysis should include only those costs that are related to the intervention or whether it should include 'unrelated' costs as well (Meltzer 1997; Garber 2000).

Performing a gold standard evaluation is most feasible when it is easy to identify when services are provided (e.g. hospital-based studies). Feasibility is also enhanced when resource use and cost data are already being collected, for example in an administrative data base, and when researchers have ready access to these data once they are collected. Traditionally, hospital-based studies have been considered as some of the best candidates for gold standard studies (because of the closed nature of the hospital, and because of the large amounts of record keeping that are done there). However, as episodes of care increasingly continue after discharge from the hospital, and when some types of resource use are not collected as part of the administrative record (e.g. physician costs in the USA), even these studies fail to meet the standard.

Gold standard assessments carry several drawbacks. For example, there may be contradictions between the goal related to conducting the trial in naturalistic settings and the one related to providing information within a time frame that informs important decisions. The information from trials that are performed early in the life of a therapy (e.g. during phases II and III of the drug development process) may aid decisions about early adoption and diffusion of the therapy. If the therapy is dramatically effective, these trials may also be one of the last chances one has to randomize patients to receive the therapy (i.e. once information about a therapy's clinical effectiveness is available, patients may not be willing to participate in experiments simply to evaluate its value for the cost). These early trials, however, may not reflect the costs and effects that would be observed in usual practice, in part because, due to regulatory needs, the trials may affect usual practice and in part because clinicians may not yet know how to use the therapy efficiently.

Trials that are performed later (e.g. post-marketing studies in the drug development process) are more capable of reflecting usual practice (although it is possible that – due to formal protocols – such trials reduce observed variation in practice). However, information from these trials may be too late to inform important early decisions about the adoption and diffusion of the therapy, and as noted above, if the therapy is shown to be clinically effective, patients may be unwilling to enrol in them. To address some, but not all, of these issues, ideally, one would evaluate new therapies throughout the development process, to inform early decisions and to re-evaluate economic findings once the therapy is in common use.

Gold standard studies also pose a large number of feasibility issues. They may require a larger number of study subjects than the investigators or funders are willing to enrol, or they may require a lengthened follow-up (e.g. the economic impacts of therapy may not end at 28 days, but regulatory agencies may accept clinical endpoints measured at 28 days as evidence of clinical efficacy). Some investigators may have difficulty collecting the clinical data required by a trial, and the additional burden of economic data collection may exacerbate this problem. Reconstructing the equivalent of a patient bill in the case report form is burdensome. Finally, investigators may have limited access to information on services provided to study subjects from providers and in centres that are unaffiliated with the trial. Because of these limitations, investigators often make trade-offs between the ideal economic assessment and assessments that are most feasible (with the presumption that imperfect information is better than none).

6.2 Nine study design issues

When designing a study, one needs to consider a number of issues. These include: (1) What preplanning should be done in preparation for the trial? (2) What proportion of the total costs should be collected in the trial? (3) In what delivery settings should the data be collected? (4) How should utilization in non-study sites be identified? (5) Among which study subjects should the data be collected? (6) In what form should the data be collected? (7) Which unit cost estimates should be used for the study? (8) Should follow-up be discontinued if study subjects fail therapy? (9) For time-limited trials of lifetime therapies: How should long-term results be projected?

6.2.1 Preplanning

A number of preplanning activities should be performed when designing an economic assessment within a clinical trial. These include, but are not limited to, identifying appropriate economic endpoints (e.g. length of follow-up); estimating means, variances and correlations for costs, health-related quality-of-life and preferences; identifying the types of medical services used by study subjects; pilot testing data collection instruments and procedures; and gauging levels of patient interest in the study.

Identifying appropriate economic endpoints (e.g. length of follow-up)

Economic assessments conducted as part of randomized trials are meant to allow decision-makers to use the results of the trial to reach conclusions about the economic benefits of the therapy under investigation. One design issue that may limit the interpretability of the economic data collected within the trial is the study's time horizon. Although clinical efficacy may be demonstrated when a difference in clinical endpoints is observed between study arms, from an economic perspective the appropriate time horizon for a trial would include all (or a substantial portion) of the time when there is resource use related to the illness under study. The economic time horizon that would best inform decision-makers about the value for the cost of a therapy thus need not be the same as the one adopted for answering the clinical question.

A number of approaches are available for identifying an appropriate economic time horizon for a clinical trial. One approach is to identify the economic episode of care. As defined in the literature, an episode of care is the period initiated by patient presentation with a diagnosis of a clinical condition (in the case of a randomized trial, initiated by randomization) and concluded when the condition is resolved (Hornbrook *et al.* 1985; Hornbrook 1995; Keeler 1992; Steinwachs 1992). For definition of the clinical episode, resolution may refer to the acute clinical condition; for definition of the economic episode, it may refer to the return of costs to the level that would have existed had the clinical condition not been present (Brainsky *et al.* 1997).

Mehta *et al.* (1999) and Schulman *et al.* (1999) have used episode of care methodology to define economic episodes of care for diabetic foot ulcers (Mehta *et al.* 1999) and migraine headaches (Schulman *et al.* 1999). These authors quantified the length of an economic episode by comparing differences in mean daily costs and differences in the proportion of patients with costs before and after an index diagnosis of foot ulcer and migraine headache: the episode was said to last until the initially elevated mean costs per day (proportion of patients with costs) after the diagnosis returned to their level prior to the diagnosis.

Figure 6.2 shows the mean daily cost for 60 days prior to an index diagnosis of migraine (days -60 to -1), the mean cost during the day of the index diagnosis (day 0), as well as mean daily cost for the 60 days after the index diagnosis (days 1 to 60). Analysis of the data suggested that costs from a migraine headache may remain elevated for three weeks (Schulman *et al.* 1999), which is markedly longer than clinical time horizons for migraine therapies, which often can be as short as 30 to 120 minutes. Given that the economic evaluation is meant to identify both the clinical and economic impacts of therapies (in this case for the treatment of migraine), one would be more likely to capture the latter effects by lengthening the time horizon of the trial and studying the entire period of time when costs are elevated.

Decision analysis represents a second approach that can be adopted for identifying an appropriate economic time horizon for a clinical trial (Glick *et al.* 1994). For example a decision analytic model that simulates the disease and the effects of therapy might demonstrate that life expectancy among individuals who would have died without the intervention but now live because of it has a substantial impact on the economics of the drug. In this case, the time horizon of the trial could be adjusted so that one is able to assess these gains in life expectancy, or one could ensure that data are collected that would allow the prediction of life expectancy after the trial.

Estimating means, variances, and correlations for costs, health-related quality-of-life, and preferences

Means, variances, and correlations for costs, health-related quality-of-life, and preferences provide the information necessary for assessing the sample size required to answer the economic questions posed in the study. Enrolment size for randomized trials often is based on the minimum number of study subjects needed to address

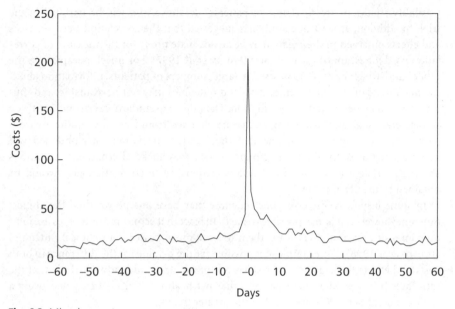

Fig. 6.2 Migraine costs
Source: Pennsylvania Medical data

the clinical questions. However, the number of subjects required for the economic assessment may differ from that needed for the clinical evaluation.

Prior to the development of the literature that described confidence intervals for cost-effectiveness ratios (van Hout *et al.* 1994; O'Brien *et al.* 1994; Chaudhary and Stearns 1996; Willan and O'Brien 1996; Polsky *et al.* 1997), a common approach to sample size calculation for economic analysis in trials was to select the larger of the sample sizes needed for estimating pre-specified cost and effect differences (i.e. what sample size was required to identify a $1000 difference in costs, and what was required to identify a 10 per cent reduction in mortality).

Once the literature on confidence intervals developed, however, it became clear that the goal of economic evaluations in trials was to determine the likelihood that the therapy represented good value for the cost. Thus, current sample size methods base their calculations on the number of study subjects needed to rule out unacceptably high upper confidence limits for the cost-effectiveness ratio (alternatively, to rule out that the net health benefits of the intervention are less than 0) (Al *et al.* 1998; Briggs and Gray 1998; Laska *et al.* 1999; Willan and O'Brien 1999).

These methods generally require more information than is needed for estimating sample sizes for clinical outcomes or for cost differences alone. Basic data for such calculations include the magnitude of the incremental costs and outcomes one expects to observe in the trial; the standard deviations for costs and outcomes in each of the treatment groups; and the correlation between costs and outcomes.

Where does one obtain this information? If both therapies are already in use, expected differences in outcomes and standard deviations can be derived from feasibility studies or from records of patients like those who will be enrolled in the trial. In addition, at least one study has suggested that the correlation between costs and effects observed in these data may be an adequate proxy for the measure of correlation used for estimating sample size (Polsky *et al.* 1997). For novel therapies, on the other hand, which have yet to be used in large numbers of patients, information about the magnitude of the incremental costs and outcomes may not be available, and thus may need to be generated by assumption. Data on the standard deviations for those who receive usual care/placebo again may be obtained from feasibility studies or from patient records (one may assume that the standard deviation thus obtained will apply equally to both treatment groups, or one may make alternative assumptions about the relative magnitudes of these deviations). The correlation also would be obtained from such data.

In some instances, the economic outcome may have less power than the clinical outcome; however, it is also possible – due to the fact that economic outcomes are joint outcomes of cost and effect – for them to have more power than clinical outcomes (Brown *et al.* 1998). For example, it is possible for the *p*-value for the difference in both costs and effects to be greater than 0.05, yet for one to confidently conclude that the ratio falls below $60,000 (alternatively, that net health benefits – calculated using a ceiling ratio of $60,000 – are significantly greater than 0).

Identifying the types of medical services used by study subjects

A third preplanning activity is to identify the types of medical services that are likely to be used by study subjects. One can do so by reviewing medical charts or administrative data sets; having patients keep logs of their health care resource use; or by asking patients and experts about the kinds of care received by those with the condition under study. This information will help identify areas that will need the most intensive data-collection efforts, particularly if, because of the burden of economic data collection, only a subset of medical services are to be recorded in the case report forms. While analysis of administrative data may provide good estimates of resource use in current practice, one must also be prepared to collect data on additional services to account for the fact that the new therapy may change practice (e.g. by causing adverse outcomes that require different kinds of services than are used by study subjects in usual practice).

Pilot testing data collection instruments and procedures

As with any other forms and procedures used in clinical trials, those used to collect economic data should be pilot tested for their efficiency, clarity, and ease of use. Poorly designed forms can lead to low quality data that will jeopardize one's ability to draw useful conclusions from the study.

Gauging levels of patient interest in the study

Substantial amounts of data may be collected from study subjects (e.g. resource use from providers and in centres that are unaffiliated with the trial, quality-of-life data, and patient preferences), and the amount that it is feasible to collect will depend on the level of the study subjects' interest in the study. This level of interest potentially varies from disease to disease. Gauging patient interest allows the investigators to better estimate how much data collection the study subjects will tolerate.

6.2.2 What proportion of the total costs should be collected in the trial?

In a trial that provides ready access to administrative data (e.g. from insurers, government agencies, or hospitals), few if any trade-offs need to be made about the proportion of total costs that should be included in the study. However, if data on resource use will be collected prospectively in study case report forms, then the goals are: (1) to measure services that make up a large portion of the difference in treatment between study subjects randomized to the different therapies under evaluation (to obtain an estimate of the new therapy's impact on the cost of care) and (2) to measure services that make up a large portion of the total costs of care. The latter services provide a measure of overall variability of costs. In addition, failure to measure a large portion of the total costs of care leaves the study open to criticisms that differences in measured services observed between therapies may have been offset among services that were not measured in the study.

The best approach is to measure as many services as possible, because minimizing the services that go unmeasured reduces the likelihood that differences among them will lead to study artefacts. However, there are no *a priori* guidelines about how much data are enough, nor are there data on the incremental value of specific items in the economic case report form. Decisions about those procedures that will be recorded within the case report form and those that will not should take into account the expense of collecting particular data items.

Admission to Hospital or Unit	Unit (*)					
	ICU	CCU	Step-down	General care	OTHER	
						Specify Unit

Fig. 6.3 CRF: site of care in hospital

Identification of the types of medical services used by study subjects during the preplanning activities for the trial can provide information to guide these decisions, by documenting the types of services used by study subjects with the disease that is being studied. In general, however, substantially more experience with various medical problems and interventions will be needed before we know which data are essential to document in an economic case report form.

Figure 6.3 is an example of a case report form for prospectively collecting data on the hospital site of care during a trial. Across the top of the form is a list of hospital units, such as intensive care, step-down and general care. On the left is a column for recording dates. The research staff uses this form to list the dates when a study subject is transferred between hospital units. A tick mark is placed in the column corresponding to the unit where the study subject was admitted. In this format, the final entry on the form is the study subject's day of discharge. The length of stay in each unit is calculated by subtracting the dates recorded on each line.

Figure 6.4 is an example of a case report form that is used to collect the same data but in a different format. In this form, unit types are listed along the left side of the form, and each column represents a different study day. A research staff member places a tick mark on each day that the study subject is in a particular unit. On days when the study subject was in more than one location, fractions may be recorded or a preselected time, such as 12:00 p.m. (noon), may be used to determine where the study subject was that day. Forms like these can also be used for recording other services as well.

There is still ongoing discussion about a number of issues related to determining the proportion of total costs that should be collected within the trial. The method described above assumes that one identifies types of services that will be documented within the case report form (e.g. hospitalization) and then one collects all of these

	Pretreatment		Postreatment					
	Day −2	Day −1	Day 1	Day 2	Day 3	Day 4	Day 5	...
	_/_	_/_	_/_	_/_	_/_	_/_	_/_	...
Type of bed (at noon)								
Intensive care unit								
High care unit								
General care unit								
Other care unit								
Discharged								

Fig. 6.4 CRF: site of care in hospital

services independent of their cause (as in the gold standard, allowing randomization to determine which are and which are not related to the study therapy). An alternative strategy that has been proposed for rationalizing the number of services that are collected in the case report form is to record only those services that health care providers deem are related to the illness or therapy under study.

Limiting data collection via this latter method may succeed in reducing the cost of the trial, and in reducing the variability that is introduced by collecting all services of certain types, independent of the reason for these services. However, there potentially are several problems with this latter strategy. For example, there is little if any evidence about the accuracy, reliability or validity of such judgements. Much of medical practice is multifactorial. In a trial for heart failure, a patient with more severe heart failure may be hospitalized for a comorbid condition, whereas a patient with the same comorbidity, but with milder heart failure may not be hospitalized. Answering counterfactuals such as this (i.e. would the patient have been hospitalized had his or her heart failure been other than it is) is the role of randomized trials, and it is unclear that provider judgement is any better at answering questions about the reasons for treatment than they are at answering questions about treatment efficacy.

In addition, for patients with complicated conditions, procedures ordered for the diagnosis and treatment of one condition may be complements or substitutes for procedures ordered for other conditions. Thus, even if providers are certain that they are ordering tests or procedures for the illness or therapy under study, it is possible that the same tests or procedure would have been ordered later for different reasons.

6.2.3 In what delivery settings should the data be collected?

It is relatively easy to collect information when study subjects see a study physician in a study centre. It is more difficult to collect data on services from providers and in centres that are unaffiliated with the trial. Given the relatively higher cost of collecting data in the latter settings compared with the former, some may propose to eliminate collection of data from non-study providers and sites. However, ignoring the cost of non-study centre care may lead to the conclusion that one treatment group has higher costs than another, when in truth costs among the groups are similar, but incurred in different settings. Thus, if large amounts of care are provided in these settings, or if there are reasons to believe that utilization in these settings will differ among treatment groups, one should consider extending data collection efforts to these settings.

6.2.4 How will utilization in non-study sites be identified?

If the study is designed to collect data on service use from providers and in centres that are unaffiliated with the trial, then a strategy should be in place to identify when study subjects receive such services. This information may be easy to collect if administrative data (e.g. insurance records) are available for the study population. In other cases, however, the data will have to come from study subject self-reporting (which is sometimes fallible) or from reporting by the study subject's proxies.

If the data come from study subjects or proxies, a decision should be made about how often study subjects will be contacted. The more frequently they are interviewed, the less perishable their data; however, the cost of data collection is higher and the burden on study subjects and proxies is greater. The less frequently they are interviewed, the cost of the data is lower and the burden is lessened. The data, however, are more perishable. For example, one study found that 10 per cent of patients failed to report that they had been hospitalized when they were interviewed approximately five months after their discharge; another found that 50 per cent failed to report them 10 to 11 months after their admission (Cannell 1977).

Even if study subjects remember that they have seen a physician or have gone to a hospital, they often will not know what services they received. Options for identifying these services include contacting the care providers directly or assuming a standard set of services, such as the marginal cost for a usual visit to a family physician. Standard sets of services might be assigned differentially to account for differences by indication (e.g. diagnosis related groups); differences in duration (e.g. brief versus intermediate office visits), or the presence of an intensity marker such as a major diagnostic study.

When collecting data from study subjects, another issue is whether to simply rely on their memory or whether to have each study subject use a memory aid, such as a diary. Diary forms can be actual pages in the case report form. More commonly, they are aids that are provided to the patient which are reviewed or abstracted by study personnel so the information can be coded on the case report form. If diaries are used, the investigators should decide how often to contact each study subject with a reminder to use the diary.

Lastly, who will collect these data: the research staff at the study site or a contract research organization. Contract research organizations can provide interviewers and computerized interview scripts with built-in skip logic and on-line data entry. On the other hand, the study-site research staff sometimes is wary of having people from outside organizations contacting their patients, particularly if the patients have a stigmatizing disease. However, these same staff may be pleased to avoid having to interview their patients about resource use on a regular basis.

6.2.5 Among which study subjects should the data be collected?

In general, data should be collected from all study subjects in a trial. At a minimum, the data should come from a random sample of all study subjects. However, organizers of many studies (e.g. phase III drug studies) usually are under pressure to minimize the time it takes to complete them. One of the determinants of a trial's duration is the time it takes to enrol the required number of study subjects. Therefore, clinical investigators may have an incentive to enrol study subjects who agree to participate in a clinical trial but are unwilling to cooperate with the economic assessment. This approach is problematic because self-selection by study subjects places the validity of the economic study in jeopardy. The economic assessment could end up comparing an estimate of effects from the entire study population with an estimate of costs derived from a relatively small and non-random subset of the population.

Another approach is to limit the economic assessment to the study centres that elect to participate. This option reduces the burden on investigators by giving them the opportunity to opt out of the economic assessment. But this approach also can lead to difficulties. In one study that used voluntary data collection (Glick *et al.* 1998), the average length of stay among study subjects at centres that provided supplementary data was not the same as the average stay from non-responding centres. This difference made the data analysis substantially more complex (i.e. we could not analyse length of stay in the ICU directly, but instead had to impute it based on total length of stay in the hospital and other explanatory factors).

6.2.6 In what form should the data be collected?

Access to administrative data may allow simultaneous collection of data about numbers of procedures as well as costs. However, if administrative data are not available, then a decision should be made about how to collect the economic data. In most studies, health professionals record the resources used by the study subject, such as the number of x-ray examinations or complete blood counts. Costs are then calculated by multiplying the resources used by unit cost estimates for those resources, which are often collected independently from the trial.

One reason that this strategy is adopted, rather than one where health professionals record the total costs of services used, is that the people who collect clinical data often are uncomfortable about collecting cost data, because cost information is not readily available. In addition, discrepancies between health care prices and actual costs are widespread in the United States (Finkler 1982) and other countries. The clinical research staff may not be sufficiently familiar with economic principles to decide whether the price data they receive are adequate proxies for costs.

6.2.7 Which unit cost estimates should be used for the study?

Sources of proxies for unit costs differ by country. For example, in the United States, there are a number of publicly-available sources of cost data, including: hospital charges adjusted using cost to charge ratios; data from internal hospital costing systems; diagnosis related group (DRG) payments for hospitalizations (Department of Health and Human Services 1991); and resource-based relative value units for physician services (Department of Health and Human Services 1991; Hsiao *et al.* 1992).

Readily available data in Europe (and in some other parts of the world) may include (depending on the country): fee schedules; data from DRG studies; and data from hospital costing systems. In some cases, data have been obtained from a limited number of centres which have cost accounting systems or from administrative data bases that recently have been developed in some countries (Schulman *et al.* 1998).

It may also be possible to develop trial-specific costing exercises (e.g. analysis of accounting data (Bridges and Jacobs 1986; Granneman *et al.* 1986), time and motion studies (Finkler 1980), or cost allocation projections for expensive experimental capital equipment).

When one has unit cost data from more than one study centre or country, one also needs to decide whether to apply centre-specific unit costs to resource use observed at that centre or whether to average the unit costs from all study centres into a single set of unit costs (this decision is similar to the one about whether, in multicentre studies in a single country, one should use centre-specific unit cost estimates or whether one should attempt to identify a single set of national costs estimates). Rationales for such averaging may include: (1) that by reducing the variance associated with different prices in different centres, one may reduce the overall variance in the cost outcome; and (2) that results based on an average set of unit cost estimates might be more representative (the validity of this latter rationale is unclear, given that it is possible that no individual centre makes purchasing/production decisions based on the averaged unit costs).

These rationales notwithstanding, because relative prices can affect quantities of services provided, and because in the face of variations in practice, the treatment's effects on resource use and outcome can differ, whenever feasible, one should multiply centre-specific unit cost estimates times centre-specific quantities (i.e. one should not use an averaged set of unit cost estimates). This practice will avoid potential biases that can arise due to substitution effects in different countries; in some cases, it may also appropriately increase the variance in the cost outcome that is being evaluated.

For centres and countries for which unit cost data are not available, ideally, one would use unit cost estimates from similar centres and countries (e.g. in a single country, use of unit costs from academic medical centres if costs are unavailable for an academic medical centre; in multinational studies, use of unit costs from countries which have similar health care expenditure data as documented by agencies such as the Office for Economic Coordination and Development (OECD 1998)). Practically, however, many investigators use a single set of unit costs reflecting the average of the available unit costs (Schulman *et al.* 1998).

6.2.8 Should follow-up be discontinued if study subjects fail therapy?

In some clinical studies (e.g. some antibiotic trials), clinical follow-up of study subjects is discontinued when they fail therapy. However, given that failure often is associated with higher costs (e.g. due to initiation of alternative therapies and the potential elongation of the duration of the episode of care), discontinuation of these patients from the economic study is likely to bias the results of an economic analysis that is conducted as part of the trial. In general, bias related to follow-up is least likely to occur if all study subjects are followed for a fixed time period (e.g. all study subjects are followed for one year after randomization or until death, whichever is sooner). Another design which is unbiased – but which requires the use of analytic methods for addressing censored data – is to end follow-up on a given calendar date (e.g. when the 500th death is observed in the trial). The latter designs have been used in a number of long-term cardiovascular trials (SOLVD 1991; SSSSG 1994).

Box 6.1 **Substitution effects and averaging of unit cost estimates**

Should one multiply centre-specific quantities times centre-specific unit cost estimates? Or alternatively, should one multiply these quantities times a single set of unit costs that represents the average of the unit costs from all study centres? The following example indicates the potential problems that can arise from the latter strategy.

Assume that you are conducting a trial in two centres. In centre 1, the relative costs of a day in an intensive care unit (ICU) compared with a day in a routine care unit are high and in centre 2, the relative costs of a day in the ICU are low. Assume that institutions respond to these differences in relative cost, and more care in the ICU is used in centre 2 with its lower relative costs of ICU. In this case, one would expect that using the average of the prices from the two centres to evaluate all resource use in the trial would lead to a biased result.

Table B6.1 Data on length of stay

| Unit | Centre 1 | | Centre 2 | |
	Treatment 1	Treatment 2	Treatment 1	Treatment 2
ICU	3	3	8	4
Routine	16	8	10	6

Table B6.1 provides hypothetical data on length of stay for the four patients who are enrolled in the trial (two in treatment group 1 and two in treatment group 2). As indicated in the assumptions, above, patients treated in centre 2 remain longer in the ICU and shorter in routine care units than do those treated in centre 1.

Table B6.2 Unit cost data

| | | | | Treatment-specific Weighted average | |
	Centre-specific	Simple average	Weighted average	Treatment 1	Treatment 2
Centre 1					
ICU	1000	750	667	636	714
Routine	250	325	310	308	314
Centre 2					
ICU	500	750	667	636	714
Routine	400	325	310	308	314

Table B6.2 shows the hypothetical centre-specific unit costs (column 1). The observed differences in costs are meant to represent differences in the relative price

Box 6.1 **Substitution effects and averaging of unit cost estimates** *(continued)*

of inputs or in the relative intensity of services that are being provided in what is being called ICU and routine care units. They are not meant to reflect differences in pricing strategies that are unrelated to input prices or intensity of service.

The table also shows several potential averages of the unit costs that might instead be used to value resource use of individuals in the trial. These include the simple average (column 2). For example, the ICU estimate of $750 was calculated as follows: (1000 + 500)/2. They also include a weighted average, with weights based on the centre-specific total number of days in each unit (column 3). For example, the ICU estimate of $667 was calculated as follows: ([1000 × 6] + [500 × 12])/18. Finally, a third possibility is a set of treatment-specific weighted average unit cost estimates, in which separate weighted average unit cost estimates are derived for each treatment group (columns 4 and 5). For example, the $636 estimate of ICU costs for treatment group 1 was calculated as follows: ([1000 × 3] + [500 × 8])/11.

Table B6.3 shows the treatment group specific estimates of mean and standard deviation for hospital costs derived using the different unit cost estimation strategies. Using the centre-specific data, the means ± SD for treatment groups 1 and 2 were $7500 ($707) and $4700 ($424), respectively. The difference was $2800 (SE, $583).

Table B6.3 Estimated means and standard deviations derived using the four sets of unit cost estimates

Unit cost estimate	Treatment group 1		Treatment group 2		Difference	
	Mean	SD	Mean	SD	Mean	SE
Centre-specific	7500	707	4700	424	2800	583
Simple average	8350	1273	4900	71	3450	901
Weighted average	7697	1042	4503	33	3193	737
Treatment-specific weighted average	7500	944	4700	61	2800	669

Use of the simple average of the unit costs yielded estimates of the means and differences that were all greater than those that were estimated using the centre-specific data (e.g. a mean difference of $3450, SE, $901). Use of weighted average unit costs yielded a higher estimate of mean costs for those in treatment group 1, a lower estimate for those in treatment group 2, a higher estimate of the incremental costs (e.g. a mean difference of $3193, SE, $737). Finally, use of the treatment-specific weighted average unit costs yielded point estimates that were the same as those derived using centre-specific costs (i.e. by definition use of these costs leaves the univariate estimate of incremental costs unchanged); however, even in this case, use of an averaged set of unit costs led to mixed results for the standard deviations in the point estimates, and a larger standard error for the difference in costs ($669).

> **Box 6.1 Substitution effects and averaging of unit cost estimates** *(continued)*
>
> Thus, in the example, use of averaged unit cost estimates generally led to biased estimates of the treatments' effects on costs, and there was no consistent reduction in the standard deviations of the estimates (i.e. one of the purported reasons for using averaged unit cost estimates).
>
> In actual practice, when one calculates costs by multiplying estimates of resource use times centre-specific unit cost estimates, the results can be affected by both substitution and income effects (i.e. more well-to-do centres may buy more of all services, whereas less well-to-do centres may buy fewer of all services). In two trials that we have analysed (unpublished data), we found less consistency in the direction of the impacts of the use of centre-specific versus averaged unit cost estimates than would be suggested by the example above. While in some instances the estimates of incremental costs were biased upwards, there were also instances where they were biased downwards. In addition, in some cases, the standard deviations that resulted from the use of pooled unit cost estimates were lower than those that resulted from using centre-specific unit cost estimate.
>
> There are good theoretical reasons to multiply centre-specific unit cost estimates times centre-specific resource use. While use of pooled unit cost estimates may reduce variance in the resulting cost estimate, it may also increase it. Also, given that unit costs may affect practice, and that the average practice reflected in the trial is unlikely to reflect practice in any other set of specific centres, it is unclear that use of an averaged set of unit costs makes the results more representative.

6.2.9 For time-limited trials of lifetime therapies: how will long-term results be projected?

Finally, many trials that evaluate therapies for chronic conditions end study follow-up before the study medication would be discontinued in usual practice (in some cases, it would only be discontinued when the study subject dies). For such a trial, it is good practice to evaluate the costs and outcomes that were observed during the trial. In such a 'within-trial' evaluation, one should maintain the same time horizons for costs and outcomes observed in the trial (e.g. if follow-up for the trial was for one year, then costs and effects should be measured for one year).

For such trials, however, it is unclear whether the relative magnitude of incremental costs and outcomes observed during the trial are reflective of the relative magnitude that would have been observed had the trial been continued until all study subjects discontinued therapy or died. A number of investigators have developed decision analytic models that use data from the trial and, in some cases, data from clinical registries and other sources, to attempt to address this issue (Glick *et al.* 1995; Mark *et al.* 1995; Cook *et al.* 1998). (Note: As with the 'within-trial' evaluation, one should maintain the same time horizons for the projections of costs and outcomes.) At a minimum, for trials that end follow-up before therapy would have ended, one needs to make plans for credibly assessing longer-term costs and outcomes.

6.3 Analysis and reporting of the results of economic assessments conducted as part of randomized trials

Analysis of economic data from randomized trials shares many features with analysis of the clinical data from these trials, and in most instances, good practice for the economic analysis parallels good practice for the clinical analysis. For example, the analysis should be guided by a pre-specified analysis plan; intention-to-treat principals should be adopted; and where appropriate, blinding of treatment groups should be maintained in the analysis. Many analytic techniques are also shared between the clinical and economic analysis. However, because of the skewed nature of cost data, the repeated observations of resource use, and because of statistical properties of the cost-effectiveness ratio, specialized analytic techniques may also need to be adopted for the analysis of economic data. In what follows, we briefly address some of the challenges and potential solutions to the analysis of economic data.

6.3.1 An analysis plan for an economic assessment

An important feature in the trial design is the development of an analysis plan prior to performing the analysis. Table 6.2 identifies a set of tasks that should be addressed in such a plan. One should describe the study design (e.g. reporting if the trial is randomized and double-blind; identifying the randomization groups; outlining the recruitment strategy (e.g. rolling admission and a fixed stopping date); describing the study subject evaluability criteria (i.e. what is a protocol violation and how will violations be handled); etc.) and any implications the design has for the analysis of costs (e.g. how one will account for recruiting strategies such as rolling admission and a fixed stopping date?).

One should specify study hypotheses and objectives. One should also define primary and secondary endpoints (as well as exploratory endpoints) and, for costs and

Table 6.2 Analysis plan outline

1	Study design/summary
2	Study hypothesis/objectives
3	Definition of endpoints
4	Covariates
5	Prespecification of time periods of interest
6	Statistical methods
7	Types of analyses
8	Hypothesis tests
9	Interim analyses
10	Multiplicity issues
11	Subgroup analysis
12	Power/sample size calculations

outcomes such as quality-adjusted life years, a description of how the endpoints will be constructed (e.g. multiplying resource use measured in the trial times a set of unit costs measured outside the trial). In addition, one should identify (potential) covariables that will be used in the analysis and specify the time periods of interest (e.g. costs and clinical outcomes at six months might be the primary outcome while costs and clinical outcomes at 12 months might be a secondary outcome).

One should identify the statistical methods that will be used and how hypotheses will be tested (e.g. a p-value cut-off or a confidence interval for the difference that excludes 0). Methods for addressing missing cost and outcome data should be identified as should methods for addressing uncertainties in the results (e.g. stochastic uncertainty, or whether or not the pooled (average) result from the trial reflects the result that would be observed in individual centres in the trial).

One should also pre-specify whether or not interim analyses are planned; indicate how issues of multiple testing will be addressed (including specifically stating that they will not be addressed); and predefine any subgroup analyses that will be conducted. Finally, one should perform power and sample size calculations.

If there are separate analysis plans for the clinical and economic evaluations, efforts should be made to make them as consistent as possible (e.g. shared use of an intention-to-treat analysis, shared use of statistical tests for variables used commonly by both analyses, etc.) At the same time, the outcomes of the clinical and economic studies may differ (e.g. the primary outcome of the clinical evaluation might focus on event-free survival while the primary outcome of the economic evaluation might focus on quality-adjusted survival). Thus, the two plans need not be identical.

The analysis plan should also indicate the level of blinding that will be imposed on the analyst. Most if not all analytic decisions should be made while the analyst is blinded to the treatment groups (i.e. fully blinded rather than being simply blinded to treatment A versus treatment B). Blinding is particularly important if you do not precisely specify the models that will be estimated, but instead rely on the structure of the data to help make decisions about these issues.

6.3.2 Analysis of cost data

When one analyses cost data (and outcomes such as quality-adjusted life years) derived from randomized trials, one should report means of costs for the groups under study as well as the difference in the means, measures of variability and precision, such as the standard deviation and quantiles of costs (particularly if the data are skewed), and an indication of whether or not the costs are likely to be economically meaningfully different from each other.

The approaches to the analysis of cost data that are described below are applicable to these data independent of the perspective from which costs are assessed (e.g. society, the payer, the provider, or the patient). The issue of perspective affects either the unicost estimates or the resource use that are used in the construction of the cost outcome. Once this outcome is constructed, however, the analysis of the resulting costdata is unaffected by the issue of perspective.

Analysis plans for economic assessments routinely include univariate and multi-variable methods for analysing the trial data (Barber and Thompson 1998, 2000). Univariate analyses are used for the predictors of economic outcomes, such as data on study subject demographic characteristics, clinical history, length of stay, and other resource use before entry of study subjects into the trial. Univariate and multivariable analyses are also used for the economic outcome data, such as total costs, hospital days, and quality-adjusted life years.

Traditionally, the determination of a difference in costs between the groups has been made using Student's *t*-tests or analysis of variance (ANOVA) (univariate analysis) and ordinary least squares regression (multivariable analysis). Recently, a growing number of methods have been used for make such determinations.

Univariate analysis

A basic assumption underlying t-tests and ANOVAs (which are parametric tests) is that cost data are normally distributed. Given that the distribution of these data often violates this assumption, a number of analysts have begun using transformations of the cost data (e.g. log transformation) or nonparametric tests such as the Wilcoxon rank-sum test (a test of median costs) and Kolmogorov–Smirnov test (a test for differences in the cumulative cost distributions) which make no assumptions about the underlying distribution of costs.

Use of statistical tests of the log of costs or of the median of costs to determine whether costs differ between the treatment groups may lead to a potential confusion about the outcome that is important for the analysis of the value for the cost of the new therapy (e.g. the cost-effectiveness ratio). No matter which statistical test one uses to make this determination, the outcome used in the numerator of the cost-effectiveness ratio should be the difference in mean costs. In other words, if for technical reasons one statistically assesses differences in the log of costs or differences in medians to determine whether costs differ between two treatment groups, the outcome of interest should still be the difference in mean costs and should not be the difference in the log or median of costs.

Multivariable analysis

Regression analysis is often used to assess differences in costs, in part to overcome potential problems related to a lack of statistical power that may occur if the study is structured to produce a statistically significant clinical outcome but potentially is too small to produce a statistically significant economic outcome. The use of additional economic predictors (e.g. non-treatment-related characteristics of patients or their providers) that were measured when study subjects entered the study may reduce variability in the economic outcomes and allow the detection of statistically significant differences that were not detectable by the univariate tests. These analyses may also account for potential imbalances among covariables in the treatment groups as well as providing information about the determinants of the outcomes.

Traditionally, ordinary least squares regression has been used to predict costs (or their log) as a function of the treatment group while controlling for covariables such as disease severity, costs prior to randomization, etc. (Use of the log of costs as the outcome variable simply to avoid statistical problems posed by untransformed costs leaves one with the problem that we are not interested in this outcome itself; rather we are interested in the difference in untransformed costs. In addition, the retransformation of the predicted difference in the log of costs into an estimate of the predicted difference in costs is not trivial (Duan 1983; Manning 1998; Ai and Norton 2000).)

Whereas an underlying assumption of univariate t-tests and ANOVAs is that the cost data are normally distributed, one of the underlying assumptions of ordinary least squares regression is that the error terms from the prediction of costs are normally distributed. A number of features about cost data lend themselves to the potential violation of this assumption. These include: the cost data are routinely skewed to the right (i.e. they never go below 0, and a small fraction of patients have very high costs); there may be a substantial proportion of observations with 0 costs; and there may be censoring of data, due to patients dropping out of the trial or being lost to follow-up (Lipscomb et al. 1998).

Because of the potential violation of the assumption that the errors are normally distributed, a number of alternative multivariable methods have recently been proposed for analysing costs. These include: nonparametric Hazard Models (Dudley et al. 1993; Fenn et al. 1995, 1996; Schulman et al. 1996; Lin et al. 1997), parametric failure time models (Dudley et al. 1993), Cox semiparametric regression (Harrell et al. 1996), two-part (or 'mixture') models (Mullahy 1998; Ai and Norton 2000) and joint distributions of survival and cost (Lancaster and Intrator 1995). A number of nonlinear models may also be appropriate for analysing cost data. These include additive models (Hastie and Tibshirani 1990), multivariate adaptive regression splines (Friedman 1991) and local regression (Cleveland and Grosse 1991; Loader 1999). The relative merits of several of these methods have been compared by Dudley et al. (1993) and by Lipscomb et al. (1998); however, there is little conclusive evidence regarding which model is best in which analytic circumstance.

Missing or censored data pose substantial challenges to the analysis of costs (and outcomes such as quality-adjusted life years) observed in randomized trials. Rubin (1976) has defined three types of censoring mechanisms. Data may be missing completely at random; they may be missing at random; or they may be nonignorably missing. The first two mechanisms are referred to as ignorable, because the process which generates the missing data does not alter the medical costs between people who are observed and those who are not observed.

When data are missing completely at random (often referred to as MCAR), patients who have incomplete follow-up are similar to those with complete follow-up, except for random differences. When data are missing at random (often referred to as MAR), patients who have incomplete follow-up are similar to those with complete follow-up within predictable categories, except for random differences (i.e. their missingness is predictable). Finally, the third mechanism is present when the values for the missing observations are conditional on the mechanism that created the missing value. Rubin (1976) has pointed out that the appropriate strategy for analysing censored costs depends on mechanisms that give rise to missing data.

A number of authors have begun to address the issue of missing cost data (Schulman et al. 1996; Lin et al. 1997; 2000; Polsky and Glick 1999; Carides et al. 2000;

Bang and Tsiatis 2000). A common approach has been to partition costs into a set of intervals (e.g. months), and predict these costs using data from patients who are alive and available for observation. The costs in each partition are then weighted by the probability a patient is alive in the interval. In some cases, authors have proposed a single weighting (i.e. the method assumes that the censoring mechanism is MCAR) (Lin *et al.* 1997); in others, weighting also depends on the probability of being missing (i.e. the method assumes that the censoring mechanism is MAR) (Polsky and Glick 1999; Bang and Tsiatis 2000; Carides *et al.* 2000).

6.3.3 Addressing uncertainty in economic analyses

Those interpreting the economic results of trials are confronted by a number of sources of uncertainty that need to be addressed, including: (1) sampling error, (2) whether the results can be generalized to the individual sites (in multicentre trials) or to other practice settings; (3) whether the value for the cost observed in short or intermediate length trials of lifetime therapies adequately represent the value that would have been observed had the trial been conducted for the longer periods of time (including the lifetime of study subjects); and (4) parameters used in the analysis that are measured without variation (e.g. procedure costs and discount rates).

Sampling error

The point estimates of cost and effect differences observed in trials are the result of a single sample drawn from a population. One would anticipate that if the trial were repeated many times, the point estimates would vary. Traditionally, researchers have used one- and two-way sensitivity analysis (potentially using the 95 per cent confidence intervals for costs and for effects) to address this uncertainty. Recently, a number of methods have been developed for addressing this uncertainty. These methods focus on the development of confidence intervals for cost-effectiveness ratios (van Hout et al. 1994; O'Brien et al. 1994; Chaudhary and Stearns 1996; Willan and O'Brien 1996; Polsky et al. 1997) and net health benefit calculations (Stinnett and Mullahy 1998) that account for the uncertainty in the ratios related to sampling error. The development of these methods offers new options for presenting data to decision-makers about the value for the cost of new therapies (e.g. depicting the results on the cost-effectiveness plane (Black 1990)).

Generalizability

There are a number of sources of uncertainty related to whether what was observed in the trial as a whole is applicable to any particular practice setting. First, the pooled result of the trial may not represent the result observed in any single centre or country that participated in the trial (e.g. in some centres or countries the therapy might be poor value for the cost; in others it might save money and improve outcomes; yet the pooled result might indicate that it is simply good value for the cost). Second, it is unclear if any of the results observed in the trial (either the pooled result or the results for individual centres) are descriptive of the results that would be observed in centres that did not participate in the trial. Third, it has been suggested that practice in trials may differ from what would have been observed had the same study subjects been treated outside the setting of a trial (Glick 1995). In that case, the trial may be producing little if any useful information.

As with the discussion of sampling error, there is a growing literature that addresses these issues of generalizability (Drummond *et al.* 1992; O'Brien 1997; Willke *et al.* 1998). A recent proposal has been to estimate country-specific cost-effectiveness ratios (net health benefits) and evaluate their homogeneity. One would use the more precise pooled ratio (net health benefits) for the overall study to represent these countries' ratios only if: it appears that there is no country-by-ratio (country-by-net health benefits) interaction; and if the minimum detectable difference was small enough to be economically important. A second proposed approach has included decomposing the treatment's effect on costs (through its effect on clinical outcome (e.g. by reducing the probability of death], and through its effect on cost when outcome is held constant) (Willke *et al.* 1998). A third has been to use decision analysis to address the problem (Drummond *et al.* 1992). These issues are discussed in greater detail in Chapter 11.

Projection beyond the trial

Uncertainty exists as to whether the relative magnitude of costs and outcomes observed within short and intermediate-term trials of lifetime therapies for chronic diseases are descriptive of the relative magnitudes that would be observed had the trials continued for the study subjects' lifetime. Thus there may be a need to project these costs and effects for longer periods, potentially for the lifetime of the study participants (sometimes referred to as a lifetime projection). These projections are made using decision-analytic models (which are described in greater detail in Chapter 7). They should incorporate the uncertainties addressed above; in addition, they create additional uncertainty related to the assumptions that are made in the development of the projections. These uncertainties need to be addressed if these models are to provide information to decision-makers.

Parameters measured without variation

A number of parameters used in economic evaluations, such as procedure costs (which in some cases are multiplied times counts of procedures to obtain estimates of total costs) and discount rates, often are measured without variation. Nevertheless, there may be uncertainty surrounding these parameter estimates (e.g. what is the precise discount rate that should be used?) Traditionally, this source of uncertainty has also been addressed using sensitivity analysis, and it still needs to be addressed this way. These analyses, however, may be incorporated into the evaluation of the confidence intervals (i.e. an assessment of how the confidence intervals change as the parameter values are varied in the sensitivity analysis).

6.4 **Conclusion**

Many opportunities exist for incorporating economic assessments into the randomized trials assessing medical therapies. When these assessments are conducted during the drug development process, they provide data about a drug's value early in its product life, and these data can be used by policy makers, drug manufacturers, health-care providers and patients when the drug is first introduced in the market. Better data about a drug's economic effect potentially can be collected after marketing begins, but for making an early decision, data from phase III studies are the best that are available.

Undertaking an economic assessment requires a substantial effort by those organizing the studies, the clinical investigators, and the study subjects in the trial. This effort includes collecting data before a trial is begun and investing in the trial itself. A successful economic assessment requires cooperation and coordination among everyone involved in the trial, including the organizers, the clinical team from the company, the clinical researchers, and the study subjects. Disinterest or dissatisfaction among any of these groups can lead to collection of flawed data and can undermine the study.

This chapter has presented a broad overview of some of the current practices and methodologic issues that are part of an economic assessment. However, a wide diversity exists in the design and implementation of economic assessments. Some who organize economic assessments limit participation to study subjects for whom large amounts of computerized billing data are available. Others focus on collecting hospitalization data in the form of electronic records from participating centres, thereby avoiding the need to deal with paper records. Another group of organizers prefers to collect the economic data from case report forms. This last option may be particularly useful for multinational trials, where the availability of electronic data may differ from country to country.

Economic analyses conducted within randomized trials share many design and analysis issues with traditional clinical trials, but they have unique issues as well. Means for addressing the latter set of issues is undergoing rapid development, and the methods for doing these studies are continuing to evolve.

References

Ai, C. and Norton, E. C. (2000). Standard errors for the retransformation problem with heteroscedasticity. *Journal of Health Economics*, 19, 697–718.

Al, M. J., van Hout, B. A. and Rutten, F. F. H. (1998). Sample size calculations in economic evaluations. *Health Economics*, 7, 327–35.

Bang, H. and Tsiatis, A. A. (2000). Estimating medical costs with censored data. *Biometrika*, 87, 329–43.

Barber, J. A. and Thompson, S. G. (1998). Analysis and interpretation of cost data in randomised controlled trials: review of published studies. *British Medical Journal*, 317, 1195–200.

Barber, J. A. and Thompson, S. G. (2000). Open access follow up for inflammatory bowel disease. Would have been better to use t test than Mann-Whitney U test. *British Medical Journal*, 320, 1730.

Black, W. C. (1990). The CE plane: a graphic representation of cost-effectiveness. *Medical Decision-Making*, 10, 212–14.

Brainsky, A., Glick, H., Lydick, E. *et al.* (1997). The economic cost of hip fractures in community-dwelling older adults: a prospective study. *JAGS*, 45, 281 7.

Bridges, M. and Jacobs, P. (1986). Obtaining estimates of marginal cost by DRG. *Healthcare Financial Management*, (10), 40–6.

Briggs, A. H. and Gray, A. M. (1998). Power and sample size calculations for stochastic cost-effectiveness analysis. *Medical Decision-Making*, 18, S81-S92.

Brown, M., Glick, H.A., Harrell, F. *et al.* (1998). Integrating Economic Analysis into Cancer Clinical Trials: The NCI-ASCO Economics Workbook. *Journal of the National Cancer Institute Monographs*, No. 24, 1–28.

Cannell, C. F. (1997). A Summary of Research Studies of Interviewing Methodology, 1959–1970. *Vital and health statistics: Series 2, Data evaluation and methods research*, Number 69, DHEW Publication; Number (HRA) 77–1343. U.S. Government Printing Office, Washington DC.

Carides, G. W., Heyse, J. F. and Iglewicz, B. (2000). A regression-based method for estimating mean treatment cost in the presence of right censoring. *Biostatistics*, 1, 1–15.

Chaudhary, M. A. and Stearns, S. C. (1996). Estimating confidence intervals for cost-effectiveness ratios: an example from a randomised trial. *Statistics and Medicine*, 15, 1447–58.

Cleveland, W. S. and Grosse, E. (1991). Computational methods for local regression. *Statistics and Computing*, 1, 47–62.

Cook, J.R., Glick, H.A., Gerth, W. *et al.* (1998). The cost and cardioprotective effects of enalapril in hypertensive patients with left ventricular dysfunction. *American Journal of Hypertension*, 11, 1433–41.

Department of Health and Human Services, Health Care Financing Administration. (1991a). Medicare program: hospital inpatient prospective payment systems. *Federal Register*. August, 56, 4821.

Department of Health and Human Services, Health Care Financing Administration. (1991b). Medicare program: fee schedule for physicians' services: final rule. *Federal Register*. (Addendum B) 25 November, 56, 59502–811.

Detsky, A. S. and Naglie, I. G. (1990). A clinician's guide to cost-effectiveness analysis. *Annals of Internal Medicine*, 113, 147–54.

Drummond, M. F., Bloom, B. S., Carrin, G. *et al.* (1992). Issues in the cross-national assessment of health technology. *International Journal of Technology Assessment in Health Care*, 8, 671–82.

Duan, N. (1983). Smearing estimate: a nonparametric retransformation method. *Journal of the American Statistics Association*, 78, 605–10.

Dudley, R. A., Harrell, F. E., Smith, L. R. *et al.* (1993). Comparison of analytic models for estimating the effect of clinical factors on the cost of coronary artery bypass graft surgery. *Journal of Clinical Epidemiology*, 46, 261–71.

Eisenberg, J. M. (1989). Clinical economics. a guide to the economic analysis of clinical practice. *Journal of the American Medical Association*, 262, 2879–86.

Fenn, P., McGuire, A., Phillips, V. *et al.* (1995). The analysis of censored treatment cost data in economic evaluation. *Medical Care*, 33, 851–61.

Fenn, P., McGuire, A., Backhouse, M. *et al.* (1996). Modelling programme costs in economic evaluation. *Journal of Health Economics*, 15, 115–25.

Finkler, S. A. (1980). Cost finding for high-technology, high-cost services: current practice and a possible alternative. *Health Care Management Review*, XX, 17–29.

Finkler, S. A. (1982). The distinction between cost and charges. *Annals of Internal Medicine*, 96, 102–9.

Food and Drug Administration. (1995). *Draft guidance for submitting pharmacoeconomic claims to the FDA*. (Unpublished proceedings from the FDA workshop, Comparing Treatments: Safety, Effectiveness, and Cost-Effectiveness). Washington, DC.

Friedman, J. H. (1991). Multivariate adaptive regression splines. *Annals of Statistics*, 19, 1–14.

Garber, A. M. (2000). Advances in cost-effectiveness of health interventions. In: A.J. Culyer and J.P. Newhouse (eds). *Handbook of health economics* Volume 1A. North-Holland, Amsterdam.

Glick. H. (1995). Strategies for economic assessment during the development of new drugs. *Drug Information Journal*, 29, 1391–403.

Glick, H., Cook, J., Kinosian, B. *et al.* (1995). Costs and effects of enalapril therapy in patients with symptomatic heart failure: an economic analysis of the Studies of Left Ventricular Dysfunction (SOLVD) Treatment trial. *Journal of Cardiac Failure*, 1, 371–80.

Glick, H., Kinosian, B. and Schulman, K. (1994). Decision analytic modelling: some uses in the evaluation of new pharmaceuticals. *Drug Information Journal*, 28, 691–707.

Glick, H., Willke, R., Polsky, D. *et al.* (1998). Economic analysis of tirilazad mesylate for aneurysmal subarachnoid hemorrhage: economic evaluation of a Phase III clinical trial in Europe and Australia. *International Journal of Technology Assessment in Health Care*, 14, 145–60.

Gold, M. R., Siegel, J. E., Russell, L. B. *et al.* (eds). (1996). *Cost-effectiveness in health and medicine*. Oxford University Press, Oxford.

Granneman, T. W., Brown, R. S. and Pauly, M. V. (1986). Estimating hospital costs. A multiple-output analysis. *Journal of Health Economics*, XXX, 107–27.

Harrell, F., Lee, K. and Mark, D. (1996). Multivariable prognostic models: issues in developing models, evaluating assumptions and adequacy, and measuring and reducing errors. *Statistics in Medicine*, 15, 361–87.

Hastie, T. and Tibshirani, R. (1990). *Generalised additive models*. London; Chapman and Hall.

Hornbrook, M.C. (1995). Definition and measurement of episodes of care in clinical and economic studies. In: M. C. Grady and K. A. Weis (eds), *Conference proceedings: cost analysis methodology for clinical practice guidelines*. DHHS Pub. No. (PHS)95–001. Agency for Health Care Policy and Research, Rockville, MD.

Hornbrook, M. C., Hurtado, A. V. and Johnson, R. E. (1985). Health care episodes: definition, measurement, and use. *Medical Care Review*, 42, 163–218.

van Hout, B. A., Al, M. J., Gordon, G. S. *et al.* (1994). Costs, effects, and C/E ratios alongside a clinical trial. *Health Economics*, 3, 309–19.

Hsiao, W. C., Braun, P., Dunn, D. L. *et al.* (1992). An overview of the development and refinement of the resource-based relative value scale. *Medical Care*, 30(suppl), NS1-NS12.

Keeler, E.B. (1992). Using episodes of care in effectiveness research. In: M. L. Grady and H. H. Schwartz, *Medical effectiveness research data methods*. DHHS Pub. No (PHS)92–0056. Agency for Health Care Policy and Research, Rockville, MD, pp. 161–72.

Kim, J., Morris, C. B. and Schulman, K. A. (2000). The role of the Food and Drug Administration in pharmacoeconomic evaluation during the drug development process. *Drug Inf. J*, 34, 1207–1213.

Lancaster, T. and Intrator, O. (1995). *Panel data with survival: hospitalization of HIV patients*. Brown University Department of Economics Working Paper Series, No. 95–36.

Laska, E. M., Meisner, M. and Seigel, C. (1999). Power and sample size in cost-effectiveness analysis. *Medical Decision-Making*, 19, 339–43.

Lin, D. Y. (2000). Linear regression analysis of censored medical costs. *Biostatistics*, 1, 35–47.

Lin, D. Y., Feuer, E. J., Etzioni, R. *et al.* (1997). Estimating medical costs from incomplete follow-up data. *Biometrics*, 53, 113–28.

Lipscomb, J., Ancukiewicz, M., Parmigiani, G. *et al.* (1998). Predicting the cost of illness: a comparison of alternative models applied to stroke. *Medical Decision-Making*, 18, S39–56.

Loader, C. (1999). *Local Regression and Likelihood*. New York: Springer-Verlag.

Manning, W. G. (1998). The logged dependent variable, heteroscedasticity, and the retransformation problem. *Journal of Health Economics*, 17, 283–95.

Mark, D. B., Hlatky, M. A., Califf, R. M. *et al.* (1995). Cost-effectiveness of thrombolytic therapy with tissue plasminogen activator as compared with streptokinase for acute myocardial infarction. *New England Journal of Medicine*, 332, 1418–24.

Mehta, S. S., Suzuki, S., Glick, H. A. *et al.* (1999). Determining an episode of care using claims data. Diabetic foot ulcer. *Diabetes Care*, 22, 1110–15.

Meltzer, D. (1997). Accounting for future costs in medical cost-effectiveness analysis. *Journal of Health Economics*, 16, 33–64.

Mullahy, J. (1998). Much ado about two: reconsidering retransformation and the two-part model in health econometrics. *Journal of Health Economics*, 17, 247–81.

O'Brien, B. S. (1997). A tale of two (or more) cities: geographic transferability of pharmacoeconomic data. *American Journal of Managed Care*, 3, S33-S40.

O'Brien, B. J., Drummond, M. F., Labelle, R. J. *et al.* (1994). In search of power and significance: issues in the design and analysis of stochastic cost-effectiveness studies in health care. *Medical Care*, 32, 150–63.

Office of Economic Cooperation and Development. (1998). *OECD health data 98*. OECD Electronic Publications, Paris, France.

Polsky, D. and Glick, H. (1999). Estimating medical costs from incomplete follow-up data. *Value in Health*, 2, 229.

Polsky, D. P., Glick, H. A., Willke, R. *et al.* (1997). Confidence intervals for cost-effectiveness ratios: a comparison of four methods. *Health Economics*, 6, 243–52.

Rubin, D. B. (1976). Inference and missing data. *Biometrika*, 63, 581–92.

Scandinavian Simvastatin Survival Study Group. (1994). Randomised trial of cholesterol lowering in 4444 patients with coronary heart disease: the Scandinavian Simvastatin Survival Study (4S). *Lancet*, 344, 1383–9.

Schulman, K., Burke, J., Drummond, M. *et al.* (1998). Resource costing for multinational neurologic clinical trials: methods and results. *Health Economics*, 7, 629–38.

Schulman, K. A., Buxton, M., Glick, H. *et al.* (1996). Results of the economic evaluation of the FIRST study. *International Journal of Technology Assessment Health Care*, 12, 698–713.

Schulman, K. A., Yabroff, K. R., Kong, J. *et al.* (1999). Claims data approach to defining an episode of care. *Health Services Research*, 34, 603–21.

The SOLVD Investigators. (1991). Effect of enalapril on survival in patients with reduced left ventricular ejection fractions and congestive heart failure. *New England Journal of Medicine*, 325, 293–302.

Steinwachs, D. M. (1992). Episode of care framework: utility for medical effectiveness research. In: M. L. Grady and H. A. Schwartz (eds), *Medical effectiveness research data methods*. DHHS Pub. No (PHS)92–0056. Rockville, MD: Agency for Health Care Policy and Research.

Stinnett, A. A. and Mullahy, J. (1998). Net health benefits: a new framework for the analysis of uncertainty in cost-effectiveness analysis. *Medical Decision-Making*, 18, S68-S80.

Willke, R. J., Glick, H. A., Polsky, D. *et al.* (1998). Estimating country-specific cost-effectiveness from multinational clinical trials. *Health Economics*, 7, 481–93.

Willan, A. R. and O'Brien, B. J. (1996). Confidence intervals for cost-effectiveness ratios: an application of Fieller's theorem. *Health Economics*, 5, 297–305.

Willan, A. R. and O'Brien B. J. (1999). Sample size and power issues in estimating incremental cost-effectiveness ratios from clinical trials data. *Health Economics*, 8, 203–211.

Chapter 7

Modelling in economic evaluation

Karen M. Kuntz and Milton C. Weinstein

Economic evaluations depend on evidence on the costs and health effects of medical and public health interventions. This evidence can be derived from clinical trials, observational studies, meta-analysis, databases, administrative records and case reports. Because the evidence required on consequences and costs of interventions is never present in a single source, practitioners of cost-effectiveness analysis use analytical structures – or mathematical models – to synthesize data on the costs and benefits of alternative clinical strategies. These mathematical representations can be used to simulate a patient's or a population's life experience under a variety of intervention scenarios. A model synthesizes data from multiple sources by making explicit assumptions about the incidence and/or prognosis of a disease, the magnitude and duration of risks and benefits of prevention and/or treatment, the determinants of utilization of health-care resources, and of health-related quality-of-life. Of particular value to clinicians and policy makers, a model allows one to investigate how cost-effectiveness ratios might change if the values of key parameters in a model, which are often unobservable in primary data, are changed. Typical outputs from a model are life expectancy, quality-adjusted life expectancy, and lifetime costs.

The use of models in economic evaluations has been the subject of considerable debate. While many national guidelines for economic evaluation of pharmaceuticals recognize that complete effectiveness data are generally not available and permits appropriate modelling techniques based on sound pharmacoepidemiology (Canadian Coordinating Office for Health Technology Assessment 1994; Commonwealth of Australia 1995), the Food and Drug Administration has taken a less favourable view of models in its regulation of promotional pharmacoeconomic claims under Section 114 of the 1997 Food and Drug Administration Modernization Act (Food and Drug Administration 1995). Concerned about the discretionary nature of modelling, the editors of *The New England Journal of Medicine* have placed restrictions on the publication of cost-effectiveness studies, similar to those placed on reviews and opinion pieces (Kassirer and Angell 1994). The US Panel on the Cost-Effectiveness in Health and Medicine support the use of modelling as a necessary and valid component of cost-effectiveness analyses (Gold *et al.* 1996).

This chapter gives an overview of the use of models in performing cost-effectiveness analyses. We give special attention to state-transition models, including Markov models, because they are the most frequently used in health economic evaluations.

We also describe methods available to modellers for estimating model parameters from clinical and epidemiological data.

7.1 Models used for economic evaluations

7.1.1 What is a model?

The term 'model' is a broad one and has been used in a number of contexts. For example, a regression analysis using primary data represents a statistical model of the relationship between a dependent outcome variable and several independent predictor variables. In the context of economic evaluations of medical interventions, however, a model is any mathematical structure that represents the health and economic outcomes of patients or populations under a variety of scenarios. For example, a simple decision tree, or probability tree, is a representation of a model. For this chapter, we will focus our attention more on the use of state-transition models, specifically Markov models.

7.1.2 Modelling versus trials

This chapter will focus on the use of models that synthesize secondary data sources, and not the use of models for economic evaluations that are 'piggy backed' on to clinical trials. Trial-based economic evaluations are typically based not only on data collected in a clinical trial but also on models that are used to extrapolate clinical trial findings beyond the study time horizon or to other populations, to evaluate relevant comparators not evaluated in the trial, or to interpolate interventions (e.g. screening frequency, dosage). Although many of the issues discussed in this chapter are equally relevant to trial-based models, we draw our examples from decision-analytic models based on existing data, mostly from the medical and public health literature.

The construction of a model based entirely on data from the literature and existing databases is often the best or only approach available. Clinical trials are not always feasible because of ethical considerations or sample size requirements. For example, because the follow-up cystoscopy schedule for low-grade superficial bladder cancer has been established as the standard of care (although without clinical trial evidence) (National Bladder Cancer Collaborative Group A 1977), conducting a trial today to compare standard of care with a less aggressive follow-up strategy would not be ethical. Using a decision-analytic framework, Kilbridge and colleagues (1995) estimated that compared with less frequent cystoscopy, standard practice gains only 10 days of life expectancy for 65-year-old men with superficial transitional cell carcinoma of the bladder and costs approximately $450,000 per life year saved in 1996 US dollars.

Trials that involve the comparison of two diagnostic tests typically require very large sample sizes because the majority of the trial population will be accurately diagnosed and treated in both arms. Kent and colleagues used a decision-analytic model to evaluate various preoperative diagnostic strategies for symptomatic patients with suspected carotid stenosis and found that a combination of duplex ultrasonography and magnetic resonance angiography, with contrast angiography reserved for patients having disparate results on the first two tests, had an incremental cost-effectiveness ratio of $22,400 per quality-adjusted life year saved in 1993 US dollars (Kent *et al.* 1995).

Trials that involve the comparison of screening strategies not only require large sample sizes but also would require long follow-up periods in order to measure differences in health outcome and long-term cost. For example, no single trial could provide all the necessary information for an economic evaluation comparing fecal occult blood testing, sigmoidoscopy, and colonoscopy at various screening intervals, but several models have been used for that purpose (Eddy 1990; Wagner *et al.* 1996; Loeve *et al.* 1999; Frazier *et al.* 2000).

7.1.3 Concerns about modelling

There are a number of valid concerns about the use of models. The data that are used to operationalize the model are from diverse sources, many of which are subject to varying degrees of bias due to confounding variables, patient selection, or method of analysis. For any modelling endeavour, a number of key assumptions have to be made regarding the underlying disease process, data extrapolations, and mathematical relationships between risk factors and clinical outcomes. Often, the best outcome data available relate to surrogate markers (e.g. serum cholesterol levels for coronary heart disease (CHD); tumour regression for cancer; viral load for HIV/AIDS), and the analyst must make the assumption that the surrogate marker is directly linked to a clinical endpoint.

Prior to the clinical trials that demonstrated a reduction in CHD-related mortality with cholesterol lowering drugs, the only information available regarding the effectiveness of these drugs was in terms of their effect on lowering serum cholesterol. Using a decision-analytic model that was based on the relationship between cholesterol level and CHD event derived from the Framingham Heart Study (US Department of Health and Human Services 1987), Goldman and colleagues (1991) estimated the cost-effectiveness of cholesterol lowering drugs. These early results have since been corroborated with economic analysis performed alongside the clinical trials that used hard clinical endpoints (Johannesson *et al.* 1997). Morris (1997) has also shown similar results for the cost-effectiveness of cholesterol-lowering pharmacotherapy for primary prevention based on clinical trial data compared with CHD risk equations derived from the Framingham Heart Study. If we had waited for the long-term endpoints trial in this therapeutic area, potential benefits would have been lost. Models in other therapeutic areas, however, have been less successful. For example, even the 'conservative assumption' regarding the long-term benefit of zidovudine therapy in a decision-analytic model (Schulman *et al.* 1991) was later shown to be too speculative once longer-term follow-up data was collected (Concorde Coordinating Committee 1994).

Another common concern of models is their lack of transparency. Decision analysts face a trade-off between building a complicated model that accurately reflects all of the important aspects of a disease and its treatment, and building a simple model that is more transparent. Decision-analytic models are often criticized as being 'black boxes'.

Many of these concerns can be addressed by careful documentation of the input probabilities, utilities, and costs, as well as the key assumptions that underlie the model. Of greater concern is the degree of freedom that the modeller has in deciding upon the model inputs and assumptions. The choice of one parameter over another, or one assumption over another, can bias the model in favour of, or against, a particular strategy. Concerns about investigator bias increase, the more an economic evaluation relies on models to supplement clinical trial outcomes. Performing extensive sensitivity analysis on the model parameters, as well as on structural model assumptions, such as the linkage between surrogate markers and health outcomes, can help to address those concerns of bias of the base case analysis.

Even with their recognized limitations, models are unavoidable. Economic evaluations that have been piggy-backed on these trials often require almost as much modelling in order to extend the time horizon, with the consequence that variations in results across these studies can be attributed as much to differences in their modelling assumptions as to differences in the primary clinical results from the trials themselves. If one fails to consider the health and economic outcomes that may occur beyond the time-frame of the observed data, there is an implicit assumption being made that all arms of the trial are equivalent. For example, if a patient in the treatment arm would have died had they been in the placebo, the 'stop and drop' analysis assumes that this person dies immediately at the end of the trial follow-up period.

7.1.4 Benefits of modelling

With or without direct evidence from a well-designed clinical trial with both economic and health endpoints, there is still a need to make informed decisions. For example, even though there are no clinical trials with economic analyses of colorectal cancer screening strategies, policy makers still have to decide whether or not to implement a such a programme, as well as deciding which screening tests to use and at what frequencies. A well-designed model is essentially a tool that can be used to simulate a clinical trial based on the available medical literature and publicly available data sources. Even in situations where a clinical trial does exist, models are often used to incorporate the benefits and costs beyond the time horizon of the trial. A good example of this is the cost-effectiveness analysis alongside the Scandinavian Simvastatin Survival Study (Johannesson *et al.* 1997), where the authors used a previous model of CHD to project beyond the five-year horizon of the study. Clinical trials can also be limiting because they evaluate only a limited number of strategies. In economic evaluations we typically want to be able to consider all available options simultaneously. For example, an analysis of a clinical trial of annual fecal occult blood testing (FOBT) versus no testing, such as the Minnesota Colon Cancer Control Study (Mandel *et al.* 1993), could be supplemented with strategies of annual FOBT with five-year sigmoidoscopy, as recommended by the American Cancer Society (Byers *et al.* 1997). Other examples relate to head-to-head, or incremental, economic evaluations of drugs that have been studied clinically only in placebo controlled trials. A model can also be used to incorporate data from multiple sources. Because clinical trial populations are typically not representative of the general population, population-based studies can be used to represent the placebo group with the clinical trial used only to inform the treatment effect. In an analysis of donepezil for the treatment of Alzheimer's disease, Neumann and colleagues used a population-based registry of patients (Morris *et al.* 1989) to represent the prognosis of patients who are not treated, and then used clinical trial data to estimate the relative reduction in the rate of progression of disease severity (Neumann *et al.* 1999).

It is important to stress that models should not be used as the sole basis for making policy but only as part of the process. As aids to decision-making, models often support and strengthen the decisions that would have been made in the absence of the model. In circumstances where the model results are not anticipated, they allow for a detailed investigation of the model parameters and model assumptions through sensitivity analysis.

7.2 Decision trees

7.2.1 Elements of a decision tree

Cost-effectiveness analyses can be performed with a decision tree that has one decision node at the root. The branches off the initial decision node represent all of the strategies that are to be compared. Embedded, or downstream, decision nodes are not useful in cost-effectiveness analyses because the optimal branch cannot be determined when folding back the tree without an explicit decision rule for comparing costs and consequences. A series of probability nodes off of each strategy branch can be used to reflect uncertain events, usually within a relatively short time frame. The outcomes at the end of each pathway are values that reflect both the cost and the health effect associated with that pathway. In cost-effectiveness analyses, these outcomes are typically grouped into two sets: health states that can be combined into a utility measure such as quality-adjusted life years, and units of resource utilization which can be combined into a monetary measure of cost. Most often, Markov cycle trees are attached to the terminal nodes of a decision tree for the purpose of calculating cumulative lifetime events such as life expectancy, quality-adjusted life expectancy, and lifetime costs. As in any decision tree the method of analysis is to average out and fold back the tree. In a cost-effectiveness analysis, the analyses are done separately for costs and health outcome. Several textbooks and articles are available on decision analysis at various levels of methodologic sophistication and health application. (See, for example: Sox *et al.* 1988; Clemen 1996).

7.2.2 Example of a decision tree used in a cost-effectiveness analysis

Magid and colleagues (1992) used a decision tree to evaluate the costs, outcomes and cost-effectiveness of strategies to prevent Lyme disease after tick bites. They reported their incremental cost-effectiveness ratios in terms of cost per major complication prevented and found that empirical treatment of patients with tick bites is a reasonable strategy when the probability of infection is greater than 0.01. Because the time frame for this analysis is short and mortality was not a factor, a simple decision tree with short-term outcomes was appropriate. However, if the clinical course of the disease of interest has an extended time horizon, or if the mortality of patients differs across strategies, a lifetime model is more appropriate.

7.3 Markov models

7.3.1 Uses of Markov models

Markov models are analytical structures that represent key elements of a disease and are commonly used in economic evaluations (Sonnenberg and Beck 1993). They are particularly useful for diseases in which events can occur repeatedly over time such as acute myocardial infarction for patients with stable angina, or cancer recurrence in patients with localized breast cancer. The cyclic nature of Markov models is also useful for depicting predictable events that occur over time such as sigmoidoscopy screening tests for colorectal cancer every five years. By assigning numeric values to a series of health states over time, Markov models allow for the synthesis of data on costs, effects, and health-related quality-of-life of alternative clinical strategies through the calculation of life expectancy, quality-adjusted life expectancy, and lifetime costs. Quality-adjusted life expectancy is the recommended health outcome for a reference case analysis by the Panel on Cost-Effectiveness in Health and Medicine (Gold *et al.* 1996).

7.3.2 Principal elements

A Markov model is comprised of a set of mutually exclusive and collectively exhaustive health states. Each person in the model must reside in one and only one health state at any point in time. At fixed increments of time known as the Markov cycle length (e.g. monthly, yearly), persons transit among the health states according to a set of transition probabilities. Transition probabilities can be either constant over time or time-dependent. Health states can be transient (persons can revisit the state at any time), temporary (a person can stay in the state for only one cycle), or absorbing (once people enter the state they can never exit). All persons residing in a particular health state are indistinguishable from one another – both in current clinical and demographic attributes and in terms of historical attributes. To operationalize the Markov structure, values are assigned to each health state that represent the cost and utility of spending one cycle in that state.

A key limitation of Markov models is the Markovian assumption, which states that the transition probabilities depend only on current health state residence and not on past health states. One can circumvent this assumption by expanding the number of health states so that each state represents a unique health-state history. This permits one to make the event rates dependent on clinical history, but increases the number of parameters to be estimated and may tax the memory capacity of available software. If the required number of state descriptions gets too large, it becomes preferable to use a stochastic (Monte Carlo) simulation rather than a cohort simulation that tracks the expected number of patients in each state over time. (We return to these computational options later, in Section 7.3.4.)

7.3.3 Constructing a Markov model

The structure and complexity of a Markov model will depend on the clinical application, the available data and how many simplifying assumptions are made. However, there are a number of basic steps to follow when constructing a Markov model. These steps will be illustrated by a simple model of breast cancer treatment for women newly diagnosed with localized breast cancer, designed to evaluate the cost-effectiveness of treatments that improve breast cancer prognosis.

To construct a Markov model for a particular application, one must first specify the Markov states. These health states should not only reflect all the relevant states of health associated with the disease and treatment over time, but should also include all relevant clinical history. One possible model for breast cancer treatment would be one with four states: (1) localized cancer; (2) localized recurrence; (3) metastatic disease; and (4) dead. Although the first two Markov states represent women with localized breast cancer, they are defined as separate states because the prognosis is different for women with a first cancer compared with women with a localized recurrence. The costs and utilities might be different as well.

The second step in building a Markov model is to choose a cycle length, which must be a constant increment of time. The choice of cycle length will depend on the timing of events in the disease process and the life expectancy of the population (shorter cycles should be used with shorter life expectancies). For our simple breast cancer treatment model, the selected cycle length is one year.

Next, a set of transition probabilities must be specified. Let $A = (a_{ij})$ be a $n \times n$ matrix, where n represents the number of Markov states and a_{ij} represents the probability that a person in health state i will transit to health state j within one cycle. By definition, $\sum a_{ij} = 1$ for all i. Transition probabilities can be equal to 0, meaning that the particular transition is not allowed. Moreover, the transition probabilities can be functions of time. For transition probabilities that vary with time, there will be a different matrix A_k for each cycle k. Note, however, that for this purpose, 'time' is defined in terms of the running index of cycles, k, and cannot be linked to a particular event without incorporating the elapsed time after an event into the state descriptors. (The device for accomplishing this is called 'tunnel states', and we return to this later, in Section 7.3.5. pp. 152–3)

For the breast cancer treatment model we will assume that all transition probabilities are constant and equal to the following:

$$A = \begin{bmatrix} 0.945 & 0.006 & 0.014 & 0.035 \\ 0 & 0.913 & 0.052 & 0.035 \\ 0 & 0 & 0.607 & 0.393 \\ 0 & 0 & 0 & 1 \end{bmatrix}$$

The first row of A indicates that women can transit from state 1 (localized cancer) to any of the other three states, or remain in that state through the year with a probability of 0.945. The last row represents an absorbing state (dead) in that persons cannot transit out of this state. All rows must sum to 1. This matrix represents the prognosis of localized breast cancer without the treatment of interest. A different transition probability matrix would need to be specified to reflect the prognosis of women with breast cancer who are compliant with the treatment under investigation. Suppose that there were a treatment that was shown to decrease recurrence by 50 per cent for those with an initial diagnosis of breast cancer. This implies that the transition probability from the localized cancer state to both the recurrent cancer state and the metastatic disease state (since this is a form of recurrence) should be divided by two (the transition probability of remaining in localized cancer is then adjusted so that the row of probabilities sum to 1). For this treatment, the transition probability matrix is:

$$A = \begin{bmatrix} 0.955 & 0.003 & 0.007 & 0.035 \\ 0 & 0.913 & 0.052 & 0.035 \\ 0 & 0 & 0.607 & 0.393 \\ 0 & 0 & 0 & 1 \end{bmatrix}$$

When estimating transition probabilities, it is important to be mindful of the cohorts or target populations that are to be analysed. One can have a number of different transition probability matrices that are specific for different cohorts defined by demographic or clinical variables. For the breast cancer treatment model, there would be different matrices for women with node-negative breast cancer versus women with node-positive breast cancer. Because nodal status is a characteristic of the starting cohort (i.e. women with newly diagnosed localized breast cancer), it affects the transition probability matrix values and not the health state descriptions. However, if one were interested in distinguishing localized recurrence by nodal status, then there would have to be separate node-negative and a node-positive recurrent cancer states.

The final step is to assign a cost and utility to each health state. If a utility of 1 is assigned to all states except dead (which is assigned a value of 0), then the model will calculate life expectancy. If the utilities represent a health-related quality adjustment for each health state, then the model will calculate quality-adjusted life expectancy. To calculate discounted life expectancy or quality-adjusted life expectancy the utilities are divided by $(1+r)^k$, where r is the discount rate corresponding to the cycle length, and k is the cycle index. Utility values can be useful in calculating other outcome measures as well. If all values are 0 except for a single state (e.g. metastatic breast cancer) then the outcome of the Markov model would be the average time a person in the cohort spends in the metastatic state (also known as 'residency time'). Suppose that the metastatic state is split into two states, the first being a temporary state where patients spend only their first year with metastatic disease and the second being a state for the second year on until death. If all utilities were set to 0 except for the first metastatic state then the model outcome would represent the proportion of the initial cohort who ever experienced metastatic disease. To calculate quality-adjusted life expectancy

Table 7.1 Health state values for breast cancer treatment Markov model

Markov State	Cost ($)	Utility
Localized cancer	500	0.95
Recurrent cancer	5000	0.80
Metastatic disease	20,000	0.40
Dead	0	0.00

and lifetime costs for our breast cancer treatment model, we will assign the following values shown in Table 7.1 for each state.

We now have a relatively simple Markov model to simulate the prognosis of women diagnosed with localized breast cancer. There are a number of simplifying assumptions that could be eliminated by constructing a more detailed model (e.g. adding more health states or incorporating time-dependent probabilities, utilities, or costs). For example, the first year with localized breast cancer (either the initial or subsequent diagnosis) is most certainly different from subsequent years in terms of utilization of health-care resources and health-related quality-of-life. To incorporate this detail, the localized state would have to be duplicated, with one state for the first year and the other state for subsequent years with localized breast cancer.

The events that can happen during a cycle can be modelled with a decision tree structure known as a Markov cycle tree. Often the cycle-specific transition probabilities are comprised of a series of transitions that take place during the cycle. The tree structure shown in Figure 7.1 is one possible Markov cycle tree for the localized cancer state (i.e. State 1). Note that patients who begin a cycle in State 1 pass through this tree once during that cycle, and the path probabilities from the tree are represented by the transition probabilities from State 1 to each of the four states. For example, the transition probability of localized cancer to metastatic disease is equal to the probability of surviving the year, multiplied by the probability of experiencing a recurrence given that the patient did not die from other causes, multiplied by the proportion of first recurrences that present as metastatic.

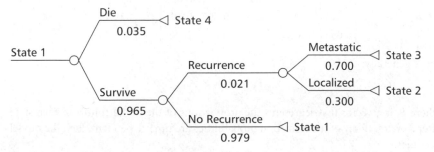

Fig. 7.1 A possible Markov cycle tree for the localized cancer state (State 1) in the breast cancer treatment model

7.3.4 Methods of evaluation

There are two methods of evaluation that are commonly used. Cohort simulation tracks a hypothetical cohort of patients simultaneously through the model. Monte Carlo simulation (first order) randomly selects a patient from the hypothetical cohort, and each patient transits through the model one at a time. The advantages of cohort simulation are that it is a faster method of evaluation and that it is easier to debug (more transparent). The primary disadvantage of cohort simulation is that it requires each state definition to describe all relevant current and past clinical information, which can result in a very complex model structure (and most available software packages have limits to the size of a Markov model). The advantage of a Monte Carlo simulation is that it only requires that health states describe the current clinical situation because it allows past information to be tracked specifically for each patient transitioning through the model. The disadvantages of a Monte Carlo simulation are that it takes much longer to run the model and that it is not as transparent.

To run a Markov model under either evaluation method, one must first 'seed' the model with an initial cohort. This is done by specifying a $1 \times n$ starting vector P_0, which specifies the probability of starting in each state. For the breast cancer treatment model, if we assume that the initial cohort is women who are newly diagnosed with breast cancer, then the starting vector is |1 0 0 0|. Alternatively, if we were considering a population of women with any localized breast cancer, then we would distribute the women between the first two states based on the proportions observed in the applicable clinical setting. The proportion of the initial cohort in each of the four states after one cycle (P_1) can be calculated by multiplying P_0 by A:

$$
\begin{vmatrix} 1 \\ 0 \\ 0 \\ 0 \end{vmatrix}^{T}
\begin{vmatrix} 0.945 & 0.006 & 0.014 & 0.035 \\ 0 & 0.913 & 0.052 & 0.035 \\ 0 & 0 & 0.607 & 0.393 \\ 0 & 0 & 0 & 1 \end{vmatrix}
=
\begin{vmatrix} 0.945 \\ 0.006 \\ 0.014 \\ 0.035 \end{vmatrix}^{T}
$$

Multiplying P_1 by A yields a vector P_2 that shows the distribution of the initial cohort among the four states at the end of the second cycle:

$$
\begin{vmatrix} 0.945 \\ 0.006 \\ 0.014 \\ 0.035 \end{vmatrix}^{T}
\begin{vmatrix} 0.945 & 0.006 & 0.014 & 0.035 \\ 0 & 0.913 & 0.052 & 0.035 \\ 0 & 0 & 0.607 & 0.393 \\ 0 & 0 & 0 & 1 \end{vmatrix}
=
\begin{vmatrix} 0.893 \\ 0.011 \\ 0.022 \\ 0.074 \end{vmatrix}^{T}
$$

More generally:

$$ P_k = P_{k-1} \times A $$

where P_k is a vector that represents the proportions of the initial cohort in each state after k cycles. If any of the transition probabilities are time-dependent, then the model becomes:

$$ P_k = P_{k-1} \times A_k $$

where A_k is the matrix of transition probabilities for cycle k. The sum of the elements of P_k must be equal to 1 for all k.

Cohort simulation

A cohort simulation produces a *Markov trace*, which shows the movement of a cohort through the health states and the cumulative utilities and costs assigned. Table 7.2 illustrates the Markov trace for the first five cycles for the breast cancer treatment model, along with their cumulative utilities. Column 1 shows the cycle number (i.e. k), Columns 2–5 show the proportion of the cohort in each of the four states at each cycle (i.e. P_k), Column 6 shows the utility (or cost) contribution of each cycle, and the last column shows a running sum of Column 6. The contribution of each cycle to expected utility (or cost) is calculated by summing the products of the health state utilities (given in Table 7.1) with the probabilities of being in each state. For example, the expected cycle utility for the first cycle is calculated as follows:

$$(0.945)(0.95) + (0.006)(0.80) + (0.014)(0.40) + (0.035)(0) = 0.908$$

On average, the cohort contributes 0.908 quality-adjusted life years during the first cycle. The maximum utility in a cycle is 1. Note that at time 0 (i.e. cycle 0) the utility is multiplied by 0.5, which is known as the half-cycle correction factor and implies that persons transition in the middle of a cycle. Thus, the maximum utility at time 0 is 0.5.

The Markov model is typically run until essentially all of the initial cohort reside in the dead state (e.g. the cycle utility is less than 0.0001). At this cycle the cumulative expected utility represents the quality-adjusted life expectancy of the cohort. If costs were used as state values instead of health-state utilities, then the cumulative 'utility' in the last cycle would represent the average lifetime costs of the cohort. Summing the health state probabilities of a particular state for all cycles results in the residency time for that Markov state, or the average length of time that the cohort spent in that state. To obtain discounted expected utility or expected cost, one would simple divide the cycle utility in each row by its discount factor $(1+r)^k$ before adding it into the cumulative utility.

Table 7.2 Five-cycle Markov trace for the breast cancer treatment model

Cycle	Localized cancer	Recurrent cancer	Metastatic disease	Dead	Cycle utility	Cumulative utility
0	1	0	0	0	0.475	0.475
1	0.945	0.006	0.014	0.035	0.908	1.383
2	0.893	0.011	0.022	0.074	0.866	2.249
3	0.844	0.016	0.026	0.114	0.825	3.074
4	0.797	0.019	0.029	0.155	0.784	3.858
5	0.754	0.022	0.030	0.194	0.746	4.604

Monte Carlo simulation

The alternative method of evaluation is to use a first order Monte Carlo simulation. The four-state breast cancer treatment model can also be evaluated by this method. Instead of a cohort of women transitioning through the model as seen in the Markov trace, one woman at a time would transition through the model. The first woman would start in the localized cancer state (based on P_0). If and where she moves during the first cycle depends upon a random number drawn from a Uniform [0, 1] distribution. If the number is in the [0, 0.006] range she moves to the recurrent cancer state (with 0.006 probability), if it's in the [0.006, 0.020] range she moves to the metastatic disease state (with 0.014 probability), if it's in the [0.020, 0.055] range she moves to the dead state (with 0.035 probability), and if it's in the [0.055, 1] range she remains in the localized cancer state (with probability 0.945). The analysis simulates a cohort (e.g. 1000 women), one at a time, and records the quality-adjusted life span for each woman depending on the particular pathway she took through the health states prior to dying. Quality-adjusted life expectancy can be calculated by taking the average of all of the quality-adjusted life spans in the sample. If the sample is large enough, this average should be very close to the value calculated by the cohort simulation. The variance of the quality-adjusted life spans can also be estimated from the simulation results, which reflects the variability of the patient-level quality-adjusted life spans (as opposed to the variability of the population-level quality-adjusted life expectancy) of the cohort. It is important to select the sample size for a Monte Carlo simulation large enough so that the variability in the estimate of the sample means (for utility and cost) is small compared to the differences of interest between strategies. The standard error of the sample mean can be estimated from a preliminary sample of, say $n = 1000$. Since the standard error is approximately proportional to $\sqrt{n}$, the standard error with sample size N would be estimated to be approximately $S_n \times (n/N)^{1/2}$. The required sample size N depends on the magnitudes of the transition probabilities, the differences in utilities between states, and the effect sizes of interest. One HIV model uses $N = 1,000,000$ in order to obtain reliable estimates of cost-effectiveness ratios (Freedberg *et al.* 1997).

The primary advantage of a Monte Carlo analysis is the ability to capture clinical history without expanding the Markov state space. For the breast cancer treatment model it would be possible to reduce the number of states to three: localized cancer, metastatic disease and dead. A binary variable could then be defined to distinguish between an initial cancer (variable set to 0) and a recurrence (variable set to 1). The probability of metastatic disease could then be a function of the binary recurrence variable so that it would be higher if the patient had experienced a recurrence.

7.3.5 Methodological challenges

Tunnel states

As stated previously, one of the biggest limitations of Markov models is the Markovian assumption. However, there are ways of getting around this assumption. The most common of these is to expand the state space to define not only the current states of health that are possible for the cohort of interest but also all the possible historical pathways that are relevant. This approach is useful to the point where the number of states becomes unreasonable. Consider the four-state breast cancer treatment model. The annual probability that a woman with a localized recurrence will present with metastatic disease depends on how long it's been since her recurrence. For example, suppose that the annual probability decreases monotonically for the first ten years after diagnosis, and then is constant thereafter. In order to capture this, the recurrent cancer state would have to be split into 11 states: one state for each of the ten years and an additional one to reflect all years beyond the tenth year. These 11 states are called 'tunnel' states in that persons transition from one state to the next as if in a tunnel (unless they exit to metastatic disease or death before they reach the end of the tunnel).

Heterogeneity

Another methodological challenge is adequately adjusting for heterogeneity. Because the assumption in a Markov model is that all persons residing in a health state are identical, any degree of heterogeneity within a state will cause some degree of bias. As an extreme example, consider a health state that consists of persons with and without an underlying (hypothetical) Syndrome X. Persons with Syndrome X face an annual probability of death of 95 per cent, while those without Syndrome X have an annual probability of death of only 5 per cent. If 10 per cent of the population has Syndrome X, then the observed chance of death in one year for this population is 14 per cent. Assigning a constant annual probability of 14 per cent to this population will greatly overestimate mortality because the people with Syndrome X will be exiting the state 19 times faster than those without Syndrome X. A more realistic example of heterogeneity would be in accounting for human papillomavirus (HPV) status in a model of cervical cancer, as women with HPV have a much greater incidence of cervical lesions than women without HPV. In practice, when issues of heterogeneity are believed to be important, health states should be defined according to the underlying heterogeneity factor. For example, the health states in a cervical cancer model would be defined to capture the underlying HPV status of the women in the model (even though the HPV status is unknown).

7.4 Survival analysis and hazard rates

7.4.1 Introduction

Survival analysis refers to statistical methods that are used to analyse data that can be used to estimate the probability distribution of time to an event. The event of interest is often mortality but can be a nonfatal event as well. In order to model the prognosis of a disease in the framework of a Markov model it is important to have a fundamental understanding of survival curves and their underlying hazard functions.

7.4.2 Survivorship function

Let T be a random variable that denotes time of death. A survivorship function, or survival curve, is a function that expresses the probability that an individual survives longer than time t:

$$S(t) = P(T > t)$$

$S(0)$ is always equal to one and is a non-increasing function that approaches 0 as t approaches ∞. The hazard function, $h(t)$, describes the instantaneous failure rate at time t. There is a direct relationship between the survivorship function and the hazard function:

$$S(t) = \exp\left(-\int_0^t h(u)\, du\right)$$

There are a number of parametric survival distributions (Lee 1992), the most simple of which is the exponential distribution, which assumes that the hazard function (μ) is constant with respect to time:

$$S(t) = \exp(-\mu t)$$

7.4.3 Rates versus probabilities

Consider a study where 100 patients are followed for two years and 50 patients die during the study. Suppose you want to estimate an *annual* transition probability of dying for these patients, where the two-year probability is 0.50 (50/100). To calculate an annual probability, it is not correct to simply divide the two-year probability by two (i.e. 0.25). This is because the one-year transition probability reflects a *conditional* probability of dying during the year given that the person is alive at the beginning of the year. For example, if a 0.25 probability were applied to 100 patients at time 0, then 75 patients would be alive at the end of the first year. Applying the 0.25 probability to those 75 patients results in 56 patients being alive at the end of the second year. Hence an annual probability of 0.25 implies a two-year probability of 0.44 ($1 - 56/100$), not 0.50. Using this logic the one-year transition probability can be calculated by:

$$(100)(1 - p)(1 - p) = 50$$

$$p = 0.2929$$

In practice, a t-year probability can be converted to a u-year probability by calculating the underlying hazard rate. A hazard rate is defined as the instantaneous failure rate, or force of mortality, per unit time. If we assume that there is a constant annual hazard rate μ over the study time horizon, then the probability that the event occurs during the t years can be expressed by an exponential cumulative distribution function $P(t)$, where

$$P(t) = 1 - \exp(-\mu t)$$

Note that $P(t)$ is just $1 - S(t)$. Thus, if we know the value of μ we can calculate the probability that an event will occur by time t. In this example, we know $P(2)$ and are interested in estimating μ. The general equation to solve for μ is

$$\mu = \frac{-\ln[1 - P(t)]}{t}$$

In this example, $\mu = 0.3466$. Because t is expressed in years, μ is an annual hazard rate. The annual transition probability is then:

$$P(1) = 1 - \exp(-0.3466) = 0.2929$$

Not coincidentally, this is identical to the result obtained before. Unlike a probability, a hazard rate can be multiplied or divided by a factor to convert to different time intervals. For example, a monthly hazard rate can be obtained from a yearly hazard rate by dividing by 12. Then a monthly transition probability (probability of dying each month conditional on being alive at the beginning of the month) can be easily obtained from the monthly rate.

7.4.4 Defining and estimating life expectancy

Life expectancy is the average life span of a population. For example, a life expectancy of 31.4 years for 50-year-old women in the USA means that while some of these women will live much fewer than 31.4 years and some will live much more than 31.4 years, the number of remaining years lived on average for a cohort of 50-year-old women is 31.4. In cost-effectiveness analysis, the effectiveness measure of interest is often life expectancy or quality-adjusted life expectancy. Before discussing the incorporation of health-related quality-of-life, we will discuss the derivation of life expectancy, which is equal to the area under the survival curve:

$$\text{life expectancy} = \int_0^\infty S(t)\, dt$$

In the case of an exponential survival curve, life expectancy is equal to $1/\mu$.

A simple approximation to life expectancy

Because life expectancy is such an important component of decision-making for physicians, Beck and colleagues developed a simple approximation of life expectancy for a person who has one or more diseases (Beck *et al.* 1982a, b). While primarily a tool to be used by clinicians 'at the bedside' (or in 'back of the envelope' calculations), the declining exponential approximation to life expectancy (the 'DEALE') provides a preliminary framework for estimating disease-specific life expectancy. The DEALE approach is based on the assumption that the underlying survival curve is exponential; thus, life expectancy can be represented as $1/\mu$, where μ is the constant mortality (hazard) rate over time. The average mortality rate of a 'healthy' person, μ_{AS} (or μ_{ASR}), is defined as the reciprocal of the age-, sex- (and race)-specific life expectancy obtained from life tables. For example, a 50-year-old woman with a life expectancy of 31.4 years has a μ_{AS} of 0.0318 (1/31.4). This component of mortality accounts for the fact that diseased persons can die of causes other than their disease. If the patient has a disease that confers additional mortality risk, he or she is exposed to the competing risks of the disease-specific mortality in addition to the age-, sex- (and race)-adjusted mortality. Survival studies of patients with the particular disease of interest can be used to calculate disease-specific mortality, or μ_D. To do this, one has to derive the compound mortality rate from the study (e.g. from a five-year survival probability) and subtract the age-, sex- (and race)-specific mortality of the study population, based on the age, sex, (and race) of the study population. If the disease of interest is a major component of mortality (e.g. CHD) then the disease-specific component of μ_{AS} (or μ_{ASR}) should be subtracted out.

To illustrate, suppose that you want to estimate the life expectancy benefit of a 54-year-old man with congestive heart failure and reduced left ventricular ejection fraction. The Studies of Left Ventricular Dysfunction (SOLVD) (SOLVD investigators 1991) estimated four-year survival probabilities of 63 per cent and 58 per cent for the enalapril and placebo arm, respectively, among a cohort of primarily men (92 per cent) with an average age of 61 years, and a risk reduction of overall mortality of 16 per cent. From the US life tables we know that the life expectancy of a 'healthy' 61-year-old is 18.3 years, which implies an age- and sex-specific mortality of 0.0546 (μ_{pop}) observed in the trial. The compound mortality rate (mortality associated with all causes of death, μ_C) for the placebo arm can be estimated using the exponential survival distribution and solving for the rate parameter:

$$\mu_C = \frac{-\ln (0.58)}{4} = 0.1362$$

To estimate the disease-specific mortality rate for the placebo group, the age- and sex-specific mortality rate must be subtracted off of the compound mortality rate: $0.1362 - 0.0546 = 0.0815$ (number off slightly due to rounding). Now, to estimate the life expectancy of the 54-year-old male patient if untreated, the *patient-specific* μ_{AS} must be added to the disease-specific mortality rate that was just calculated. From the US life tables, the life expectancy of a 54-year-old 'healthy' man is 23.7 years, which implies that μ_{AS} is 0.0422 and his total mortality rate is: $0.0422 + 0.0815 = 0.1237$. Thus, an approximation of the life expectancy for this patient is $1/(0.1237) = 8.08$ years. Applying a 16 per cent risk reduction to μ_C of the placebo arm yields a compound rate of 0.1144 (0.1362×0.84) for the enalapril arm. The disease-specific mortality rate for the enalapril group is: $0.1144 - 0.0546 = 0.0597$. The life expectancy of the 54-year-old male patient if treated is: $0.0422 + 0.0535 = 0.1019$. Thus, an approximation of the life expectancy for this patient is $1/(0.1019) = 9.81$ years, and an approximation of the life expectancy benefit due to treatment is 1.73 years.

Using life tables

While other closed-form approximations do exist that make more reasonable assumptions than the DEALE method about how the underlying mortality rate varies with age (Keeler and Bell 1992), a Markov model is an ideal tool for estimating life expectancy. A simple two-state Markov model (with 'alive' and 'dead' states) can be used to estimate life expectancy based on annual probabilities of death that vary with time. Estimates of annual age-, sex- and race-adjusted mortality rates as a function of time can be obtained from the US life tables. For cohorts defined by sex and race, the life tables provide estimates of the number of persons alive at each age up to 85 years out of 100,000 born. These numbers can be used to calculate the probability of dying in the following year conditional on being alive at the beginning of that year. For example, if 72,391 persons are alive at age 70 and 71,496 are alive at age 71, the probability of a 70-year-old person dying in his or her 71st year is 0.0124 [(72,391 − 71,496)/72,391]. This annual probability can then be converted into an annual rate to establish a table of annual mortality rates by age (up to age 85). To extrapolate beyond age 85 (as approximately one-third of the population is still alive), one can rely on the fact that age versus the natural logarithm of the annual hazard rate is approximately linear for ages 45 to 85. The Gompertz survivorship function has this property and, for that reason, is often used to parameterize life table data (Gompertz 1825).

Approximating life expectancy with a Markov model

The simplest Markov model has two states, one of which is absorbing. Its transition probability matrix can be described by a single nontrivial parameter – mortality. Let h_t represent the hazard rate for cycle t that is consistent with the cycle length (e.g. annual hazard rates for one-year cycles). Consider a Markov model with two states ('alive' and 'dead') with a cycle-specific probability of dying (p_t) that is equal to:

$$1 - \exp{(-h_t)}$$

The proportion of the initial cohort residing in the 'alive' state at each cycle t in the Markov trace will reflect the t-year survival probability, $S(t)$. If the state utility assigned to the 'alive' state is equal to 1, then the cycle utility of the Markov trace will equal the proportion of the cohort alive in each cycle. Life expectancy is then the cumulative utility of the final cycle (when $S(t)$ is essentially equal to 0). In Figure 7.2, the first rectangle is only one-half of a year wide with an area of 0.5 and represents the half-cycle correction factor. All of the other rectangles have areas that are equal to the

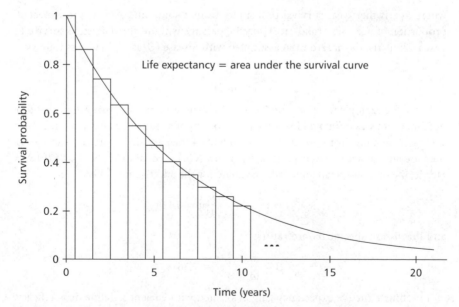

Fig. 7.2 Survivorship curve with approximating rectangles

proportion of the cohort that is alive at each year. Thus, life expectancy, which is equal to the area under the survival curve, is equal to the sum of the areas of the rectangles shown in the figure, or the sum of all of the cycle utilities in a Markov trace.

Additive versus multiplicative mortality relationship for calculating disease-specific mortality

The mortality rate h_t can be represented as a step function of a time-dependent age-, sex- (and race)-specific component, b_t, and a disease-specific component, where the steps are equal to the cycle length. The relationship between background mortality (b_t) and disease-specific mortality can be either additive or multiplicative (Kuntz and Weinstein 1995). In the additive model, the assumption is that the disease-related mortality confers an excess hazard (λ) over that of the time-dependent baseline rate:

$$h_t = b_t + \lambda$$

Alternatively, the multiplicative model assumes that the effect of disease on the baseline hazard rate (β) is proportional:

$$h_t = b_t \times \beta$$

The disease-specific parameters can be estimated from the literature, for example, from a five-year survival probability. The excess hazard rate (λ) is estimated by subtracting out age-, sex-, (and race)-specific mortality based on the *time-dependent* function:

$$\lambda = -\left(\frac{1}{t}\right) \ln\left(\frac{S(t)}{N(t)}\right)$$

where $S(t)$ is the t-year survival probability from a study, and $N(t)$ is the 'expected' proportion of age-, sex- (and race)-specific persons without the disease to survive to year t. Similarly, the hazard ratio associated with disease (β) is estimated as follows:

$$\beta = \frac{\ln S(t)}{\ln N(t)}$$

Recall the example from Section 7.4.4, p. 156 where a four-year survival probability of 58 per cent was estimated from the placebo arm of a study of 61-year-old men (on average). We know from the life tables that 80,864 men are alive at age 61 and 75,097 men are alive at age 65 (four years later). Thus, $N(4)$ is equal to 75,097/80,864(0.93). Hence, the disease-specific mortality estimate for the additive model is

$$\lambda = -\left(\frac{1}{4}\right) \ln\left(\frac{0.58}{0.93}\right) = 0.118$$

and the disease-specific hazard ratio is

$$\beta = \frac{\ln (0.58)}{\ln (0.93)} = 7.36$$

To estimate the life expectancy gain associated with enalapril, define drug efficacy, γ, as the reduction of *disease-specific* mortality, where a value of 0 indicates no efficacy and a value of 1 indicates complete reduction of disease-related mortality. The additive model with efficacy incorporated is thus:

$$h_t = b_t + \lambda(1 - \gamma)$$

and the multiplicative model is

$$h_t = b_t[1 + (\beta - 1)(1 - \gamma)]$$

Let $S_p(t)$ and $S_r(t)$ be the t-year survival probabilities for the placebo and treatment arms of a clinical trial, respectively. The estimated risk reduction of disease-related mortality is:

$$1 - \frac{\ln\,[S_r(t)/N(t)]}{\ln\,[S_p(t)/N(t)]} * 100\%$$

The four-year survival probability for the enalapril arm in SOLVD was 63 per cent, yielding an efficacy estimate of 18 per cent, which is slightly greater than the 16 per cent reported in the study as the reduction in *all-cause* mortality. Note that the survival models could also be specified with an efficacy parameter that pertains to the reduction in all-cause mortality. Using a simple two-state Markov model to calculate the life expectancy gain of a 54-year-old man with congestive heart failure and reduced left ventricular ejection fraction yields values of 1.29 and 1.02 years under the additive and multiplicative assumptions, respectively. (Recall, the DEALE approach estimated a gain of 1.73 years.) Another benefit of using a Markov model approach is that the modeller can make different assumptions about treatment efficacy over time (e.g. allowing treatment efficacy of a surgical procedure to stop or decline at some point in time).

Kuntz and Weinstein observed a predictable pattern for these two survival models when used to extrapolate to other ages assuming that the estimates of λ and β were independent of age (Kuntz and Weinstein 1995). Specifically, life expectancy gains decrease monotonically with age under the additive assumption, whereas they tend to be ∩-shaped under the multiplicative assumption. Similarly, incremental cost-effectiveness ratios increase monotonically with age under the additive assumption, and tend to be ∪-shaped under the multiplicative assumption. Evidence of whether or not a multiplicative model is appropriate in a specific disease can be gleaned from studies that report proportions of disease-specific deaths across different age groups. If these proportions are constant across age groups then the use of a multiplicative model to describe the relationship between disease-specific mortality and background mortality is appropriate. For example, a multiplicative model is appropriate for patients after acute myocardial infarction (Kuntz and Weinstein 1995, Kuntz *et al.* 1996).

7.5 Estimating probabilities from the literature

7.5.1 Data sources

Although a number of economic evaluations are performed when the analyst has access to primary data, most cost-effectiveness studies rely on the medical literature, publicly available databases, or as a last resort, expert opinion. When utilizing studies from the literature as sources for estimating model parameters it is important to attempt to collect all relevant studies that inform a particular probability, utility, or cost. Randomized trials are ideal for determining the *relative* effect of an intervention; if several randomized trials have been done, then a meta-analysis of all trials is desirable. Using the outcomes of a placebo arm of a clinical trial to represent the natural history (i.e. absence of intervention) of a disease, however, has limitations in that it is typically not representative of the population of interest. Cohort studies or disease registries can provide valuable information regarding the natural history of a disease in the general population.

7.5.2 Converting cumulative probabilities into transition rates

Suppose a study reports a five-year cumulative probability (or cumulative incidence), $P(t)$, of an event and you want to estimate an annual probability of the event. Assuming that the annual event rate over the five years is constant (r) it can be estimated as follows:

$$r = \frac{- \ln [1 - P(t)]}{5}$$

If you did not want to assume that the annual probability of the event was constant over time you would need to estimate the cumulative incidence of the event at different time intervals. Cumulative incidence of breast cancer by age for women with a strong family history (i.e. age of onset of mother 20–29, age of onset of maternal aunt 30–39) is shown in Table 7.3 (Claus *et al.* 1996). A reasonable assumption would be that the probability of breast cancer prior to the age of 19 is 0 per cent. Thus, there is a 43.7 per cent chance of breast cancer over a period of 60 years. Using only this 60-year cumulative incidence would yield a constant probability of 0.0096. However, using the ten-year estimates we can estimate annual probabilities as a step function of age, constant within ten-year intervals. To do this we have to first estimate the conditional probability of a woman getting breast cancer during each decade given that she is free

Table 7.3 Cumulative incidence of breast cancer among women who have a strong family history[a]

Age (a)	Pr(breast cancer < a)
29	0.018
39	0.062
49	0.148
59	0.265
69	0.371
79	0.437

Note: [a] From Claus *et al.* (1996)

Table 7.4 Calculation of annual probabilities from cumulative incidence of breast cancer[a]

Age (a)	Pr(BCA < a)	Conditional 10-year probability (p)[b]	Annual rate (r)[c]	Annual probability[d]
19	0	0.018	0.0018	0.0018
29	0.018	0.045	0.0046	0.0046
39	0.062	0.092	0.0096	0.0096
49	0.148	0.137	0.0148	0.0147
59	0.265	0.144	0.0156	0.0155
69	0.371	0.105	0.0111	0.0110
79	0.437	[e]	[e]	[e]

Notes:

[a] BCA = breast cancer

[b] $p = Pr(a < BCA < a + 10 \mid BCA > a)$

[c] $r = [-\ln(1 - p)/10]$, for ages a to $a+10$

[d] $1 - \exp(-r)$, for ages a to $a+10$

[e] Risk beyond age 79 is unknown

from breast cancer at the beginning of the decade. These ten-year conditional probabilities are shown in the third column of Table 7.4. For example, the ten-year conditional probability of breast cancer for 49-year-old women is: $(0.265 - 0.148)/(1 - 0.148) = 0.137$. We can then treat these ten-year conditional probabilities as a ten-year cumulative incidence for each cohort to calculate annual rates by the method described in Section 7.4.3, shown in the fourth column of the table. These derived annual rates and their corresponding annual probabilities are shown in the last column. Thus, the annual risk of breast cancer increases by age until a women enters her seventh decade.

7.5.3 Relative-reduction parameters

The effect of an intervention is often modelled as a relative reduction in a particular transition probability, whether it be a transition to a dead state or an event state. Depending on the statistical analysis used in the study that is informing these relative reductions, they will be reported in a variety of manners. In this section we will review three relative reduction parameters – the hazard ratio, the relative risk and the odds ratio – for situations where the relative-reduction parameter is less than one (i.e. the risk with the treatment lower than the risk without treatment).

A hazard ratio is a ratio of the rate of an event with treatment to the rate of an event without treatment. This measure is most often referred to as a relative risk in the clinical trial literature, and is estimated by survival analysis techniques such as Kaplan–Meier methods or Cox proportional hazards models. Suppose the annual transition probability from A to B without treatment is 10 per cent and the hazard ratio associated with treatment is 0.8. To estimate the transition probability for a treated cohort, one must first calculate the annual transition rate: $-\ln(1-0.1) =$

0.1054. This rate is then multiplied by the hazard ratio to obtain the transition rate with treatment, which is then converted back to a probability: $1 - \exp(-0.1054^*0.8)$ = 0.0808.

A relative risk is a ratio of the t-year probability of an event with treatment to the t-year probability of an event without treatment. It is important to note that unlike the hazard ratio, the relative risk varies depending upon the time frame of the analysis. For example, a relative risk with one-year probabilities will be less than a relative risk with five-year probabilities when underlying rates are constant. Relative risks are larger than hazard ratios (i.e. closer to 1) and approach the hazard ratio as t approaches 0. Thus, applying a five-year relative risk to an annual transition probability would underestimate the treatment effect and bias the model against treatment.

An odds ratio is a ratio of the t-year odds of an event with treatment to the t-year odds of an event without treatment, where the odds of an event is a function of the probability of the event: $p/(1-p)$. Odds ratios will also vary depending upon the time frame of the analysis, where an odds ratio with one-year probabilities will be greater than an odds ratio with five-year probabilities. Odds ratios are smaller than hazard ratios (and relative risks) and approach the hazard ratio as t approaches 0. Thus, using an odds ratio to approximate a relative risk will bias the model towards treatment, and this bias gets larger when probabilities approach 1.

7.5.4 Risk equations

Risk equations, obtained from prospective population-based cohort studies using regression analytic techniques, can be used to model the risk of an event conditional on a variety of clinical and demographic variables. One of the more commonly used risk equations come from the Framingham Heart Study (Anderson *et al.* 1991). These equations estimate the 10-year risk of CHD for a person or population based on age, sex, diabetes status, diastolic blood pressure, smoking status, serum cholesterol level, and the presence of left ventricular hypertrophy on the electrocardiogram. A risk equation can also predict the decline in 10-year CHD risk due to a decline in, for example, serum cholesterol levels. Other population-based cohort studies, such as the Nurses' Health Study, have also been used to generate risk functions related to cancer incidence (Rosner and Colditz 1996).

7.5.5 Some tricks

Teasing out parameters of interest

Suppose you want to estimate the annual probability of CHD among smokers, $P(C|S)$, and non-smokers, $P(C|N)$, but the only information you have is the overall probability of CHD each year for the cohort of interest, $P(C)$, the relative risk of CHD for smokers compared with non-smokers (RR), and the prevalence of smokers in the population of interest, $P(S)$. From the available data you know the following:

$$P(C) = P(C|S) \times P(S) + P(C|N) \times P(N)$$

and

$$RR = \frac{P(C|S)}{P(C|N)}$$

Using these two equations, one can solve for $P(C|S)$ and $P(C|N)$:

$$P(C|N) = \frac{P(C)}{1 - P(S) + RR \times P(S)};$$

$$P(C|S) = \frac{RR \times P(C)}{1 - P(S) + RR \times P(S)}$$

The annual transition probability of CHD for smokers versus non-smokers can be entered into a model directly as these equations to ensure that the overall annual probability of CHD remains at $P(C)$ unless specifically varied in a sensitivity analysis. For example, if a sensitivity analysis were done on RR, the overall annual probability of CHD would not change, only the CHD probabilities that are specific for smokers and non-smokers.

Using 'on-the-side' models

There are some clinical examples where it is necessary to 'back into' probabilities when there is no direct evidence available. One example of this is modelling colorectal cancer screening. One of the goals of screening is to identify and remove precancerous lesions (or polyps) in order to interrupt the polyp–cancer sequence of the disease process. Thus, one has to model the progression of underlying disease to model the ultimate effects on cancer incidence and mortality. However, because most persons in the general population are not screened regularly – and those that are screened are a biased population – there are no direct data available to infer the progression from polyp to cancer. Using data from autopsy studies on the underlying prevalence of polyps and data from the Surveillance Epidemiology and End Results (SEER) programme on colorectal cancer incidence (Ries *et al.* 2000), one can use a Markov model to calibrate to the SEER data and thus infer a reasonable estimate for the progression from polyp to cancer.

Suppose that you want to assign a one-time cost to an event (e.g. diagnosis of cancer) that reflects the present value of all of the current and downstream costs. There are a number of situations like this for which the construction of a Markov model 'on the side' can be useful. For the case of estimating the present value of the lifetime costs for a cancer diagnosis, a simple model can be built to represent the prognosis of the cancer based on published survival curves with initial, continuing and final costs incorporated into the health states.

Estimating parameters from longitudinal, cross-sectional data

Suppose you want to estimate the transition probabilities for a three-state model with states describing the nature of chest pain as none, mild, or severe, and the only data available are cross-sectional analyses of a population at different points in time (e.g. time 0, 1, 3 and 5 years). As an example, consider the data in Table 7.5 estimated from a quality-of-life study for patients with three-vessel CHD who are treated with medical

Table 7.5 Distribution of angina over time among a cohort of patients with triple-vessel coronary artery disease treated with medical therapy[a]

| Angina level | Time point | | | |
	Baseline	1 year	3 years	5 years
None	0.22	0.35	0.41	0.40
Mild	0.78	0.57	0.54	0.53
Severe	0	0.08	0.05	0.07

Note: [a] From CASS (1983)

therapy (CASS 1983). The goal is to estimate a 3×3 transitional probability matrix A such that if P_0 is equal to $|0.22 \ 0.78 \ 0|$, then P_1, P_3, and P_5 will be 'close' to $|0.35 \ 0.57 \ 0.08|$, $|0.41 \ 0.54 \ 0.05|$ and $|0.40 \ 0.53 \ 0.07|$, respectively.

While there is not a single approach to this estimation problem, one approach is to simulate a Markov trace with a series of possible A matrices and calculate some measure of model error. For example, one measure of error would be to minimize the absolute values of the observed proportions minus the expected proportions (as predicted by a particular Markov trace, using clinically plausible ranges for the transition probabilities) at each time period (1, 3 and 5 years) and each state (no, mild and severe angina). Using this approach yields the following estimate:

$$A = \begin{vmatrix} 0.67 & 0.32 & 0.01 \\ 0.24 & 0.72 & 0.04 \\ 0.14 & 0.19 & 0.67 \end{vmatrix}$$

Table 7.6 shows that the predicted distributions of patients among the three health states at each time point is not much different from the observed, and the largest differences are observed at one year.

Table 7.6 Comparison of the observed versus predicted angina distribution over time

| Angina level | Time Point | | | | | |
| | 1 year | | 3 years | | 5 years | |
	Observed	Predicted	Observed	Predicted	Observed	Predicted
None	0.35	0.33	0.41	0.40	0.40	0.41
Mild	0.57	0.63	0.54	0.54	0.53	0.52
Severe	0.08	0.03	0.05	0.06	0.07	0.07

Applying relative hazards to a 'canonical' transition matrix

Suppose you have estimated a transition matrix for a 'base case' scenario, such as the natural history of a disease, or the course of disease on some standard treatment. You may have accomplished this by using a combination of public health data and clinical trial data. This transition matrix may evolve over time, according to a variety of modelling assumptions regarding parameters such as age-, sex- (and race)-specific mortality.

Embedded within this matrix are a small number of key parameters that are influenced by interventions of interest, such as the monthly probability of disease progression from a latent stage to an active stage of hepatitis, or from a stage of treatment response to disease relapse in cancer. An example might be the transition from treatment response to treatment failure in patients receiving antiretroviral therapy for HIV disease. There may be several of these 'failure probabilities' within the baseline transition matrix, in which the monthly probability of failure depends on the patient's immune state and viral load. A key objective of economic evaluation might be to assess how reductions in these failure probabilities affect the cost-effectiveness of an antiretroviral treatment strategy. The challenge is how to estimate transition matrices for various interventions that have different sets of failure probabilities, without having to re-estimate the entire transition matrix for each intervention. Another challenge is how to perform sensitivity analysis with respect to a single or small number of parameters that reflect the proportional reduction in the failure probabilities.

The device that can be used in this context is to define a standard, or 'canonical' transition matrix, and to parameterize it in terms of a small number of parameters. One such parameter for the HIV treatment example might be the 'proportional reduction in the probability of failure relative to baseline'. Suppose that p_{i3} represents the probability of failure ($j = 3$) for a patient who begins the month in state i (where $i = 1, 2, \ldots, n$ for n states, $i \neq 3$). Let k be the proportional reduction in these probabilities, for a particular intervention. Then p_{i3} would be reduced to $(1-k)p_{i3}$ for all i. The other transition probabilities from state i would therefore have to increase. One possible assumption for reallocating this probability mass would be to allocate the residual probability mass kp_{i3} to the other transition probabilities p_{ij} ($j \neq 3$) in proportion to their baseline values. Thus, each of these probabilities would increase from p_{ij} to:

$$p_{ij} + kp_{i3}\left(p_{ij} / \sum_{j\neq 3} p_{ij}\right)$$

Alternatively, the residual probability could be reallocated to transitions from only a subset of the remaining states, the others remaining fixed. In any case, the parameter k can be used as a summary measure of the 'relative effectiveness' of an intervention and can be used in sensitivity analysis.

7.6 Model calibration

Often there are multiple targets for calibration, and these targets are known with varying degrees of precision themselves. Moreover, there may be several parameters within the model, each one estimated with varying levels of precision, which can be 'dialled up or down' to try to achieve calibration. While statistical methods can, in principle, be used to achieve optimal calibration in terms of a specified loss function, or in terms of maximizing the likelihood function for the observed data given a set of parameter values, in practice the process of calibration is more art than science.

One form of calibration is to use the model to simulate an external source of data. Using a model developed to evaluate the use of laparotomy for early-stage Hodgkin's disease, Ng and colleagues (1999) simulated a cohort of patients similar to that of a cohort study with long-term results (and a study that was not used as a model input). The model predictions of 10-, 15-, and 20-year survival probabilities were very similar to the actuarial survival probabilities estimated from the study cohort.

A more complex example of model calibration arose in connection with the CHD Policy Model, a state-transition model of the US population whose states correspond to coronary risk factors and disease history (Weinstein *et al.* 1987). Key transition probabilities included the age- and sex-specific incidence of CHD, the age- and sex-specific prevalence of CHD in the baseline year ($t = 0$), the probabilities of surviving a cardiac arrest or myocardial infarction, and the relative risks of event survival by age. These did not comprise a complete set of model parameters – far from it! – but they were selected as instruments for calibration because they could be estimated only with limited precision and from multiple and disparate sources. The target variables for calibration included the number of deaths from CHD by age and sex, and the numbers of hospitalizations for myocardial infarction. These were far from 'gold standards', as the International Classification of Disease (ICD), used for the number of deaths, has changing and often arbitrary rules for assigning deaths to a CHD cause. For example, deaths from 'congestive heart failure' (ICD-9 410) may or may not have been due to complications of CHD. Even worse, the numbers of admissions from the US Hospital Discharge Survey are subject to uncertainty about the true cause of admission, since it is common practice to record myocardial infarction as an admission diagnosis if a myocardial infarction had occurred within 30 days. Through a process of trial and error, the combination of input parameters was found that minimized the sum of the percentage deviations in all of the age- and sex-specific target variables, subject to the constraint that none of these deviations exceeded 10 per cent. The resulting set of parameters was then established as the default values for subsequent applications of the model.

7.7 Individual versus population models

7.7.1 Open versus closed cohort

Markov models are state-transition models that are 'closed' in that they keep track of a single cohort over time (i.e. no one enters or exits the model at any time). State-transition models can also be dynamic ('open') in that they allow people to enter or exit the model over time. Dynamic models look at populations cross-sectionally over time and are useful for studying the nature of epidemics or disease trends over time. Closed models follow a cohort of persons over time and are useful for evaluating the outcomes of competing medical interventions or programmes.

Population models are open models that keep track of the members of a population as they enter and leave the population, and as they transition among states, over time. Often population models keep track of the population of a country, stratified into health states defined by age, risk factors for disease, and disease status. If the model includes persons of all ages, the number of persons entering the first year of age in a given year is equal to the number of live births in that year, which may in turn be a function of the current number of women of child-bearing age and a parameter related to the fertility rate. If the model includes persons from a given age (e.g. 18 years) onward, then the number of person entering their 18th year of age in a given calendar year may be determined from exogenous age-specific population projections. (Such projections are available for the USA from the Department of the Census.) At the other end of the model, persons may exit because of endogenous mortality or, if there is an upper limit on the ages tracked within the model (e.g. 85 years), they exit when they reach that age. The CHD Policy Model, mentioned earlier in Section 7.6, is an example of an open population model of person in the US population from ages 35 to 84 years.

Modelling interventions in a population model can be challenging, because, unlike cohort models, calendar time and age are not synchronous. Transient effects of initiating an intervention in a population in which many members have already missed the opportunity to receive the intervention is one problem. For example, a simulation of an intervention to reduce blood pressure from age 35 onward would actually affect the members of a population for different lengths of time. Those who were 80 initially would receive the intervention only from that point forward, with the result that the consequences and costs for them would be limited to the years of life past 80. Those who entered the model (e.g. at age 35) in subsequent years would begin receiving the intervention immediately, but depending on the time horizon for the analysis, may receive the intervention for only a limited period of time. Thus, the incremental costs and consequences of an intervention that are modeled in a population model really reflects a sort of weighted average of incremental costs and consequences across different cohorts. The result may be useful as an aggregate summary of the overall economic and health impacts on a population, cross-sectionally or over time, and it certainly lends itself more to calibration against public health data than a cohort model, but it cannot be interpreted in the same way as a longitudinal intervention in a cohort.

Because of entry to and exit from population models, results can be quite sensitive to the time horizon of analysis. While there may be reasons to be cautious about extrapolating into the too-distant future, failure to extend the horizon out to reasonable 'steady state' may have the effect of overweighting the transient phenomena, such as inadequately sustained interventions in young people, or tardy implementation of interventions in older people.

7.7.2 Same starting characteristics versus distributions

When seeding a Markov model with a cohort, the modeller must specify which state or states the cohort resides in at the start of the model. Often, the cohort will start in a single state, for example, a 'disease-free' state or a 'responded-to-treatment' state. Typically, a cohort (or 'closed') model is seeded with a cohort of patients who 'look' similar. The starting cohort may be distributed among various states based on either events that occurred in a decision tree preceding the Markov model, or on underlying clinical factors that cannot be observed. An example of the former case is when a decision tree is used to model the outcomes of a diagnostic test. Hence, the distribution of a cohort of true-positive patients will be different from that of false-negative patients. An example of the latter case is a Markov model used to evaluate cervical cancer screening. The cohort might be 20-year-old women who have never been screened previously, yet the health states should reflect the chance that some of these women will have undiagnosed precancerous lesions or invasive cancer and are not all truly 'disease-free'. Patient characteristics that are evident, such as the presence of family history of cancer, are not typically captured in health-state descriptions but accounted for in defining the starting cohort. In other words, instead of defining health states for women with or without a family history of cervical cancer and allowing the starting distribution to reflect the percentage of women with a family history, the model would be run twice – once with a cohort of women without a family history and once with a cohort with a family history. The starting cohort in population-based models, on the other hand, tends to capture both the observed and unobserved heterogeneity of a cohort of persons and should reflect all clinical and demographic characteristics within the population of interest.

7.8 **Software**

Currently there are three software packages that are commonly used to construct Markov models and perform cost-effectiveness analysis (DATA, Decision-Maker, SMLTREE). Although there are advantages and disadvantages to all of these programs, they are all capable of building fairly complex decision trees with multiple Markov models to perform incremental cost-effectiveness analysis. Other options for performing the same analyses are to program the model in a spreadsheet program, or to use a programming language such as C++. Very large models, such as the CHD Policy Model mentioned in Section 7.6 or the HIV model mentioned in Section 7.3.4 (p.152) are too large for existing software and have been programmed individually.

7.9 **Conclusion**

While clinical trials can provide important information about cost and health-related quality-of-life measures for new technologies, there often exist data from other sources that can and should be incorporated into an economic analysis. In addition, the time frame of clinical trials is often too short to obtain adequate estimates of the number of quality-adjusted years of life saved by an intervention. For these reasons, the use of models is an important and necessary component of cost-effectiveness analysis. In this chapter, we provide a framework for the construction and implementation of state-transition models. While decision-analytic models are invaluable tools in evaluating the relative effects of an intervention on health and economic outcomes, it is also important that the limitations of modelling are appreciated.

References

Anderson, K. M., Wilson, P. W., Odell, P. M. *et al.* (1991). An updated coronary risk profile: a statement for health professionals. *Circulation*, 83, 356–62.

Beck, J. R., Kassirer, J. P. and Pauker, S. G. (1982a). A convenient approximation of life expectancy. (The 'DEALE'). I. Validation of the method. *American Journal of Medicine*, 73, 883–8.

Beck, J. R., Pauker, S. G., Gottlieb, J. E. *et al.* (1982b). A convenient approximation of life expectancy. (The 'DEALE'). II. Use in medical decision-making. *American Journal of Medicine*, 73, 889–97.

Byers, T., Levin, B., Rothenberger, D. *et al.* (1997). American Cancer Society guidelines for screening and surveillance for early detection of colorectal polyps and cancer: update 1997. *CA Cancer. J. Clin.*, 47, 154–60.

Canadian Coordinating Office of Health Technology Assessment (CCOHTA). (1994). *Guidelines for economic evaluation of pharmaceuticals: Canada.* CCOHTA, Ottawa.

CASS Principal Investigators and their Associates. (1983). Coronary Artery Surgery Study (CASS): a randomised trial of coronary artery bypass surgery. Quality-of-Life in patients randomly assigned to treatment groups. *Circulation*, 68, 951–60.

Claus, E. B., Schildkraut, J. M., Thompson, W. D. *et al.* (1996). The genetic attributable risk of breast and ovarian cancer. *Cancer*, 77, 2318–24.

Clemen, R. T. (1996). *Making hard decisions. An introduction to decision analysis*, 2nd edn. CA: Duxbury Press, Pacific Grove.

Commonwealth of Australia, Department of Health, Housing and Community Services. (1995). *Guidelines for the pharmaceutical industry on preparation of submissions to the Pharmaceutical Benefits Advisory Committee.*

Concorde Coordinating Committee (1994). Concorde: MRC/ANRS randomised double-blind controlled trial of immediate and deferred zidovudine in symptom-free HIV infection. *Lancet*, 343, 871–81.

Eddy, D. M. (1990). Screening for colorectal cancer. *Annals of Internal Medicine*, 113, 373–84.

Food and Drug Administration, Division of Drug Marketing, Advertising, and Communications. (1995). *Principles for the review of pharmacoeconomic promotion* (draft).

Frazier, A. L., Colditz, G. A., Fuchs, C. S. *et al.* (2000). Cost-effectiveness of screening for colorectal cancer in the general population. *Journal of the American Medical Association*, 284, 1954–61.

Freedberg, K. A., Scharfstein, J. A., Seage, C. R. *et al.* (1997). The cost-effectiveness of preventing AIDS-related opportunistic infections. *Journal of the American Medical Association*, 279, 130–6.

Gold, M. R., Siegel, J. E., Russell, L. B. *et al.* (1996). *Cost-effectiveness in health and medicine.* Oxford University Press, New York.

Goldman, L., Weinstein, M. C., Goldman, P. A. *et al.* (1991). Cost-effectiveness of HMG-CoA reductase inhibition for primary and secondary prevention of coronary heart disease. *Journal of the American Medical Association*, 265, 1145–51.

Gompertz, B. (1825). On the nature of the function expression of the law of human mortality. *Philosophical Transactions of the Royal Society London*, 115, 513–85.

Johannesson, M., Jonsson, B., Kjekshus, J. *et al.* (1997). Cost-effectiveness of simvastatin treatment to lower cholesterol levels in patients with coronary heart disease. *New England Journal of Medicine*, 336, 332–6.

Kassirer, J. P. and Angell, M. (1994). The journal's policy on cost-effectiveness analyses [editorial]. *New England Journal of Medicine*, 331, 669–70.

Keeler, E. and Bell, R. (1992). New DEALEs: Other approximations of life expectancy. *Medical Decision-Making*, 12, 307–11.

Kent, K. C., Kuntz, K. M., Patel, M. R. *et al.* (1995). Perioperative imaging strategies for carotid endarterectomy: an analysis of morbidity and cost-effectiveness in symptomatic patients. *Journal of the American Medical Association*, 274, 888–93.

Kilbridge, K. L., Kuntz, K. M., Kagan, A. R. *et al.* (1995). Evaluation of frequent follow-up cystoscopy in superficial bladder cancer [Abstract]. *Medical Decision-Making*, 15, 421.

Kuntz, K. M., Tsevat, J., Goldman, L. *et al.* (1996). Cost-effectiveness of routine coronary angiography after acute myocardial infarction. *Circulation*, 94, 957–65.

Kuntz, K. M. *et al.* (1995). Life expectancy biases in clinical decision modelling. *Medical Decision-Making*, 15, 158–69.

Lee, E. T. (1992). *Statistical Methods for Survival Data Analysis*, 2nd edn. John Wiley & Sons, Inc., New York.

Loeve, F., Boer, R., van Oortmarssen, G. J. *et al.*. (1999). The MISCAN-COLON Simulation Model for the evaluation of colorectal cancer screening. *Computers and Biomedical Research*, 32, 13–33.

Magid, D., Schwartz, B., Craft, J. *et al.* (1992). Prevention of Lyme disease after tick bites. A cost-effectiveness analysis. *New England Journal of Medicine*, 327, 324–41.

Mandel, J. S., Bond, J. H., Church, T. R. *et al.* (1993). Reducing mortality from colorectal cancer by screening for fecal occult blood. Minnesota Colon Cancer Control Study. *New England Journal of Medicine*, 328, 1365–71.

Morris, J. C., Heyman, A., Mohs, R. C. *et al.* (1989). The Consortium to Establish a Registry for Alzheimer's Disease (CERAD). Part I: Clinical and neuropsychological assessment of Alzheimer's disease. *Neurology*, 39, 1159–65.

Morris, S. (1997). A comparison of economic modelling and clinical trials in the economic evaluation of cholesterol-modifying pharmacotherapy. *Health Economics*, 6, 589–601.

National Bladder Cancer Collaborative Group A. (1977). Development of a strategy for the longitudinal study of patients with bladder cancer. *Cancer Research*, 37, 2898–906.

Neumann, P. J., Hermann, R. C., Kuntz, K. M. *et al.* (1999). Cost-effectiveness of donepezil in the treatment of mild or moderate Alzheimer's disease. *Neurology*,52, 1138–45.

Ng, A. K., Weeks, J. C., Mauch, P. M. *et al.* (1999). Laparotomy versus no laparotomy in the management of early-stage, favorable-prognosis Hodgkin's disease: a decision analysis. *Journal of Clinical Oncology*, 17, 241–52.

Ries, L. A. G., Eisner, M. P., Kosary, C. L. *et al.* (2000). *SEER Cancer Statistics and Review, 1973–1997*. National Cancer Institute, Bethesda, MD.

Rosner, B. and Colditz, G. A. (1996). Nurses' health study: log-incidence mathematical model of breast cancer incidence. *Journal of National Cancer Institute*, 88, 359–64.

Schulman, K. A., Lynn, L. A., Glick, H. A. *et al.* (1991). Cost-effectiveness of low-dose zidovudine therapy for asymptomatic patients with human immunodeficiency virus (HIV) infection. *Annals of Internal Medicine*, 114, 798–802.

The SOLVD investigators. (1991). Effect of enalapril on survival in patients with reduced left ventricular ejection fractions and congestive heart failure. *New England Journal of Medicine*, 325, 293–302.

Sonnenberg, F. A. and Beck, J. R. (1993). Markov models in medical decision-making: a practical guide. *Medical Decision-Making*, 13, 322–38.

Sox, H. C., Blatt, M. A., Higgins, M. C. *et al.* (1988). *Medical Decision-Making*. Butterworth Publishers, Stoneham, MA.

Tom, E. and Schulman, K.A. (1997). Mathematical models in decision analysis. *Infection Control Hospital Epidemiology*, 18, 65–73.

US Department of Health and Human Services. (1987). *The Framingham Heart Study: an epidemiological investigation of cardiovascular disease. Some risk factors related to the annual incidence of cardiovascular disease and death using pooled repeated biennial measurements: Framingham Heart Study, 30-year follow-up.* Section 34, NIH Publication 87–2703. National Heart, Lung and Blood Institute, Bethesda, MD.

Wagner, J. L., Tunis, S., Brown, M. *et al.* (1996). Cost-effectiveness of colorectal cancer screening in average-risk adults. In: G. P. Young, P. Rozen, and B. Levin, (eds.) *Prevention and Early Detection of Colorectal Cancer*, Chapter 19. W. B. Saunders, London.

Weinstein M. C., Coxson P. G., Williams L. W. *et al.* (1987). Forecasting coronary heart disease incidence, mortality, and cost: the coronary heart disease policy model. *American Journal of Public Health*, 77, 1417–26.

Chapter 8

Handling uncertainty in economic evaluation and presenting the results

Andrew H. Briggs

8.1 Introduction

Economic evaluations of health care interventions are increasingly common, with the growth of the economic evaluation literature now widely documented (Pritchard 1998; Briggs and Gray 1999; Stone *et al.* 2000). Uncertainty in economic evaluation is pervasive, entering the evaluative process at every stage. It is useful to distinguish uncertainty related to the data requirements of a study (the resource use and health outcome consequences of a particular intervention and the data required to value those consequences) from uncertainty related to the process of evaluation.

Uncertainty in the data requirements of a study arises through natural variation in populations, such that estimates based on samples drawn from that population will always be associated with a level of uncertainty which is inversely related to sample size. At a design stage, ensuring the appropriate sample size is recruited to a study can control such uncertainty. However, at an analysis stage such uncertainty must be quantified. Where patient specific resource use and health outcome data have been collected (for example, as part of a prospective clinical trial) in a so-called stochastic analysis (O'Brien *et al.* 1994), then statistical techniques can be employed to calculate confidence intervals around point estimates of cost-effectiveness – although the methods required to estimate confidence limits around a ratio statistic are less straightforward than for many other commonly used statistics.

In practice, despite the increased use of clinical trials as a vehicle for collecting economic data, such designs still represent a minority of all published evaluations. (Pritchard 1998; Stone *et al.* 2000) More often, data are synthesized from a number of different sources – such as previously reported studies, hospital records and even clinical judgement – in a decision-analytic type framework. Moreover, even when standard statistical analysis is undertaken, the remaining levels of uncertainty that are not related to sampling variation need exploration and quantification. Thus sensitivity analysis is commonly employed for handling uncertainty not related to sampling variation or where no patient-level data on resource costs and health outcomes are directly available.

Exactly how decision-makers should incorporate that uncertainty in a way that is consistent with the economic objectives of the health system is beyond the scope of this chapter. Recent research has highlighted the strong economic arguments for adopting a value of information approach (Claxton and Posnett 1996; Felli and Hazen 1998; Claxton 1999) to incorporating uncertainty into the decision-making process together with option values (Palmer and Smith 2000), rather than adopting standard but ad hoc criteria, such as the 5 per cent rate of error commonly adopted by statisticians. However, it is clear that such approaches to decision-making are predicated on clearly quantified uncertainty in results of cost-effectiveness analysis, which allow decision-makers to appropriately incorporate uncertainty into the decision-making process.

The aim for this chapter is to describe the state of the art of methods for handling uncertainty in the economic evaluation of health care interventions, where the technique of cost-effectiveness analysis has been employed,[1] in order to determine how uncertainty should be quantified and presented to aid decision-making. A further aim is to consider how uncertainty might best be presented to decision-makers in order to give them the appropriate information on which to make a decision.

The chapter is organized as follows. The next section sets the scene by outlining the nature of the decision rules underlying cost-effectiveness analysis. The nature of uncertainty in economic analysis is described, and the methods of sensitivity analysis and statistical analysis are introduced as the principal approaches for handling uncertainty. Section 8.4 looks in detail at statistical methods for handling uncertainty due to sampling variation in stochastic cost-effectiveness analyses where patient-level data are available. The next sections look at sensitivity analysis methods for handling uncertainty where patient-level data are not available and for handling those types of uncertainty not related to sampling variation. A final section offers a summary and conclusions.

8.2 Cost-effectiveness analysis on the CE plane

O'Brien and colleagues suggest that the aim of cost-effectiveness analysis 'is to compare the costs and effects of one treatment compared to some *relevant alternative*.' (O'Brien *et al.* 1994, p. 151, emphasis added).

Suppose that we are comparing a new experimental therapy (or treatment group) with some currently provided standard (or control) therapy, which represents the most cost-effective treatment available at present. Further suppose that we know both the true mean cost of the new therapy (μ_{CT}) versus the control therapy (μ_{CC}) and the true effectiveness (in terms of health outcome) of the new therapy (μ_{ET}) versus the control therapy (μ_{EC}). O'Brien and colleagues identify four situations that can arise in relation to the incremental cost and effectiveness of the therapies (O'Brien *et al.* 1994):

---

[1] Most economic evaluations undertaken are of the cost-effectiveness form (broadly defined to include cost-utility analyses), although the principal issues covered in this chapter are directly applicable to cost-benefit analyses.

1. $\mu_{CT} - \mu_{CC} < 0$; $\mu_{ET} - \mu_{EC} > 0$; *dominance* – accept experimental therapy as it is both cheaper and more effective than existing therapy.

2. $\mu_{CT} - \mu_{CC} > 0$; $\mu_{ET} - \mu_{EC} < 0$; *dominance* – reject experimental therapy as it is both more expensive and less effective than existing therapy.

3. $\mu_{CT} - \mu_{CC} > 0$; $\mu_{ET} - \mu_{EC} > 0$; *trade-off* – consider magnitude of the additional cost of the new therapy relative to its additional cost.

4. $\mu_{CT} - \mu_{CC} < 0$; $\mu_{ET} - \mu_{EC} < 0$; *trade-off* – consider magnitude of the cost-saving of the new therapy relative to its reduced effectiveness.

These four situations are equivalent to the four quadrants of the cost-effectiveness plane, which has been advocated for the analysis of cost-effectiveness results (Anderson *et al.* 1986; Black 1990). The cost-effectiveness plane is presented in Figure 8.1. Note that the cost-effectiveness space illustrated in the figure is incremental such that the comparison therapy (control treatment in this case) is the origin in the figure and the horizontal and vertical axes therefore relate to the effect and cost *differences* respectively. Where one intervention is both more effective and less costly than the alternative treatment (situations 1 and 2 above and the SE and NW quadrants on the plane) it is said to dominate and is clearly the treatment of choice. Where one treatment is found to be both more costly and more effective (situations 3 and 4 above and the NE and SW quadrants of the plane) then a trade-off must be made between the additional health outcomes and the additional resources that must be committed to achieve those outcomes.

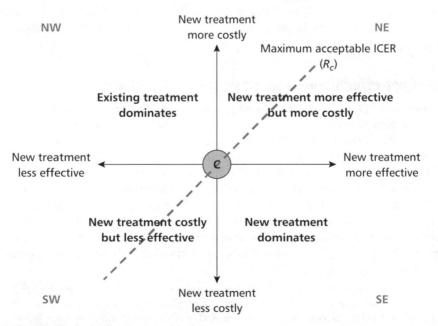

Fig. 8.1 The cost-effectiveness plane

In order to summarize this trade-off an incremental cost-effectiveness ratio (ICER) is calculated and if this ICER is less than the maximum acceptable cost-effectiveness ratio (or ceiling ratio, R_C) then the treatment is considered cost-effective. Algebraically, this decision rule can be expressed as a decision to implement the new treatment if

$$ICER = \frac{\mu_{CT} - \mu_{CC}}{\mu_{ET} - \mu_{EC}} = \frac{\mu_{\Delta C}}{\mu_{\Delta E}} < R_C$$

Note that this decision rule can be represented as a straight line on the cost-effectiveness plane that passes through the origin with slope equal to R_C. Such a line (as shown in Figure 8.1) effectively divides the plane into two: points falling to the right of the line indicate cost-effective interventions; points falling to the left of the line indicating cost-ineffective interventions (i.e. the treatment of choice is that which is currently provided).

The decision rules of cost-effectiveness analysis have been much debated over recent years (Birch and Gafni 1992, 1993; Johannesson and Weinstein 1993) and attempts to identify the value of the ceiling ratio, R_C (Laupacis et al. 1992) have been criticized as inconsistent with maximizing outcomes from a fixed budget (Gafni and Birch 1993). However, it is not the purpose of this chapter to review those arguments here. It is assumed that those analysts undertaking a cost-effectiveness analysis do so with the aim of informing decisions that are based on maximizing health outcomes. By presenting cost-effectiveness information, it is implicit that such information will be compared to the ceiling ratio (which represents the shadow price for a unit of effect). Weinstein provides a clear overview of the ways in which the outcome of a cost-effectiveness analysis can be determined as cost-effective (or not) and how the shadow price of the unit of effect can be determined (Weinstein 1995).

8.3 Uncertainty in cost-effectiveness analysis

The preceding discussion assumed that the average treatment cost and effect parameters for the eligible patient group are known with certainty. Of course, in practice this is never the case and therefore consideration must be given to how uncertainty associated with parameter estimates impacts on the results of a cost-effectiveness analysis. Before considering this impact, the types of uncertainty that exist in economic evaluation and the methods available for handling that uncertainty are identified – the taxonomy developed below will then form the basis for the structure of the discussion in the remainder of the chapter.

Briggs and colleagues (1994) developed a taxonomy of uncertainty in economic evaluation alongside clinical trials, identifying four key sources. Methodological disagreement among analysts and commentators introduces a level of uncertainty when it comes to comparing results of studies that have employed different methods. The data requirements of the study in terms of the estimated resource and health outcomes consequences together with the unit cost and quality-of-life weights add a further layer of uncertainty related to sampling variation. Extrapolation of observed results over time, or from intermediate to health outcomes introduces further uncertainty. Finally, the extent to which the reported results of an analysis can be generalized (or 'transferred') to another setting will be an important source of uncertainty for those seeking to interpret the results. The authors argued that despite the increasing use of the clinical trial as a vehicle for economic analysis, sensitivity analysis still had an important role in quantifying uncertainty since statistical analysis could only be employed to handle uncertainty relating to sampling variation where patient-level information is available.

The US panel on cost-effectiveness analysis (Gold *et al.* 1996) included a chapter on dealing with uncertainty (Manning *et al.* 1996) which adopted a slightly different taxonomy. They distinguished 'parameter uncertainty', the uncertainty in parameter inputs to a study that includes (but is not limited to) sampling variation, from 'modelling uncertainty'. This second type of uncertainty is further distinguished as uncertainty due to the model 'structure' relating to the functional form of the model employed, for example the form of the dose-response relationship assumed in the evaluation of a pharmaceutical, and the uncertainty due to the overall 'process' of the cost-effectiveness analysis.

For this chapter, a distinction is made between stochastic cost-effectiveness analyses and cost-effectiveness analyses based on decision-analytic type modelling.[2] Stochastic analyses are taken to be those studies that collect information on resource use and health outcome (usually as part of a clinical trial) and for which patient-level data on costs and effects can therefore be derived. It is important to note that it is the resource use that is truly stochastic – in general, statistical analysis of costs proceeds by employing deterministic unit costs as weights to resource items. Although unit costs will not vary at the individual patient level, they will vary between different treatment centres. The importance of considering the potential for unit costs to vary in multi-centre (Raikou *et al.* 2000) or in multinational studies (Willke *et al.* 1998) has been an area of recent research interest. The impact of deterministic unit cost weights on the potential significance of statistical tests of cost difference has also been highlighted (Rittenhouse *et al.* 1999).

Modelling type analyses are taken to be those studies that synthesize data from a number of different sources in order to estimate cost-effectiveness and are often structured around a formal decision-analytic model. Tables 8.1 and 8.2 list the types of uncertainty and the general approach to handling that uncertainty for each of these types of cost-effectiveness analyses drawing on both the taxonomies of uncertainty outlined above.

In both types of cost-effectiveness analysis, the issues surrounding methodological uncertainty and generalisability/transferability of results is the same. The suggested solution to methodological uncertainty is the use of a reference case in combination with simple one-way sensitivity analysis and this is outlined in detail below. It is clear that results may be very specific to the setting of the study (e.g. unit costs may be derived from the study centres) for both stochastic and modelling analyses. If some aspects of the study are known to be atypical (for example, if a study was undertaken

---

[2] In general, the term modelling is used broadly in this chapter to mean decision analytic type models for synthesizing information from a number of sources that may include, but are not limited to, statistical models.

Table 8.1 Methods for handling uncertainty in stochastic analyses

Type of uncertainty	Handling uncertainty
Methodological	Reference case / sensitivity analysis
Sampling variation	Statistical analysis
Extrapolation	Modelling methods
Generalisability/Transferability	Sensitivity analysis

Table 8.2 Methods for handling uncertainty in modelling-based analyses

Type of uncertainty	Handling uncertainty
Methodological	Reference case/sensitivity analysis
Parameter uncertainty	Probabilistic sensitivity analysis
Modelling uncertainty – structure – process	 Sensitivity analysis ?
Generalisability/Transferability	Sensitivity analysis

in a national teaching centre associated with both higher costs and outcomes than a typical centre) then sensitivity analysis may be useful for handling this uncertainty.[3]

In a study of the type that involves synthesizing data from a number of secondary sources into a decision-analytic framework, there will be many parameters that form the inputs to the model and these will be subject to uncertainty in their estimated value. In addition, there will be uncertainty associated with the modelling process, which may be amenable to sensitivity analysis if, for example, alternative functional forms can be assumed for relationships between parameters. However, as the US panel noted (Manning *et al.* 1996), it is not clear that the individual analyst can do much about uncertainty relating to the whole structure of the analysis. If it is felt that the decision concerning whether to implement a particular technology is sufficiently crucial, then a funding body could commission separate analyses from different teams of researchers on the understanding that the modelling were undertaken independently. In Section 8.5 below, the use of probabilistic sensitivity analysis to handle parameter uncertainty in deterministic analyses is reviewed.

For stochastic cost-effectiveness analyses, it is natural to handle the uncertainty due to sampling variation using statistical methods, although some care needs to be taken over the problems of estimating the ICER from patient-level data and a review of the

---

[3] Indeed, if the study question is broad and the study setting is known to be atypical then it may be appropriate to estimate corrections to the baseline result to cover the more general nature of the analysis. Note that this issue is broader than the issue of adjusting results for 'protocol-driven' costs incurred as part of the evaluative process (Johnston *et al.* 1999).

suggested methods is presented in Section 8.4. However, it is rare that complete information on cost-effectiveness can be obtained from a clinical trial since trials rarely extend beyond a few years and economic evaluation is concerned with the costs and benefits of treatment over the lifetime of patients. Furthermore, clinical trials will often collect information only on surrogate endpoints (such as blood cholesterol levels) that are observed in the short-term rather than on the ultimate health outcomes of interest (mortality and morbidity) that require more sustained follow-up. For this reason, modelling will often be required to extrapolate from the original data. Where this is the case, parameter and modelling uncertainty will also become important in the overall analysis. Therefore, it is important to remember that the dichotomy between stochastic and modelling-based analyses is largely one of convenience. In practice, few studies will be wholly stochastic (Buxton *et al.* 1997). However, before examining the methods for handling uncertainty in these two types of analysis are explored the case is made for handling methodological uncertainty using a reference case of methods.

8.3.1 **Methodological uncertainty: the case for a 'reference case'**

The analytic methods used in an economic evaluation consist of a range of techniques employed to measure and value costs and health outcomes together with the choice of costs and benefits to include in an evaluation. There exists, in a number of these areas, disagreement amongst practitioners about the most appropriate analytical method (Drummond *et al.* 1993). There has been considerable debate in the literature concerning the preferred way to incorporate time preference into economic evaluation, and in particular, the role of differential discounting of costs and benefits[4] (Cairns 1992; Coyle and Tolley 1992; Parsonage and Neuburger 1992; Katz and Welch 1993; Brouwer *et al.* 2000; Lipscomb 1996; Lipscomb *et al.* 1996b). Uncertainty also exists concerning the methods selected to value the resource and health outcome consequences in an evaluation. There has also been extensive debate over the choice of instruments to value health outcome (Torrance 1986; Mehrez and Gafni 1989; Donaldson 1990; Ryan 1999). Perhaps a less obvious lack of consensus exists regarding such issues as whether or not to include in economic assessments the cost of health care resources consumed, due to unrelated illness, during extra years of life generated by the intervention under evaluation (Gold *et al.* 1996; Meltzer 1997; Garber and Phelps 1997; Etzioni *et al.* 2001). Similarly, there is some debate concerning whether (and how) to include the cost of production losses from time away from work[5] and/or time losses from general activities

---

[4] For UK analysts, this issue has become all the more important recently with the updated Treasury guidelines (HM Treasury 1997), which the Department of Health has interpreted as recommending differential discounting for health outcomes in cost-effectiveness analysis (by removing the component of discounting assumed by the Treasury to relate to the combination of annual growth of income and the marginal utility of income).

[5] These costs are often referred to as indirect costs, however, this term is avoided here since Drummond and colleagues (1997) have argued that this terminology can cause confusion through the use of the same term in accountancy to mean overhead costs.

which may not receive a wage, but which may be valued by society or the individual none the less (Koopmanschap *et al.* 1995; Koopmanschap and Rutten 1996; Posnett and Jan 1996; Brouwer *et al.* 1997; Weinstein *et al.* 1997).

Russell has argued for a set of core methods to be employed to facilitate comparisons between evaluations (Russell 1986). This idea has been adopted by the recent US panel on cost-effectiveness (Gold *et al.* 1996), which recommended the use of a 'reference case' of core methods to be used by analysts when conducting economic evaluations, which could then be supplemented by additional analyses employing other methods thought appropriate by the authors. In a recent review of all published UK cost-effectiveness studies presenting cost-per-life year and cost-per-QALY results[6] this idea of a reference case was applied retrospectively in order to improve the comparability of the results presented in different studies (Briggs and Gray 1999). A similar approach has been undertaken in the US to generate a league table of 'panel-worthy' studies (Chapman *et al.* 2000).

The use of a reference case of methods has a great deal of appeal in cost-effectiveness analysis where results of a study only have meaning in comparison to the results of other studies. While sensitivity analysis may be useful for considering whether conclusions would change under the application of alternative methods, it should be clear that sensitivity analysis used at this level is different from sensitivity analysis used to examine the effects of 'unknown' parameters. In fact, it would be useful to have interval estimates accompanying point estimates of cost-effectiveness for all the methodological scenarios presented as part of a study's results.

8.4 Statistical methods for stochastic analyses

It is only relatively recently that economic information has begun to be collected alongside clinical trials and with the availability of patient-level data on costs and effects it is natural to summarize uncertainty in the ICER as a confidence interval. However, the ICER, as a ratio statistic, poses particular problems for confidence interval estimation since a non-negligible probability in the neighbourhood of zero on the denominator makes a formula for the variance of the ICER intractable.

In Section 8.2 above, the formulation of the ICER was based on knowledge of the true average costs and effects in each of the treatment and control groups. In practice, these quantities are unobservable, rather they are estimated from mean cost and effects from the treatment and control groups observed in a clinical trial-based economic evaluation, giving an estimated ICER of

$$\hat{R} = \frac{\overline{C}_T - \overline{C}_C}{\overline{E}_T - \overline{E}_C} = \frac{\Delta \overline{C}}{\Delta \overline{E}}$$

The standard errors of the difference in costs and the difference in effects (the numerator and denominator of the ICER) can be estimated as

$$se(\Delta \overline{C}) = s_{\Delta C} = \sqrt{\frac{s^2_{CC}}{n_C} + \frac{s^2_{TC}}{n_T}}$$

---

[6] This review included all published studies up to the end of 1996.

$$\text{se}(\Delta \bar{E}) = s_{\Delta E} = \sqrt{\frac{s^2_{CE}}{n_C} + \frac{s^2_{TE}}{n_T}}$$

where s^2 is the estimated variance from the sample (subscripted to represent the treatment or control and cost or effect) and n represents the sample size (subscripted for treatment and control groups). Similarly, the correlation between cost and effect differences can be estimated as

$$\rho = \frac{\rho_C s_{CC} s_{CE}/n_C + \rho_T s_{TC} s_{TE}/n_T}{s_{\Delta E} s_{\Delta C}}$$

where ρ (subscripted for treatment or control) is the correlation coefficient for cost and effect in that group.

In this section the literature on the use of statistical methods for handling uncertainty in stochastic CEA is reviewed. In the first sub-section, the focus is on the estimation of confidence intervals for cost-effectiveness ratios when uncertainty is limited to the NE quadrant of the CE plane (i.e. the new treatment under evaluation is both *significantly* more costly and *significantly* more effective. Different methods for estimating confidence intervals can give different answers and the results of large-scale simulation studies have shown which methods have the best coverage properties. In the second sub-section, the problems of interpretation when uncertainty covers more than one quadrant of the CE plane are considered. In particular, the net-benefit approach of handling uncertainty and the presentation of results as cost-effectiveness acceptability curves are argued to provide the relevant information for decision-making in such circumstances. A final sub-section offers some comments on the frequentist approaches described here and their link with the Bayesian view of probability often adopted in the interpretation of acceptability curves.

8.4.1 Confidence intervals for ICERs

Many papers in the health economics literature have offered potential solutions to the problems of confidence interval estimation for ICERs. In this section, the key methods are reviewed in approximately chronological order of their appearance in the literature. In addition, the key weaknesses of the methods are identified and finally, the results of some large scale Monte Carlo simulation studies examining the coverage properties are reviewed.

The methods discussed are illustrated employing hypothetical data that are summarized in Table 8.3. It is clear from these summary statistics that the observed cost and effect differences are significantly different from zero locating the intervention under evaluation firmly in the NE quadrant of the CE plane.

The confidence box

O'Brien and colleagues (1994) show how the cost-effectiveness (CE) plane can be used to present the confidence limits for the estimate of incremental cost effectiveness and a one-sided version of this interval has also appeared in the recent literature (Wakker

Table 8.3 Summary statistics for example to data set to be employed for calculating confidence limits for the ICER

	Control Group		Treatment Group		Difference	
	Effect	Cost	Effect	Cost	Effect	Cost
Mean	10	£40,000	11	£55,000	1	£15,000
SD	1.30	£18,000	1.5	£24,000	N/A	N/A
SE	0.13	£1,800	0.15	£2,400	0.20	£3,000
Corr	0	0	0			
ICER	£15,000 per year of life saved					
SE	N/A					

and Klaassen 1995). Figure 8.2, illustrates this representation of the data from Table 8.3 on the CE plane. The difference in effect between two therapies is shown on the horizontal axis with mean effect difference $\Delta \bar{E}$ and upper and lower confidence limits for the effect difference ($\Delta \bar{E}^U$ and $\Delta \bar{E}^L$) represented by the horizontal 'I' bar. Similarly, the difference in cost between the two therapies is shown on the vertical axis with mean cost difference $\Delta \bar{C}$, and upper and lower confidence limits for the cost difference ($\Delta \bar{C}^U$ and $\Delta \bar{C}^L$) represented by the vertical 'I' bar. These 'I' bars intersect at point ($\Delta \bar{E}, \Delta \bar{C}$), hence the ray that connects this point of intersection to the origin has a slope equal to the value of the point estimate of the ICER.

The upper and lower limits of the confidence intervals on cost and effect are calculated employing standard parametric assumptions, such that the $(1-\alpha)100\%$ confidence limits on the incremental costs and effects are given by

$$(\Delta \bar{E} - z_{\alpha/2} s_{\Delta E}, \Delta \bar{E} + z_{\alpha/2} s_{\Delta E})$$

$$(\Delta \bar{C} - z_{\alpha/2} s_{\Delta C}, \Delta \bar{C} + z_{\alpha/2} s_{\Delta C})$$

where $z_{\alpha/2}$ represents the standardized normal deviate exceeded in either direction with probability α such that for $\alpha = 0.05$, $z_{\alpha/2} = 1.96$.[7]

O'Brien and colleagues argue that combining the limits of the confidence intervals for costs and effects and the lower limit of costs divided by the upper limit of effects ($R^L = D\bar{C}^L/D\bar{E}^U$) gives the lowest (best) value of the ratio. Thus the approximation to the $(1-\alpha)100\%$ confidence interval employing this method is given by

$$\left(\frac{\Delta \bar{C} - z_{\alpha/2} s_{\Delta \bar{C}}}{\Delta \bar{E} + z_{\alpha/2} s_{\Delta \bar{E}}}, \frac{\Delta \bar{C} + z_{\alpha/2} s_{\Delta \bar{C}}}{\Delta \bar{E} - z_{\alpha/2} s_{\Delta \bar{E}}} \right)$$

---

[7] In practice, it will be appropriate to use Student's t-distribution for small sample size rate than the normal distribution to reflect the fact that the standard errors for the differences are not known, but estimated (Laska *et al.* 1997). The normal distribution assumption is used here as this reflects much of the development of the literature.

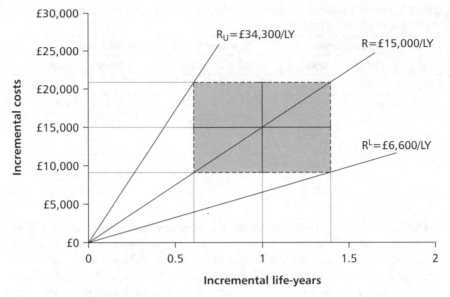

Fig. 8.2 The confidence box on the CE plane

The area of the shaded box in Figure 8.2 represents this combined area of confidence for the example data from Table 8.3. It is important to note, however, that the confidence level of this area does not correspond to the confidence level on the individual costs and effect differences where those cost and effect differences are independent. The chance of a type I error (usually represented by α) can be interpreted as the proportion of times the true parameter lies outside the estimated interval in repeated sampling. Hence, the chance that the true cost difference is contained within the estimated cost interval is $(1-\alpha)$, as is the chance that the true effect difference is contained within the estimated effect interval. Thus, the chance that both these events occur simultaneously is $(1-\alpha)^2$. Hence, combining the 95 per cent confidence limits for cost and effects individually gives a 90 per cent confidence box in terms of the number of times the true cost and effect differences will be contained by the shaded surface of Figure 8.2 in repeated sampling.

The Taylor series expansion (or Delta method)

O'Brien and colleagues recognize that the representation of uncertainty as box shaped on the CE plane is misleading since, for the case of independence, the chance of observing extreme values for both cost and effect differences simultaneously will be very low. Instead they suggest that contour lines on the cost-effectiveness plane for which the joint density is constant are likely to be elliptical in shape. However, rather than try to estimate confidence limits based on this ellipse, they favour the Taylor series approximation of the variance of a function of two random variables to estimate the variance of a ratio. They argue that the advantage of this method over the confidence box approach is that it accounts for the covariance between the numerator and denominator.

The Taylor approximation shows that where y is a function of two random variables x_1 and x_2, the variance of y can be expressed in terms of the variances and covariance of x_1 and x_2, weighted by the partial derivatives of y with respect to x_1 and x_2. The Taylor series formula is presented below

$$\text{var}(y) \approx \left(\frac{\partial y}{\partial x_1}\right)^2 \text{var}(x_1) + \left(\frac{\partial y}{\partial x_2}\right)^2 \text{var}(x_2) + 2\left(\frac{\partial y}{\partial x_1}\right)\left(\frac{\partial y}{\partial x_2}\right)\text{cov}(x_1, x_2) \quad (8.1)$$

This expression can now be solved for the case of the ICER presented in Equation (8.1) by substituting $\Delta\bar{C}$ for x_1 and $\Delta\bar{E}$ for x_2.[8] Hence the Taylor series approximation of the variance of the ratio estimator, using the sample estimates of the means and variances (since by definition the population values cannot be observed), is given as

$$\text{var}(\hat{R}) \approx \frac{1}{\Delta\bar{E}^2}\text{var}(\Delta\bar{C}) + \frac{\Delta\bar{C}^2}{\Delta\bar{E}^4}\text{var}(\Delta\bar{E}) - 2\frac{\Delta\bar{C}}{\Delta\bar{E}^3}\text{cov}(\Delta\bar{C}, \Delta\bar{E}) \quad (8.2)$$

Taking

$$\hat{R}^2 = \frac{\Delta\bar{C}^2}{\Delta\bar{E}^2}$$

outside on the right-hand side of the above simplifies the expression to

$$\text{var}(\hat{R}) \approx \hat{R}^2\left[\frac{\text{var}(\Delta\bar{C})}{\Delta\bar{C}^2} + \frac{\text{var}(\Delta\bar{E})}{\Delta\bar{E}^2} - 2\frac{\text{cov}(\Delta\bar{C}, \Delta\bar{E})}{\Delta\bar{C}\Delta\bar{E}}\right] \quad (8.3)$$

and noting that the coefficient of variation[9] for a random variable x is defined by

$$\text{cv}(x) = \sqrt{\frac{\text{var}(x)}{\bar{x}^2}}$$

and that the correlation coefficient between two random variables x and y is defined by

$$\rho = \frac{\text{cov}(x, y)}{\sqrt{\text{var}(x)\,\text{var}(y)}}$$

further simplifies the exposition

$$\text{var}(\hat{R}) \approx \hat{R}^2\left[\text{cv}(\Delta\bar{C})^2 + \text{cv}(\Delta\bar{E})^2 - 2\rho\,\text{cv}(\Delta\bar{C})\,\text{cv}(\Delta\bar{E})\right] \quad (8.4)$$

Employing standard parametric assumptions gives the confidence interval as

$$\left(\hat{R} - z_{\alpha/2}\sqrt{\text{var}(\hat{R})},\ \hat{R} + z_{\alpha/2}\sqrt{\text{var}(\hat{R})}\right) \quad (8.5)$$

---

[8] The partial derivatives of the ICER with respect to $\Delta\bar{C}$ and $\Delta\bar{E}$ are $1/\Delta\bar{E}$ and $-\Delta\bar{C}/\Delta\bar{E}^2$ respectively.

[9] For an estimator the coefficient of variation is given by the ratio of the standard error to the mean. Coefficients of variation are often defined in terms of the ratio of the standard deviation to the mean. Since this is true for any random variable (Armitage and Berry 1994) and standard errors are equivalent to standard deviations of the estimator; the coefficients of variation for the estimator can be defined in terms of the standard error.

and applying this to the example from Table 8.3 gives a confidence interval of £6,700 to £23,300 for the ICER.

O'Brien and colleagues argue that although the assumption of a normal distribution may be justified in the case of large samples, it is unlikely that the distribution of a ratio will follow a well-behaved distribution. In general they remain cautious about the use of both the Taylor series method and the confidence box method.

Even though the numerator and denominator of the ratio may follow a normal distribution, the sampling distribution of the ICER may be non-normal due to the non-negligible probability that the denominator of the ratio could take a zero value. Increasing sample sizes in a study will increase the precision of the estimated cost and effect differences, reducing their coefficients of variation and the associated probability of observing a zero value. Hence, it is true that with large sample sizes (or rather small coefficients of variation) the distribution of a ratio may be normal. However, O'Brien and colleagues are correct in remaining cautious of the Taylor series approach. A high coefficient of variation for the denominator of the ratio (i.e. a non-negligible probability of observing a zero value) means that the sampling distribution of the ICER is likely to be non-normal and that the Taylor series will give a poor estimate of variance (Armitage and Berry 1994).

The confidence ellipse

Van Hout and colleagues (1994) argue that because the ratio of two normal distributions has neither a finite mean nor a finite variance, the approach of approximating the variance of the ratio using the Taylor series and then assuming a normal sampling distribution is formally incorrect.[10] Instead, they return to the idea that the joint cost and effect density function might be elliptical in shape and they derive the formula for this ellipse by assuming that the costs and effects follow a joint normal distribution. Employing the previous notation, the joint probability density function can be expressed as

$$f(\Delta \bar{E}, \Delta \bar{C}) = \frac{1}{2\pi \sigma_{\Delta C} \sigma_{\Delta E} \sqrt{1 - \rho^2}} \exp (Q) \tag{8.6}$$

where the correlation between $\mu_{\Delta C}$ and $\mu_{\Delta E}$ is given by ρ, and Q is defined by

$$Q = -\frac{1}{2(1-\rho^2)} \left[\frac{(\mu_{\Delta C} - \Delta \bar{C})^2}{\sigma^2_{\Delta C}} + \frac{(\mu_{\Delta E} - \Delta \bar{E})^2}{\sigma^2_{\Delta E}} - \frac{2\rho(\mu_{\Delta C} - \Delta \bar{C})(\mu_{\Delta E} - \Delta \bar{E})}{\sigma_{\Delta C} \sigma_{\Delta E}} \right] \tag{8.7}$$

The elliptical contour lines on the CE plane are those lines on which the joint density is constant. It is clear that $f(\Delta \bar{E}, \Delta \bar{C})$ is constant if Q is constant and the locus

---

[10] In fact, Armitage and Berry (1994) note that the Taylor series approximation will provide a good estimate of the variance of a ratio statistic providing the coefficient of variation of the denominator of the ratio is small. The problem in using the Taylor series for the ICER is not that the ICER is the ratio of two normally distributed random variables, but that (as argued above) in practical application the coefficient of variation of the denominator of the ratio is likely to be high.

of such points is an ellipse of equal probability centred at $(\mu_{\Delta E}, \mu_{\Delta C})$. They go on to propose that such an ellipse might cover 95 per cent of the integrated probability to give a confidence surface analogous to a confidence interval. Such an ellipse is characterized by setting $Q = \ln(1-\lambda)$ where λ is the value of the integrated probability (0.95 for a 95 per cent confidence surface). An approximation of the 95 per cent confidence interval is given by those rays from the origin of the CE plane that are tangential to the ellipse. Other commentators have also presented the confidence interval of a ratio in terms of the tangents to an ellipse of equal density (Manning *et al.* 1996; Drummond *et al.* 1997).

The ellipse approach to confidence interval estimation is shown in Figure 8.3 for the example from Table 8.3 where costs and effects are independent. The advantage of this method of confidence interval estimation over the confidence box approach is that it will allow for the covariance between the numerator and denominator.

Figure 8.4(a) and (b) shows the 95 per cent confidence ellipse for (a) positive correlation between the numerator and denominator of the ICER of 0.6, and (b) negative correlation between the numerator and denominator of -0.6. These figures clearly show the dramatic difference in the width of the confidence interval for the ICER for differing levels of covariance between the numerator and denominator. Both Figures 8.3 and 8.4(a) and (b) show the confidence box in addition to the ellipse and it is worth noting that the 95 per cent confidence ellipse is not contained within the box defined by the two 95 per cent confidence intervals on cost and effect differences. There is no straightforward relationship between the ellipse and the box: it is a confidence box, constructed from two 98.6 per cent confidence intervals which just contains the 95 per cent confidence ellipse, and which itself covers 97.1 per cent of the integrated probability of the joint density function.

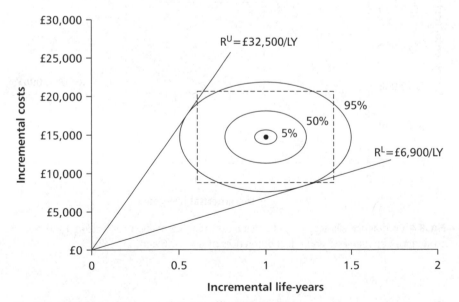

Fig. 8.3 Confidence ellipses on the cost-effectiveness plane

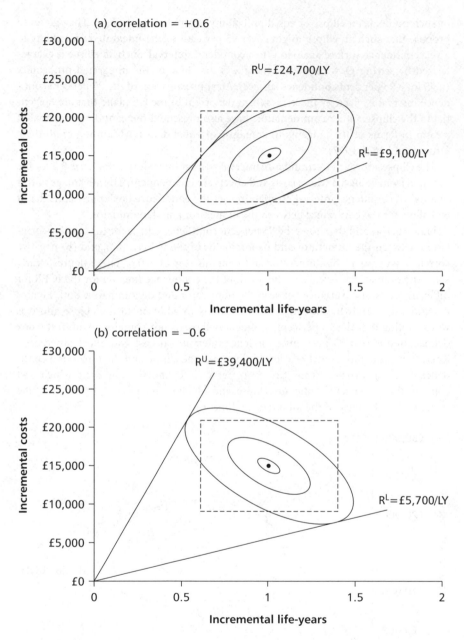

Fig. 8.4 Confidence ellipses on the CE plane assuming correlation coefficients for the covariance between cost and effect differences of (a) + 0.6 and (b) − 0.6

Fieller's theorem

As van Hout and colleagues (1994) note, the method of calculating the slope of tangents to the 95 per cent probability ellipse gives only an approximation to the 95 per cent confidence interval for the ratio. Since the area between the rays covers more than 95 per cent of the joint density function. The statistical properties of ratio statistics and an exact method of calculating confidence intervals around ratios has been described by Fieller as early as 1932 in relation to bioassay (Fieller 1932, 1954). This approach has been advocated for use in calculating confidence intervals around ICERs by both Chaudhary and Stearns (1996) and Willan and O'Brien (1996).

The advantage of Fieller's method over the Taylor series expansion is that it takes into account the potential skewness in the sampling distribution of the ratio estimator, and may not therefore be symmetrically positioned around the point estimate. In contrast to the Taylor series approximation, Fieller's theorem provides an exact solution, subject to the assumption of the method that the numerator and denominator of the ratio follow a joint normal distribution – i.e. the expression $\Delta\bar{C} - R\Delta\bar{E}$ rather than the ratio is normally distributed with zero mean. Thus by dividing through by the standard deviation, it follows that

$$\frac{\Delta\bar{C} - R\Delta\bar{E}}{\sqrt{\text{var}(\Delta\bar{C}) + R^2\,\text{var}(\Delta\bar{E}) - 2R\,\text{cov}(\Delta\bar{C}, \Delta\bar{E})}} \sim N(0, 1)$$

Setting this expression equal to $z_{\alpha/2}$ and rearranging gives the following quadratic equation in R (using the simplified notation based on coefficients of variation)

$$R^2\left[1 - z_{\alpha/2}^2\,\text{cv}(\Delta\bar{E})^2\right] - 2R\hat{R}\left[1 - z_{\alpha/2}^2\,\rho\,\text{cv}(\Delta\bar{C})\,\text{cv}(\Delta\bar{E})\right]$$

$$+ \hat{R}^2\left[1 - z_{\alpha/2}^2\,\text{cv}(\Delta\bar{C})^2\right] = 0$$

and solving for R using the standard quadratic formula[11] gives the confidence interval as

$$\hat{R}\frac{1 - z_{\alpha/2}^2\,\rho\,\text{cv}(\Delta\bar{C})\,\text{cv}(\Delta\bar{E})}{1 - z_{\alpha/2}^2\,\text{cv}(\Delta\bar{E})^2}$$

$$\pm\hat{R}\frac{z_{\alpha/2}\sqrt{\text{cv}(\Delta\bar{C})^2 + \text{cv}(\Delta\bar{E})^2 - 2\rho\,\text{cv}(\Delta\bar{C})\text{cv}(\Delta\bar{E}) - z_{\alpha/2}^2(1 - \rho^2)\,\text{cv}(\Delta\bar{C})^2\text{cv}(\Delta\bar{E})^2}}{1 - z_{\alpha/2}^2\text{cv}(\Delta\bar{E})^2}$$

Where the sampling distribution of the ratio statistic is skewed, this confidence interval will not be symmetrically positioned around the point estimate of the ICER (c.f. the Taylor series method). Applying Fieller's theorem to the example from Table 8.3 gives the estimated confidence interval for the ICER as £8,300 to £27,000.

---

[11] The solution formula for a quadratic equation of the form: $ax^2 + bx + c = 0$ is:

$$\frac{-b \pm (b^2 - 4ac)^{1/2}}{2a}$$

However, it has been argued that the assumption of joint normality may not apply, particularly where sample sizes are small (Chaudhary and Stearns 1996). In particular, health care costs will often follow a substantially skewed distribution which may cause problems for the normality assumption (Zhou *et al.* 1997; Briggs and Gray 1998).

Non-parametric bootstrapping

Given the unknown nature of the ICER's sampling distribution, there is reason to be cautious of the parametric approaches to confidence interval estimation. A number of commentators have suggested the non-parametric approach of bootstrapping (Efron and Gong 1993; Efron and Tibshirani 1993) as a possible method of estimating confidence limits for the ICER (O'Brien *et al.* 1994; Mullahy and Manning 1995; Manning *et al.* 1996; Mullahy 1996) and this approach has been successfully demonstrated using clinical trial data (Chaudhary and Stearns 1996; Briggs *et al.* 1997; Obenchain *et al.* 1997). The advantage of such intervals is that they do not depend on parametric assumptions of the sampling distribution of the ICER. Rather, the bootstrap method involves building up an empirical estimate of the sampling distribution of the statistic in question by resampling from the original data.

In the case of the ICER, where data on resource use and outcome exists for two groups of patients of size n_C and n_T receiving the control and active treatment group respectively, the bootstrap method involves a three stage process:

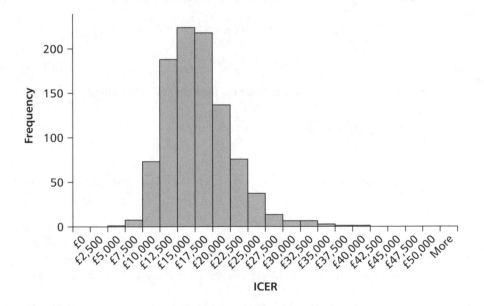

Fig. 8.5 Bootstrap estimate of the ICER sampling distribution

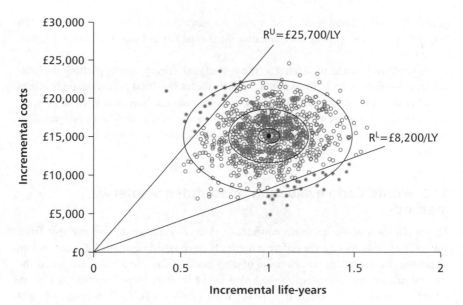

Fig. 8.6 Bootstrap replications of the cost and effect differences on the CE plane. Overlaid are the rays representing the confidence limits from the percentile bootstrap method together with the 5 per cent, 50 per cent and 95 per cent confidence ellipses

1. Sample with replacement n_C cost/effect pairs from the patients in the control group and calculate the bootstrap estimates $\bar{C}_C^*$ and $\bar{E}_C^*$ for the bootstrap sample;

2. Sample with replacement n_T cost/effect pairs from the sample of patients in the treatment group and calculate the bootstrap estimates $\bar{C}_T^*$ and $\bar{E}_T^*$ for the bootstrap sample;

3. Calculate the bootstrap replicate of the ICER given by the equation:

$$R^* = \frac{\bar{C}_T^* - \bar{C}_C^*}{\bar{E}_T^* - \bar{E}_C^*} = \frac{\Delta \bar{C}^*}{\Delta \bar{E}^*}$$

Repeating this three-stage process many times gives a vector of bootstrap estimates, which is an empirical estimate of the sampling distribution of the ICER statistic. For example, the histogram in Figure 8.5 shows the estimated sampling distribution for the ICER from Table 8.3 using this approach.

Once the sampling distribution of the ICER has been estimated in this way, several approaches exist to estimate confidence intervals using the bootstrap estimate of the sampling distribution, including methods to adjust the confidence limits for the bias that exists in the estimate of the ICER statistic (Chaudhary and Stearns 1996; Stinnett 1996; Briggs *et al.* 1997) since it is well known that ratio statistics in general are biased (but consistent) (Cochran 1977). However, for the purposes of this chapter, only the straightforward percentile method, which employs the $(\alpha/2)100$ and $(1 - \alpha/2)100$ percentiles of the empirical sampling distribution as the estimated confidence limits, is used.[12]

This approach can be illustrated on the cost-effectiveness plane by plotting the individual cost-effect pairs as in Figure 8.6 which shows the 1000 bootstrap replications from the example in Table 8.3. Note how the bootstrap method clearly shows how the ellipse method leads to an overestimate in the coverage of the confidence interval. Also notice the similarity between the results from the bootstrap and Fieller's approaches compared to the other methods.

8.4.2 Monte Carlo evaluation of confidence interval methods

The application of the different confidence interval methods to the example from Table 8.3 emphasizes how the different methods can give substantially different results. Recall that the (frequentist) definition of a 95 per cent confidence interval is that the true population parameter will be included in the interval 95 per cent of the time in repeated sampling. Although it is possible to predict which of the methods will perform best in repeated sampling from their theoretical properties, the increasing power of computers has enabled analysts to design studies to test the coverage properties of the different methods directly (Polsky *et al.* 1997; Tambour and Zethraeus 1998; Briggs *et al.* 1999; Heitjan *et al.*1999).[13] The results from these Monte Carlo simulation studies are reassuringly similar in that there is strong evidence that Fieller's method and the bootstrap method outperform the Taylor series and box methods in that the coverage probabilities were consistently closer to the chosen nominal level.The intuition for this result is that both Fieller's method and the bootstrap attempt to adjust the interval such that it contains $(1 - \alpha)100\%$ of the joint density, whereas the tangents to the ellipse and rays to the corners of the box cover more than $(1 - \alpha)100\%$ of the joint density and are therefore simply approximations. Since the Taylor series estimate of the variance is applied to the standard parametric assumption of a normal sampling distribution when there is good reason to believe the sampling distribution is non-normal, it clearly provides an inappropriate interval.

There is little to choose between Fieller's and the bootstrap methods on the basis of the Monte Carlo simulation experiments. This suggests that while the sampling distribution of the ICER is clearly non-normal, the parametric assumption of a joint normal distribution of the numerator and denominator of the ICER may be reasonable.

---

[12] This is because (as will be argued below), alternatives to confidence intervals for ICERs exist that do not require bias correction.

[13] None of the studies examined the ellipse method, perhaps due to the relative complexity of obtaining the limits.

8.4.3 Beyond the confidence interval

In the preceding section methods of confidence interval estimation for the ICER were compared using a data set that indicated that both cost and effect differences are significant. However, this is unlikely to be the case in many economic evaluations, and the problem arises of how to handle uncertainty that extends into more than one quadrant of the CE plane.

The death of cost-minimization analysis?

Drummond and colleagues present a matrix of nine possible mutually exclusive situations relating to the results of a cost-effectiveness analysis, by whether or not the results indicate the cost and effect differences of treatment compared to control are greater, the same or less (Drummond *et al.* 1997, p, 248). Implicit in this representation is the idea of testing whether there is a difference in cost and effect between the two treatments. Figure 8.7 presents the same nine possible outcomes of a cost-effectiveness analysis, but the testing of differences is explicit through the representation of uncertainty on the CE plane as the confidence box generated by the confidence intervals on cost and effect differences.

Up to this point, we have been considering confidence limits for ICERs when we are in situation 7 (or equivalently situation 8). But how should uncertainty be handled in the other situations that can arise? By extension to the original arguments of Section 2, in situations 1 and 2, where it is possible to demonstrate the dominance of one treatment over another as being significant, there is no need to calculate a cost-

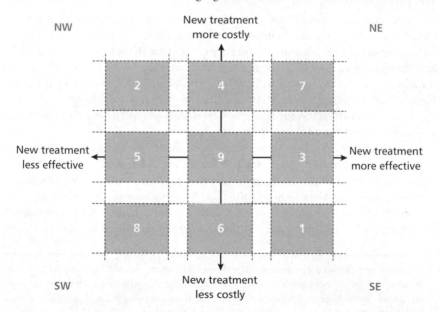

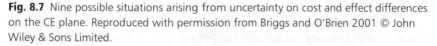

Fig. 8.7 Nine possible situations arising from uncertainty on cost and effect differences on the CE plane. Reproduced with permission from Briggs and O'Brien 2001 © John Wiley & Sons Limited.

effectiveness ratio and the treatment of choice is clear. Situations 4 and 6 correspond to what has been termed 'cost-minimization analysis' with the implication that having failed to find a difference in effect, the treatment of choice is that which has been shown to be less costly. In keeping with the symmetry of Figure 8.7, situations 3 and 5 could be termed 'outcome-maximization' with the implication that having failed to find a difference in cost, the treatment that has been shown to be most effective should be implemented. Finally, many would argue that in situation 9 nothing useful can be said about cost-effectiveness.

The problem with these interpretations of situations 3–6 and situation 9 is that there is an overemphasis on hypothesis testing of the cost and effect differences with no consideration given to the power of the study to detect such differences. In consequence, we would expect a large number of type II errors, where the null hypothesis of no difference is not rejected when in fact a difference does exist. This phenomenon has been comprehensively illustrated in the clinical literature (Freiman et al. 1978) and has been responsible for guidelines recommending confidence interval estimation rather than hypothesis testing (Gardner and Altman 1989; Altman and Bland 1995). Extending this argument to stochastic cost-effectiveness analysis would suggest that the confidence intervals for ICERs should still be calculated in situations 3–6 and 9 so that the limits of the possible cost-effectiveness can be determined. Hence, even apparently simple cost-minimization analyses may be revealed to have sufficient uncertainty that the results are consistent with positive values of the ICER (Briggs and O'Brien 2001).

The problem of negative (and positive) ICERs

Situations 3–6 and 9 are all characterized by uncertainty that includes two or more quadrants of the plane. This is important because, from Section 8. 2, the ICER was only calculated for the NE and SW quadrants where the ICER is positive. In the NW and SE quadrants the ICER is negative and its magnitude conveys no useful meaning.[14] Furthermore, negative ICERs in the Northwest quadrant of the plane (favouring the existing treatment) are qualitatively different from negative ICERs in the Southeast quadrant (favouring the new treatment) yet will be grouped together in any rank-ordering exercise.

Consider Figure 8.8 which shows bootstrap replications on the cost-effectiveness plane for an intervention with point estimate of the ICER of £15,000 per life year gained (as in the example above) but where the standard errors on life years gained and incremental costs are 0.6 and £10,000. In other words, the individual costs and effects are not statistically significant, so the example is equivalent to situation 9 from Figure 8.7. As a consequence of this lack of significance in the cost and effect

---

[14] The problem is that in the positive quadrants low CERs are preferred to high ICERs (from the point of view of the more costly more effective treatment). However, no such simple arrangement exists in the negative quadrants. Consider the three following points in the SE quadrant: A (1LY, −£2,000); B (2LYs, −£2,000); C(2LYs, −£1,000); giving negative ICERs of −£2,000/LY, −£1,000/LY and −£500/LY respectively. Therefore, in terms of magnitude, A has the lowest ICER with C the highest and B between the two. However, it should be clear that B is preferred to both A and C as it has the highest number of life years saved and the greatest cost-saving.

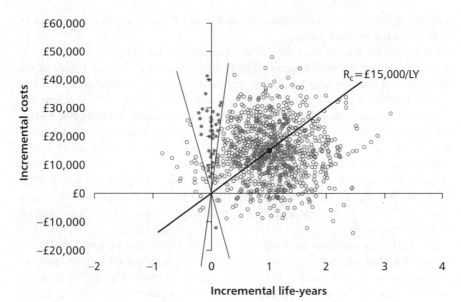

Fig. 8.8 Confidence intervals for cost-effectiveness ratios when neither costs nor effects are significant

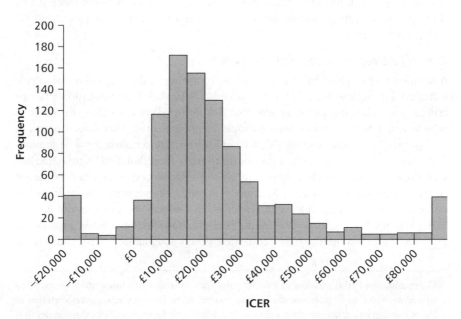

Fig. 8.9 Bootstrap estimate of the sampling distribution of the ICER from the results in Figure 8.8

differences, the bootstrap replications, while mainly falling in the NE quadrant, cover all four quadrants of the plane.

Looking at the histogram of the bootstrap estimate of the sampling distribution of the ICER under these circumstances (Figure 8.9), reveals the 'extreme' nature of the distribution due to the large number of replications with effect differences very close to zero. (Note that the histogram is truncated and does not show the full magnitude of the most positive and negative ICERs.) Although not incorrect statistically, there is a problem with the bootstrap approach of estimating confidence limits in this situation. Taking the 2.5th and 97.5th percentiles from vector of bootstrapped ICERs conflates the negative ICERs in the NW quadrant with those in the SW quadrant. The result is indicated on the CE plane in Figure 8.8: the omitted highest and lowest ICER values are indicated by the solid points and the two rays containing these points have slope equal to the estimated confidence limits. It is not clear how such an interval should be interpreted.

In addition to problems with negative ratios, it should also be noted that there is a problem with positive ratios in this example. Going back to the CE plane in Figure 8.1 it should be clear that although low ICERs are preferred to high ICERs from the point of view of the new technology on the NE quadrant, in the SW quadrant low ICERs are less favourable towards the new treatment. Where the bootstrap replications cover all four quadrants (as they do in Figure 8.8) then it turns out that the bootstrap approach to confidence intervals fails to distinguish between those ICERs (both positive and negative) that favour the new treatment from those that favour the existing treatment.

Cost-effectiveness acceptability curves

A solution to this problem can be found by returning to the original decision rule introduced in Section 8.2.[15] If the estimated ICER lies below some shadow price or ceiling ratio reflecting the maximum that decision-makers are willing to invest to achieve a unit of effectiveness then it should be implemented. Therefore, in terms of the bootstrap replications on the CE plane in Figure 8.8, uncertainty could be summarized by considering how many of the bootstrap replications fall to the right of the line with slope equal to R_C lending support to the cost-effectiveness of the intervention. Of course, the appropriate value of R_C is itself unknown, however, R_C can be varied in order to show how the evidence in favour of cost-effectiveness of the intervention varies with R_C. The resulting curve for the example shown in Figure 8.8 is presented in Figure 8.10 and has been termed a cost-effectiveness acceptability curve as it directly

---

[15] Other solutions to this problem do exist. In particular, a number of commentators have noted that if we make an angular transformation, equivalent to the conversion from cartesian to polar coordinates, then the uncertainty in the ICER can be represented as an angle, thus different quadrants of the CE plane can be successfully distinguished (Obenchain et al. 1997; Cook and Heyse 2000). While there is undoubtedly merit in such an approach, the interpretation of cost-effectiveness and associate uncertainty as an angle will provide substantial challenges for those not used to handling polar coordinates, thus in this chapter we concentrate on those solutions that retain a simple geometric interpretation in cartesian coordinates.

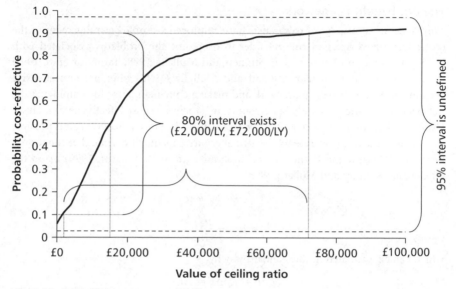

Fig. 8.10 Cost-effectiveness acceptability curve

summarizes the evidence in support of the intervention being cost-effective for all potential values of the decision rule.

This 'acceptability curve' presents much more information on uncertainty than do confidence intervals. The curve cuts the horizontal axis at the p-value (one-sided) for the cost difference since a value of zero for R_C implies that only the cost is important in the cost-effectiveness calculation. The curve is tending towards one minus the p-value for the effect difference, since an infinite value for R_C implies that effect only is important in the cost-effectiveness calculation. As well as summarizing, for every value of R_C, the evidence in favour of the intervention being cost-effective, acceptability curves can also be employed to obtain a confidence interval on cost-effectiveness. For example, by excluding 10 per cent of the probability from each end of the vertical axis and reading down from the curve at those points the 80 per cent interval on cost-effectiveness can be defined as £2000/LY to £72,000/LY. Notice that using this method, the 95 per cent confidence interval is not defined since the curve does not cross the 2.5 per cent and 97.5 per cent points on the vertical axis. This is expected since the overall uncertainty is so great that such a confidence interval is unreasonable.

The use of such acceptability curves was first proposed by van Hout and colleagues (1994) in the same paper in which they explored the ellipse approach to estimating confidence intervals. Rather than the use of bootstrapping, they estimated the curve by assuming the distribution of costs and effect differences on the CE plane to follow the joint normal distribution and then integrating over the joint density for the portion of the plane in which the intervention was cost-effective. It is only relatively recently that applied studies (rather than methodological papers) have begun to make use of acceptability curves (Raikou *et al.* 1998).

The net-benefit framework

More recently, a number of researchers have employed a simple rearrangement of the cost-effectiveness decision rule in order to overcome the problems associated with ICERs (Claxton and Posnett 1996; Stinnett and Mullahy 1998; Tambour *et al.* 1998; Claxton 1999). In particular, Stinnett and Mullahy (1998) offer a comprehensive account of the net-benefit framework and make a convincing case for employing the net-benefit statistic to handle uncertainty in stochastic cost-effectiveness analysis. Using the decision rule for cost-effectiveness analysis laid out in Section 2, it is possible to rearrange the decision-rule to give two alternative inequalities on either the monetary scale (Claxton and Posnett 1996; Tambour *et al.* 1998; Claxton 1999) or on the effect scale (Stinnett and Mullahy 1998)

$$0 < R_C \mu_{\Delta E} - \mu_{\Delta C}$$

$$0 < \mu_{\Delta E} - \frac{\mu_{\Delta C}}{R_C}$$

which can be estimated in the standard way by

$$N\hat{M}B = R_C \Delta \overline{E} = \Delta \overline{C}$$

$$N\hat{H}B = \Delta \overline{E} - \frac{\Delta \overline{C}}{R_C}$$

The advantage of formulating the cost-effectiveness decision rule in this way is that, by using the value of R_C to turn the decision rule into a linear expression, the variance for the net-benefit statistics is tractable

$$\text{var}(\hat{N}B) = R_C^2 \, \text{var}(\Delta \overline{E}) + \text{var}(\Delta \overline{C}) - 2R_C \, \text{cov}(\Delta \overline{E}, \Delta \overline{C})$$

$$N\hat{H}B = \text{var}(\Delta \overline{E}) + \frac{\text{var}(\Delta \overline{C})}{R_C^2} - \frac{2}{R_C} \, \text{cov}(\Delta \overline{E}, \Delta \overline{C})$$

and the sampling distribution of the net-benefits is much better behaved. For example, Figure 8.11 shows the bootstrap estimate of the sampling distribution for net-benefits on the monetary scale assuming $R_C = £100,000$ employing the exact same bootstrap replications from Figures 8.6 and 8.8. It is quite clear from this histogram that the net-benefit statistic is approximately normally distributed – which suggests that standard parametric assumptions can be employed.

Since the net-benefit statistic relies on the decision rule R_C to avoid the problems of ratio statistics when in fact the value of R_C is unknown, so the net-benefit can be plotted as a function of R_C. Figure 8.12 shows this for both the formulations of net-benefits and includes both 80 per cent and 95 per cent confidence intervals on net-benefits using the formula for the variance given above and assuming a normal distribution. The net-benefit curves cross the horizontal axis at the point estimate of cost-effectiveness of the intervention. Where the confidence limits on net-benefits cross the axis gives the confidence interval on cost-effectiveness. It is clear from the figure that the 95 per cent limits do not cross the axis indicating that a 95 per cent confidence interval on cost-effectiveness is not defined. The 80 per cent limits do cross

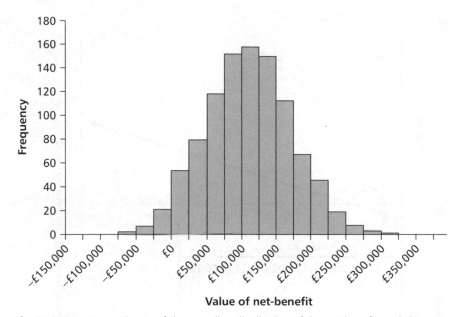

Fig. 8.11 Bootstrap estimate of the sampling distribution of the net-benefit statistic on the cost scale

the axis and yield the same interval on cost-effectiveness that was generated from the cost-effectiveness acceptability curve of Figure 8.10. Indeed, the net-benefit statistic provides a straightforward method to estimate the acceptability curve parametrically. The cost-effectiveness acceptability curve is calculated from the p-value on the net-benefits being positive. Note that an acceptability curve calculated in this way gives the exact same acceptability curve as the analysis on the CE plane suggested by van Hout and colleagues (1994), based on the joint normal distribution of cost and effect differences.

It is clear from Section 8.4.1 that there is much common ground between the net-benefit method and Fieller's theorem. Indeed, the formal equivalence of the confidence limits described from the net-benefit method and from Fieller's theorem (and by extension the limits obtained form the acceptability curve above) have recently been demonstrated (Heitjan 2000; Zethraeus and Löthgren 2000). Thus the failure of Fieller's method to produce a confidence limit for the ICER at a specified level of alpha, the type I error rate, reflects a problem not of the method itself, but of the level of uncertainty. While such an interval can be defined for net-benefits, that interval, by definition, will include zero at the specified alpha rate of error.

8.4.4 **On being Bayesian with probability**

Although a strict frequentist interpretation of cost-effectiveness acceptability curves is possible through the consideration of the P-value on net-benefits (Löthgren and Zethraeus 1999), the natural way to interpret these curves (as illustrated by the

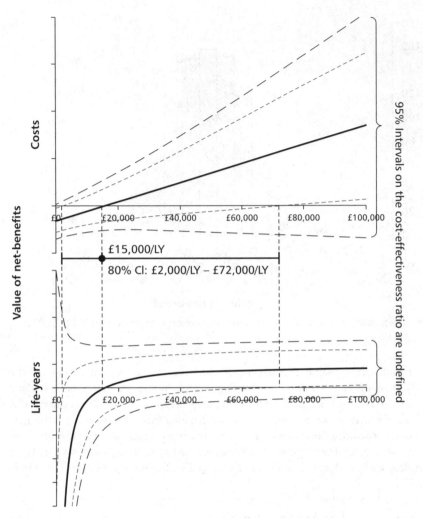

Fig. 8.12 Net benefit statistics on the cost and effect scales with 80 per cent and 95 per cent intervals.

labelling of the vertical axis in Figure 8.10) is as the probability that the intervention is cost-effective. Indeed, this is the way cost-effectiveness acceptability curves have been presented in the literature to date (van Hout *et al.* 1994; Briggs and Fenn 1998; Raikou *et al.* 1998). It has also been argued that the widespread mistaken interpretation of traditional *P*-values by researchers as a probability that the null hypothesis is false may be due to the fact that researchers want to be able to make probability statements about the null hypothesis in this way (Bland and Altman 1998). A number of commentators have stressed that such a view of probability in cost-effectiveness analysis is only possible in a Bayesian framework (Luce and Claxton 1999; Heitjan *et al.* 1999; O'Hagan *et al.* 2000).

Fundamentally, the Bayesian approach includes a learning process whereby beliefs concerning the distributions of parameters (prior distributions) are updated (to posterior distributions), as information becomes available, through the use of Bayes' Theorem. Historically, advocates of the Bayesian approach were seen to inhabit a different scientific paradigm that was at odds with the frequentist paradigm such that frequentists considered Bayes methods as subjective and highly dependent on the prior beliefs employed, while frequentist methods were objective and robust. However, the adoption of such an extreme position would be to reject a set of very powerful methods that may be of import, even for frequentists (Carlin and Louis 1996). The empirical Bayes methods and Bayesian analysis based on uninformative prior distributions are not subjective and have much to offer the frequentist analyst. Acceptability curves based on observed data, such as those presented in Figure 8.10, can be given the Bayesian interpretation assuming an uninformative prior distribution (Briggs 1999). Of course, if there is good prior information available on the cost-effectiveness of an intervention, then analysts may want to use this to formulate the prior in a Bayesian analysis.

At present, and most likely in the immediate future, health economists conducting economic analyses alongside clinical trials will have to work within the sample size constraints imposed by clinical investigators. This is likely to generate the situation where important economic differences cannot be detected at conventional levels of power and significance. A number of commentators have suggested that it may be appropriate for economic analysts to work with 'error rates' (in the frequentist sense) that are higher than those employed in clinical evaluation (O'Brien and Drummond 1994; Drummond et al. 1997). This suggestion indicates the desire of economic analysts to consider the weight of evidence relating to the cost-effectiveness of the intervention under evaluation rather than relying on showing significance at conventional levels. This is most easily achieved through the use of cost-effectiveness acceptability curves which show the weight of evidence for the intervention being cost-effective for all possible values of the ceiling ratio, R_c. Furthermore, a Bayesian view of probability allows analysts to directly address the study question: how likely is it that the intervention is cost-effective?

8.5 Probabilistic analysis of cost-effectiveness models

In most cost-effectiveness analyses, costs and outcomes are not directly observed for patients following different treatment pathways. Rather existing evidence is synthesized using a decision-analytic model in order to estimate the costs and health outcome effects of the different treatments under study. These models require information to populate them, and these informational requirements are often referred to as parameters of the model. An analogy with statistical techniques is employed to distinguish between different 'levels' of parameters: those parameters relating to analytic methods (e.g. the discount rate) employed in an evaluation; parameters that describe the characteristics of such a patient sample (e.g. age/sex composition or clinical characteristics such as blood pressure), and parameters that could in principle be sampled if an appropriate study were designed to collect the relevant data.

It has already been argued above (see Section 8.3) that parameters relating to the methods employed in an analysis should be handled through the use of a reference case with supporting univariate sensitivity analyses, and this will be demonstrated in Section 8.6 below.

Characteristics of a patient sample in the model are equivalent to covariates in a statistical analysis. For example, while age will clearly vary across different patients with the same condition, for a given patient age will be a known covariate. It is not appropriate, therefore, to consider age as an 'uncertain' parameter in the model. Rather, the function of a good cost-effectiveness study will be to examine how cost-effectiveness varies across patient characteristics such as age since patients with different demographic and clinical characteristics may well respond differently to treatment and by implication will have different cost-effectiveness ratios for the same treatment. Indeed, commentators have been stressing the importance of clear specification of patient characteristics in cost-effectiveness models for many years, due to the important implications for the cost-effectiveness results (Weinstein and Fineberg 1980; Williams 1985; Pauker and Kassirer 1987). Unfortunately, it is all too common to see known characteristics included in the sensitivity analyses of published economic evaluations.

The remaining parameters of a model will relate to: probabilities (for example conditional probabilities for branching pathways in a model and transition probabilities for movement between model states over time); the resource use and health outcome consequences of the programmes under evaluation; and the data necessary to value those consequences (unit cost/price information for resource use and quality-of-life weights for cost-utility analyses). Having carefully specified parameters relating to the characteristics of the patient group to which the results of the cost-effectiveness analysis will apply, these remaining parameters could, in principle, be estimated by sampling from patients with the specified characteristics.

In traditional sensitivity analyses analysts tend to report a range of values for parameters in their model and use this range to consider the effect of altering a parameter value either individually (a univariate sensitivity analysis) or in combination with others (in a multivariate analysis). More recently, however, there has been increasing interest in the methods of probabilistic sensitivity analysis (PSA),(Doubilet *et al.* 1985; Critchfield *et al.* 1986) as a method for handling uncertainty in CE models (O'Brien *et al.* 1994; Manning *et al.* 1996; Briggs 2000). In PSA, each parameter is assigned a distribution, and cost-effectiveness results associated with simultaneously selecting random values from those distributions are recorded in a Monte Carlo simulation of the model.

In this section, the focus is on this PSA approach to handling uncertainty in cost-effectiveness models. First, consideration is given to how distributions can be selected to represent uncertainty in parameters that could, in principle, be sampled with an emphasis on the appeal of a Bayesian approach. Next, an example of a cost-effectiveness model for beta-blocker therapy is outlined. Finally, some general considerations for cost-effectiveness modelling are outlined.

8.5.1 **Choosing distributions for parameters**

Very often, although a clinical trial may not be the primary source of data for a stochastic economic evaluation, trials and other forms of investigation may provide important patient level data on particular parameters (e.g. effectiveness of a drug in reducing clinical events) of the cost-effectiveness model. Therefore it is natural to describe the uncertainty in that parameter using the same distributional assumptions that underlie the calculation of a confidence limit in a standard statistical analysis.

Note that in standard statistical methods (such as practised in almost all clinical trials) parameters to be estimated from the data are considered to have true values and do not vary. Probabilities attached to confidence limits relate to long-run coverage probabilities of the intervals, were the same experiment to be repeated many times. In modelling the cost-effectiveness of interventions in a PSA, this approach is not taken. Parameters are considered as random variables, which can take a range of values defined by the chosen distribution. Such an approach is inherently Bayesian in nature. Explicit recognition of this fact allows analysts to exploit the existing Bayesian methodology in a way that is entirely consistent with the aims of a modelling-based CEA. Eddy and colleagues have outlined just such an approach to synthesizing data based on empirical Bayes methods that they term the 'confidence' profile technique (Eddy *et al.* 1990a, b) for health technology assessment and such methods are beginning to be applied to CEA modelling (Sendi *et al.* 1999;) (Fryback *et al.*, 2001). Attempting PSA within a Bayesian framework in order to choose distributions for parameters should lead to more defensible assumptions than without adopting a Bayesian approach. For example, the problem of describing a continuous distribution for a probability over the range zero-one when existing data are available has a straightforward Bayesian solution based on statistical theory of the Beta–Binomial relationship (Gelman *et al.* 1995). By contrast, without the benefit of Bayesian methods, solutions to the same problem appear rather ad hoc (Lord & Asante 1999; Pasta *et al.* 1999).

Note that distributions are chosen to represent uncertainty in the parameter of interest – known as second-order uncertainty – rather than variability in the underlying population from which the sample is drawn – which is known as first-order uncertainty (Stinnett and Paltiel 1997). This distinction between first- and second-order uncertainty becomes important when we consider how to handle uncertainty when sample data do not exist for the parameter of interest. In the absence of data from which to estimate a parameter we know to be important for a model, we are left with having to estimate that parameter by other means. Usually this will involve some form of review of the literature and/or consultation with medical experts. Where feasible, a number of experts should be consulted in order that the prior distribution employed in the final analysis reflects uncertainty between experts as to the distribution of the unknown parameter rather than representing the subjective beliefs of a single expert.

In summary, for those parameters of a cost-effectiveness model that could, in principle, be estimated from observed data, consideration should be given to the prior distribution of these parameters to reflect uncertainty. Where possible, this should be based on the available data from studies supplemented where necessary by expert opinion. The specified prior distributions should relate to second-order uncertainty rather than the variability between individual patients and care should be taken to ensure that the prior distributions chosen are consistent with any logical bounds on the parameter values.

In specifying prior distributions, it will be important to consider the level of generalizability required for the model. Generalizability relates to the setting of the study: for a given population of patients would the resource use and health outcome consequences observed in one hospital, region or country be replicated in other locations? This area of uncertainty is linked to known variations in clinical practice within and between countries (Wennberg and Gittelsohn 1982; Andersen and Mooney 1990; Cleary *et al.* 1991). Note that generalizability relating to setting is essentially data-driven, in that this issue can be handled by relating the specification of prior distributions to the scope of the evaluation. For example, an evaluation of a proposed national screening programme should include prior distributions for unit costs/resource use that reflect the variation between clinical centres in different parts of the country. By contrast, an evaluation of an intervention designed to inform a particular institution might have very little variation in the prior distributions related to unit costs if that institution is able to provide accurate information on those costs. These examples emphasize how cost-effectiveness modelling might be made much more dynamic than a single publication summarizing the results of a study would suggest.

8.5.2 Modelling the cost-effectiveness of beta-blockers for CHF

In order to illustrate a Bayesian approach to CEA modelling an example of a probabilistic analysis of beta-blocker treatment for congestive heart failure (CHF) is employed. A brief introduction to the model follows, full details of the model can be found elsewhere (Levy *et al.* 2001; Briggs *et al.*, 2001). For the purposes of illustration we focus on the choice of distribution for key parameters of the model and the analysis of the results. The original article contains a complete account of the cost-effectiveness estimates including the sensitivity of the results to key assumptions concerning the duration of treatment effect (Levy *et al.* 2001).

The use of beta-blocker therapy has recently been shown to be effective in reducing mortality in patients with CHF (Heidenreich *et al.* 1997; Avezum *et al.* 1998; Lechat *et al.* 1998). A recently published US study estimated the cost-effectiveness of a proprietary beta-blocker employing a Markov model to synthesize data from clinical trials of mortality benefit together with estimated costs of therapy and other treatment costs of CHF (Delea *et al.* 1999). However, generic beta-blocker therapy is also available and emerging evidence suggests that some generics may also reduce mortality at a fraction of the cost. In order to examine the relative cost-effectiveness of beta-blockers for CHF in Canada, a model was developed following the structure of previous models (Paul *et al.* 1994; Delea *et al.* 1999), but updated to include Canadian prices and to include a generic as well as the proprietary beta-blocker. A meta-analysis of the literature on the mortality effects of the two compounds was undertaken to

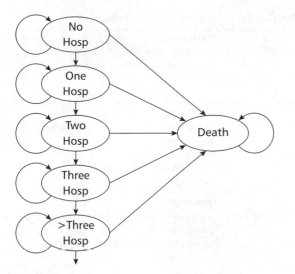

Fig. 8.13 Markov model of congestive heart failure. States are shown as ovals and transitions between states as arrows. 'Hosp' is the abbreviation for hospitalizations

estimate the relative risk reduction for each model. Benefits were estimated as life years gained from treatment.

The Markov model is presented in Figure 8.13. Patients are classified by the number of CHF hospitalizations which are represented by different Markov states since patients' hospitalization history is assumed to influence future risk of hospitalization, and therefore, death.

The choice of prior distributions

The model involves four basic types of parameters: absolute risks of death and hospitalization among patients not receiving beta-blocker therapy; relative risks of death and hospitalization among patients receiving beta-blocker therapy; resource events; and unit costs of resource events. Table 8.4 shows the description of the parameters and the assumed distributions for the CHF model. Absolute risks were assumed to follow a beta distribution, which is constrained on the interval zero-one. Relative risks were assumed to be normally distributed on the log scale, with the measure of variance estimated directly from the random-effects meta-analysis conducted as part of the original study. The average number of resource events was assumed to have a Gamma distribution, with coefficient of variation equal to 0.4. Finally unit costs were assumed to have a normal distribution again with coefficient of variation equal to 0.4.[16]

---

[16] Since no information was available on variance of mean resource event or unit cost the coefficient of variation was used to relate the variance to the mean value. Although 0.4 is an arbitrary value, it was chosen to give quite a large variance, and therefore, vague prior for the resource use and unit cost parameters.

Table 8.4 Distributional assumptions for the parameters in the CHF model

PdieHosp			**PDieHome**	
Probability of dying in hospital at age 45			*Probability of dying at home at age 45*	
Beta distribution with parameters:			Beta distribution with parameters:	
alpha	244		alpha	183
beta	1791		beta	1852

LnRRdieM			**LnRRhospM**	
Log of relative of death on Metoprolol			*Log of relative risk of hospitalization on Metroprolol*	
Normal distribution with parameters:			Normal distribution with parameters:	
Mean	−0.35		Mean	−0.68
SE	0.10		SE	0.43

LnRRdieC			**LnRRhospC**	
Log of the relative risk of death on Carvedilol			*Log of the relative risk of hospitalization on Carvedilol*	
Normal distribution with parameters:			Normal distribution with parameters:	
Mean	−0.58		Mean	−0.41
SE	0.19		SE	0.17

IpHosp45			**cpHosp23**	
Probability of initial hospitalization at age 45			*Probability of third hospitalization*	
Beta distribution with parameters:			Beta distribution with parameters:	
alpha	251		alpha	95
beta	1784		beta	270

CpHosp12			**cpHosp34**	
Probability of second hospitalization			*Probability of four or more hospitalizations*	
Beta distribution with parameters:			Beta distribution with parameters:	
alpha	288		alpha	36
beta	1768		beta	70

los45			**ucIPday**	
length of stay in hospital at age 45			*unit cost of an inpatient day*	
Gamma distribution with parameters:			Normal distribution with parameters:	
mean	9		mean	675.5
se	0.342		se	67.5

NGPvisists			**ucGPvisit**	
Number of visits to a GP per cycle			*Unit cost of a GP visit*	
Gamma distribution with:			Normal distribution with parameters:	
mean	0.333		mean	674.5
se	0.167		se	67.5

NOPvisitsH	**ucOPvisit**			
Outpatient visits following hospitalization			*Unit cost of an outpatient visit*	
Gamma distribution with:			Normal distribution with parameters:	
mean	3		mean	674.5
se	1.5		se	67.5

NOPvisitsM		
Outpatient visits for monitoring disease		
Gamma distribution with parameters:		
mean	0.167	
se	0.083	

Note that some parameters of the model were not given a distribution. For example, discount rates as methodological variables were not handled probabilistically. In addition, the prices of the drug treatments under evaluation were kept fixed at the current formulary reimbursement rates.

Results from the probabilistic analysis of the CHF model

Having chosen the distributions for the parameters of the model, values were selected from each of the distributions at random and the costs and life years associated with each of the treatment options evaluated. This process was repeated 1000 times and the results are presented on the CE plane in Figure 8.14. The results show that there is a clear difference in cost between the generic and the proprietary beta-blocker. While favouring the proprietary drug treatment, the difference in effectiveness between the two compounds is less clear. At baseline, the cost-effectiveness of a generic beta-blocker over no treatment was Can$4,100 per life year gained. The incremental cost-effectiveness of the proprietary beta-blocker over the generic is Can$8,400 per life year gained. Note that the slopes of the lines on the cost-effectiveness plane joining the treatment options are equal to the appropriate ICERs and define a cost-effectiveness frontier.

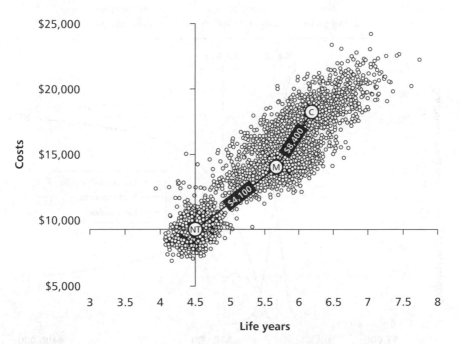

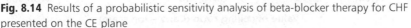

Fig. 8.14 Results of a probabilistic sensitivity analysis of beta-blocker therapy for CHF presented on the CE plane

Notes: NT – no therapy; M – generic beta-blocker; C – proprietary beta-blocker

The treatment choice from among the three options available depends on the willingness to pay for life years gained, together with attitudes to uncertainty. For each of the 1000 simulation results a similar cost-effectiveness frontier could be estimated. If the critical value of the ceiling ratio, R_c, were known then it would be possible to say for each simulation which treatment option was preferred. Therefore results illustrated on the cost-effectiveness plane can be summarized using cost-effectiveness acceptability curves by estimating the probability that the treatment is cost-effective as the proportion of times the treatment is preferred from the results of the 1000 simulations. This is illustrated in Figure 8.15. Since the choice is now between three treatment options rather than two alternatives (as was the case in the previous examples), curves for all three treatment options (no beta-blocker, generic beta-blocker, or proprietary beta-blocker) are shown. Note that at any point the probability is shared between the three treatments such that the sum of the three curves is equal to one.

The results in Figure 8.15 show that the acceptability curves intersect at the point estimates of cost-effectiveness. The favoured option shown in the figure defines ranges of the ceiling ratio over which each treatment is the treatment of choice in more than 50 per cent of the simulation results. Of course, to simply take these ranges as sufficient for decision-making would be to ignore substantial uncertainty.

The no beta-blocker curve is tending to zero emphasizing that the prediction of the model is that beta-blocker therapy is more effective than no therapy (in fact the model

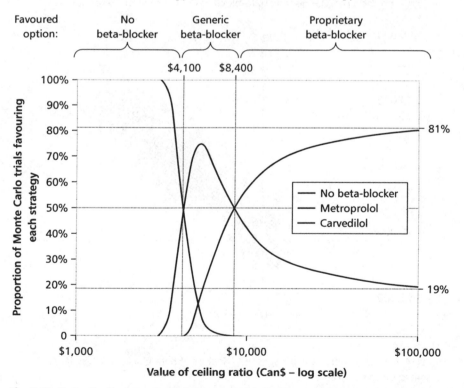

Fig. 8.15 Cost-effectiveness acceptability curves for the three treatment options for CHF

prediction is that beta-blocker therapy is significantly more effective at conventional levels if the ceiling ratio is greater than approximately Can$4,600/LYG). The generic and proprietary beta-blocker curves are tending to 0.19 and 0.81 respectively, reflecting that although the proprietary beta-blocker is predicted to be more effective, this difference is not significant at the conventional level. Whether there is sufficient evidence to justify expenditure on the more expensive beta-blocker is clearly a difficult decision, but at least the information in Figure 8.15 presents the uncertainty clearly.

8.6 Non-sampling uncertainty

Sections 8.4 and 8.5 have been concerned with estimating second-order uncertainty in cost-effectiveness analyses, that is, uncertainty arising due to sampling variation, either directly in a stochastic evaluation or indirectly in the parameters of a CE model. However, it was emphasized in Section 8.3 that there are other forms of uncertainty that arise in economic evaluation, not simply sampling variation. In particular, it was argued that a reference case of methods should be employed by analysts to improve comparability between studies. This sort of uncertainty is best handled employing univariate sensitivity analysis for the changing of assumptions combined with an acceptability curve for each underlying set of methods employed.

Just such an approach was taken by the UK prospective diabetes study group (Raikou *et al.* 1998) when looking at uncertainty in the cost-effectiveness of tight versus less tight control of blood pressure in diabetics with hypertension. Figure 8.16 shows the results of their analysis presented as cost-effectiveness acceptability curves. The base-case shows an acceptability curve under the UK Treasury's approved discount rate of 6 per cent for both costs and health outcomes. Two further curves are presented showing the effect of reducing both discount rates to 3 per cent (as recommended by the US panel on cost-effectiveness) and employing differential discounting (currently being considered by UK National Institute of Clinical Effectiveness (NICE) as a baseline requirement for submissions).

It was also emphasized in Section 8.2 that in modelling cost-effectiveness there is likely to be uncertainty related to the process of modelling. In particular assumptions concerning the specific form of relationships between parameters such as the functional form of a hazard function or a dose-response relationship. In Section 8.5, it was argued that decision models are fundamentally Bayesian in that parameters are ascribed distributions. However, in arriving at those distributions the approach adopted was empirically based with data collection informing the distributional assumptions that were designed to capture second order uncertainty related to sampling variation. Where expert opinion is required (i.e. when data are lacking), it was recommended that distributions reflect the disagreement between experts rather than being based on the subjective notions of just one expert.

However, the Bayesian approach is more widely applicable since the Bayesian notion of probability can be applied to events that have no long run frequency interpretation. Hence, if there are more than one possible formulations of a hazard function, for example, it is possible within a Bayesian framework to run the analysis under different assumptions concerning the hazard function and then to assign degrees of belief (in coherent fashion) to each model in order to give an overall estimate of

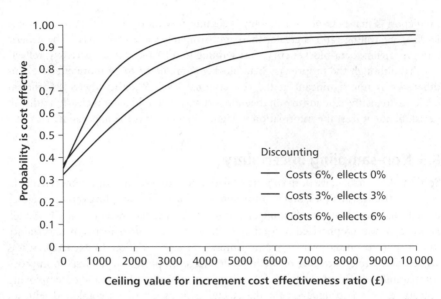

Fig. 8.16 Cost-effectiveness of tight versus less tight control of blood pressure in diabetic with hypertension. Reproduced with permission from Raikou *et al.* 1998, BMJ Publishing Group.

uncertainty that includes the functional form of the hazard function (together with other examples of process uncertainty). This approach has been demonstrated by Draper for problems as diverse as the prediction of Oil prices and predicting the space shuttle disaster (Draper 1995).

8.7 Summary

This chapter provided a comprehensive overview of methods for handling uncertainty in cost-effectiveness analyses. Uncertainty in economic evaluation is pervasive and takes a number of different forms. Since cost-effectiveness analysis is essentially a comparative approach to economic evaluation, a reference case of methods should be adopted by analysts to improve comparability between studies. Such an approach has been argued by the US panel on cost-effectiveness analysis, although it is likely that different decision-making organizations may want to adopt a different reference case for evaluations in their jurisdictions. Where economic analyses are conducted alongside clinical trials it may be possible to summarize uncertainty due to sampling variation using confidence intervals. It is clear that Fieller's theorem and the non-parametric approach of bootstrapping give the most accurate intervals of the available methods. However, analysts should be aware of the problems for representing uncertainty in cost-effectiveness analysis when uncertainty covers multiple quadrants of the CE plane. The net-benefit framework and the use of cost-effectiveness acceptability curves are important contributions to this area in that they overcome these problems and information can be presented in terms of the evidence in favour of the original hypothesis. While this necessitates a Bayesian interpretation of probability, this should not necessarily be seen as adopting a subjective approach to analysis. Principles of

Bayesian analysis can also be applied to choosing distributions for parameters in a CE modelling framework to summarize uncertainty. Repeated simulation from the distributions of the parameters of a decision model allow a probabilistic analysis of CE models and acceptability curves can be obtained in a similar way to stochastic analyses. Acceptability curves are also a convenient way in which to present uncertainty for greater than two mutually exclusive options and multiple curves can be used to present uncertainty not related to sampling variation.

Acknowledgements

I am grateful to many people for contributions to my understanding of the issues raised in this chapter. In particular, Alastair Gray, Bernie O'Brien, Paul Fenn and Mark Sculpher have all been important influences. Adrian Levy and Alistair McGuire provided detailed feedback on earlier drafts. All views and remaining errors are my own responsibility.

References

Altman, D. G. and Bland, J. M. (1995). Absence of evidence is not evidence of absence. *British Medical Journal*, 311(7003), 485.

Andersen, T. F. and Mooney, G. (1990). *The challenge of medical practice variations*. Macmillan, Basingstoke.

Anderson, J. P., Bush, J. W., Chen, M. *et al.* (1986). Policy space areas and properties of benefit-cost/utility analysis. *Journal of the American Medical Association*, 255(6), 794–5.

Armitage, P. and Berry, G. (1994). *Statistical methods in medical research*. 3rd edn. Blackwell Scientific Publications, Oxford.

Avezum, A., Tsuyuki, R. T., Pogue, J. *et al.* (1998). Beta-blocker therapy for congestive heart failure: a systemic overview and critical appraisal of the published trials. *Canadian Journal of Cardiology*, 14(8),1045–53.

Birch, S. and Gafni, A. (1992). Cost-effectiveness/utility analyses. Do current decision rules lead us to where we want to be? *Journal of Health Economics*, 11, 279–96.

Birch, S. and Gafni, A. (1993). Changing the problem to fit the solution: Johannesson and Weinstein's (mis) application of economics to real world problems. *Journal of Health Economics*, 12, 469–76.

Black, W. C. (1990). The CE plane: A graphic representation of cost-effectiveness. *Medical Decision-Making*, 10, 212–14.

Bland, J. M. and Altman, D. G. (1998). Bayesians and frequentists. *British Medical Journal*, 317(7166), 1151–60.

Briggs, A. H. (1999). A Bayesian approach to stochastic cost-effectiveness analysis. *Health Economics*, 8(3),

Briggs, A. H. (2000). Handling uncertainty in cost-effectiveness models. *PharmacoEconomics*, 17, 479–500.

Briggs, A., Sculpher, M. and Buxton, M. (1994). Uncertainty in the economic evaluation of health care technologies: the role of sensitivity analysis. *Health Economics*, 3(2), 95–104.

Briggs, A. and Gray, A. (1998). The distribution of health care costs and their statistical analysis for economic evaluation. *Journal of Health Services Research and Policy*.

Briggs, A. H., Wonderling, D. E. and Mooney, C. Z. (1997). Pulling cost-effectiveness analysis up by its bootstraps: a non-parametric approach to confidence interval estimation. *Health Economics*, 6(4), 327–40.

Briggs, A. H. and Fenn, P. (1998). Confidence intervals or surfaces? Uncertainty on the cost-effectiveness plane. *Health Economics*, 7(8), 723–740.

Briggs, A. H. and Gray, A.M. (1999). Handling uncertainty when performing economic evaluation of health care interventions. *Health Technology Assessment*, 3(2), pp.134.

Briggs, A. H., Mooney, C. Z. and Wonderling, D. E. (1999). Constructing confidence intervals for cost-effectiveness ratios: an evaluation of parametric and non-parametric techniques using Monte Carlo simulation. *Stat.Med.*, 18(23), 3245–62.

Briggs, A. H. and O'Brien, B. J. (2001). The death of cost-minimisation analysis? *Health Economics*, 10(2), 179–184.

Briggs, A. H., Levy, A. R. and O'Brien, B. J. (2001). Building probabilistic cost-effectiveness models: the case of beta-blockers for heart failure. Abstract submitted to Society for Medical Decision Making Conference, 2001.

Brouwer, W., van Hout, B. and Rutten, F. (2000). A fair approach to discounting future effects: taking a societal perspective. *J. Health Serv. Policy*, 5, 114–18.

Brouwer, W. B., Koopmanschap, M. A. and Rutten, F. F. (1997a). Productivity costs measurement through quality-of-life? A response to the recommendation of the Washington Panel. *Health Economics*, 6(3), 253–9.

Brouwer, W. B., Koopmanschap, M. A. and Rutten, F. F. (1997b). Productivity costs in cost-effectiveness analysis: numerator or denominator: a further discussion [comment]. *Health Economics*, 6(5), 511–14.

Buxton, M. J., Drummond, M. F., van Hout, B. A. *et al.* (1997). Modelling in economic evaluation: an unavoidable fact of life. *Health Economics*, 6, 217–27.

Cairns, J. (1992). Discounting and health benefits: another perspective. *Health Economics*, 1(1), 76–9.

Carlin, R.P. and Louis, A. T. (1996). *Bayes and empirical Bayes methods for data analysis.* Chapman & Hall, London.

Chapman, R .H., Stone, P. W., Sandberg, E. A. *et al.* (2000). A comprehensive league table of cost-utility ratios and a sub-table of "panel-worthy" studies. *Med. Decis. Making*, 20, 451–67.

Chaudhary, M. A. and Stearns, S. C. (1996). Estimating confidence intervals for cost-effectiveness ratios: An example from a randomised trial. *Statistics in Medicine*, 15, 1447–58.

Claxton, K. (1999). The irrelevance of inference: a decision-making approach to the stochastic evaluation of health care technologies. *Journal of Health Economics*, 18(3), 341–64.

Claxton, K. and Posnett, J. (1996). An economic approach to clinical trial design and research priority-setting. *Health Economics*, 5(6), 513–24.

Cleary, P. D., Greenfield, S., Mulley, A. G. *et al.* (1991). Variations in length of stay and outcomes for six medical and surgical conditions in Massachusetts and California. *Journal of the American Medical Association*, 266(1), 73–9.

Cochran, W. G. (1977). *Sampling techniques.* John Wiley & Sons, New York.

Cook, J. and Heyse, J.F. (2000). Use of angular transformation for ratio estimation in cost-effectiveness analysis. *Statistics in medicine*, 19, 2989–3003.

Coyle, D. and Tolley, K. (1992). Discounting of health benefits in the pharmacoeconomic analysis of drug therapies. *PharmacoEconomics*, 2(2), 153–62.

Critchfield, G. C., Willard, K. E. and Connelly, D. P. (1986). Probabilistic sensitivity analysis methods for general decision models. *Computers and Biomedical Research*, 19, 254–65.

Delea, T. E., Vera, L. M., Richner, R. E., et al. (1999). Cost-effectiveness of carvedilol for heart failure. American Journal of Cardiology, 83(6), 890–6.

Donaldson, C. (1990). Willingness to pay for publicly-provided goods: A possible measure of benefit. Journal of Health Economics, 9, 103–18.

Doubilet, P., Begg, C.B. and Weinstein, M.C., Braun, P. and McNeil, B.J. (1985). Probabilistic sensitivity analysis using Monte Carlo simulation. A practical approach. Medical Decision-Making, 5, 157–77.

Draper, D. (1995). Assessment and propagation of model uncertainty. Journal of the Royal Statistical Society, Series B, 57(1), 45–97.

Drummond, M., Brandt, A., Luce, B. et al. (1993). Standardising methodologies for economic evaluation in health care. Practice, problems, and potential. International Journal of Technology Assessment in Health Care, 9(1), 26–36.

Drummond, M. F., O'Brien, B., Stoddart, G. L. et al. (1997). Methods for the economic evaluation of health care programmes. 2nd edn. Oxford University Press, Oxford.

Eddy, D. M., Hasselblad, V. and Shachter, R. (1990a). A Bayesian method for synthesizing evidence. The Confidence Profile Method. International Journal of Technology Assessment in Health Care, 6(1), 31–55.

Eddy, D.M., Hasselblad, V. and Shachter, R. (1990b). An introduction to a Bayesian method for meta-analysis: The confidence profile method. Medical Decision-Making, 10(1), 15–23.

Efron, B. and Gong, G. (1993). A leisurely look at the Bootstrap, the Jackknife, and cross-validation. The American Statistician, 37(1), 36–48.

Efron, B. and Tibshirani, R. (1993). An introduction to the bootstrap. Chapman & Hall, New York.

Etzioni, R., Ramsey, S. D., Berry, K. et al. (2001). The impact of including future medical care costs when estimating the costs attributable to a disease: a colorectal cancer case study. Health Econ., 10, 245–56.

Felli, J. C. and Hazen, G. B. (1998). Sensitivity analysis and the expected value of perfect information. Medical Decision-Making, 18(1), 95–109.

Fieller, E. C. (1932). The distribution of an index in a normal bivariate population. Biometrika, 56, 635–9.

Fieller, E. C. (1954). Some problems in interval estimation. Journal of the Royal Statistical Society, Series B, 16, 175–83.

Freiman, J. A., Chalmers, T. C., Smith, H. Jr. et al. (1978). The importance of beta, the type II error and sample size in the design and interpretation of the randomised control trial. Survey of 71 'negative' trials. New England Journal of Medicine, 299(13), 690–4.

Fryback, D. G., Chinnis, J. O. and Ulvila, J. W. (2001). Bayesian cost-effectiveness analysis. An example using the GUSTO trial. International Journal of Technology Assessment in Health Care 17(1), 83–97.

Gafni, A. and Birch, S. (1993). Guidelines for the adoption of new technologies: a prescription for uncontrolled growth in expenditures and how to avoid the problem. Canadian Medical Association Journal, 148(6), 913–17.

Garber, A. M. and Phelps, C. E. (1997). Economic foundations of cost-effectiveness analysis. J. Health Econ. 16, 1–31.

Gardner, M. J. and Altman, D. G. (1989). Estimation rather than hypothesis testing: confidence intervals rather than P values. In: M. J. Gardner, D. G. Altman (eds). Statistics with confidence. BMJ, London.

Gelman, A., Carlin, J. B., Stern, H. S. et al. (1995). Bayesian data analysis. London: Chaapman & Hall.

Gold, M. R., Siegel, J. E., Russell, L. B. *et al*. (1996). *Cost-effectiveness in health and medicine.* Oxford University Press, New York.

Heidenreich, P. A., Lee, T. T. and Massie, B. M. (1997). Effect of beta-blockade on mortality in patients with heart failure: a meta-analysis of randomised clinical trials. *J.Am.Coll.Cardiol.,* 30(1), 27–34.

Heitjan, D. F. (2000). Fieller's method and net health benefits. *Health Economics,* 9(4), 327–35.

Heitjan, D. F., Moskowitz, A. J. and Whang, W. (1999). Problems with interval estimates of the incremental cost-effectiveness ratio. *Med. Decis. Making,* 19, 9–15.

Heitjan, D. F., Moskowitz, A. J. and Whang, W. (1999). Bayesian estimation of cost-effectiveness ratios from clinical trials. *Health Economics,* 8(3), 191–201.

HM Treasury. (1997). *Appraisal and evaluation in central government.* HMSO, London.

van Hout, B. A., Al, M. J., Gordon, G. S. *et al*. (1994). Costs, effects and C/E-ratios alongside a clinical trial. *Health Economics,* 3(5), 309–19.

Johannesson, M. and Weinstein, M. C. (1993). On the decision rules of cost-effectiveness analysis. *Journal of Health Economics,* 12, 459–67.

Johnston, K., Buxton, M. J., Jones, D. R. *et al*. (1999). Assessing the costs of healthcare technologies in clinical trials. *Health Technology Assessment,* 3(6), p. 76.

Katz, D. A. and Welch, H. G. (1993). Discounting in cost-effectiveness analysis of healthcare programs. *PharmacoEconomics,* 3(4), 276–85.

Koopmanschap, M. A., Rutten, F. F. H., Van Ineveld, B. M. *et al*. (1995). The friction cost method for measuring indirect costs of disease. *Journal of Health Economics,* 14, 171–89.

Koopmanschap, M. A. and Rutten, F. F. H. (1996). Indirect costs: the consequence of production loss or increased costs of production. *Medical Care,* 34(12 Suppl), DS59–DS68.

Laska, E., Meisner, M. and Siegel, C. (1997). Statistical inference for cost-effectiveness ratios. *Health Economics,* 6, 229–42.

Laupacis, A., Feeny, D., Detsky, A. S. *et al*. (1992). How attractive does a new technology have to be to warrant adoption and utilisation? Tentative guidelines for using clinical and economic evaluations. *Canadian Medical Association Journal,* 146(4), 473–81.

Lechat, P., Packer, M., Chalon, S. *et al*. (1998). Clinical effects of beta-adrenergic blockade in chronic heart failure: a meta-analysis of double-blind, placebo-controlled, randomised trials. *Circulation,* 98(12), 1184–91.

Levy, A. R., Briggs, A. H., O'Brien, B. J. *et al*. (2001). Cost-effectiveness of carvedilol and Metoprolol for treatment of persons with congestive heart failure. *American Heart Journal.* (in press)

Lipscomb, J. (1996). The proper role for discounting: search in progress. *Med. Care,* 34, DS119-DS123.

Lipscomb, J., Weinstein, M.C. and Torrance, G.W. (1996). Time Preference. In: Gold, M.R., Siegel, J.E., Russell, L.B. and Weinstein, M.C., (Eds.). *Cost-effectiveness in health and medicine.* Oxford University Press, New York, pp. 214–46

Lord, J. and Asante, M. A. (1999). Estimating uncertainty ranges for costs by the bootstrap procedure combined with probabilistic sensitivity analysis. *Health Economics,* 8(4), 323–33.

Löthgren, M. and Zethraeus, N. (1999). *On the interpretation of cost-effectiveness acceptability curves.* Working Paper Series in Economics and Finance No.323. Stockholm School of Economics.

Luce, B. R. and Claxton, K. (1999). Redefining the analytical approach to pharmacoeconomics (editorial). *Health Economics,* 8(3), 187–9.

Manning, W. G., Fryback, D. G. and Weinstein, M. C. (1996). Reflecting uncertainty in cost-effectiveness analysis. In: M. R. Gold, J. E. Siegel, L. B. Russell and M. C. Weinstein (eds). *Cost-effectiveness in health and medicine.* Oxford University Press, New York.

Mehrez, A. and Gafni, A. (1989). Quality-adjusted life years, utility theory, and healthy-years equivalents. *Medical Decision-Making,* 9, 142–9.

Meltzer, D. (1997). Accounting for future costs in medical cost-effectiveness analysis. *J.Health Econ.,* 16, 33–64.

Mullahy, J. and Manning, W. G. (1995). Statistical issues in cost-effectiveness analyses. In F. A. Sloan (ed.) *Valuing health care.* Cambridge University Press, Cambridge.

Mullahy, J. (1996). What you don't know can't hurt you? Statistical issues and standards for medical technology evaluation. *Medical Care,* 34(12), DS124-DS135.

Obenchain, R. L., Melfi, C. A., Croghan, T. W. *et al.* D. P. (1997). Bootstrap analyses of cost-effectiveness in antidepressant pharmacotherapy. *PharmacoEconomics,* 11, 464–72.

O'Brien, B. J. and Drummond, M. F. (1994). Statistical versus quantitative significance in the socioeconomic evaluation of medicines. *PharmacoEconomics,* 5(5), 389–98.

O'Brien, B. J., Drummond, M. F., Labelle, R. J. *et al.* (1994). In search of power and significance: issues in the design and analysis of stochastic cost-effectiveness studies in health care. *Medical Care,* 32(2), 150–63.

O'Hagan, A., Stevens, J. W. and Montmartin, J. (2000). Inference for the C/E acceptability curve and C/E ratio. *PharmacoEconomics,* 17, 339–49.

Palmer, S. and Smith, P. (2000). Incorporating option values into the economic evaluation of health care technologies. *Journal of Health Economics* 19, 755–66.

Parsonage, M. and Neuburger, H. (1992). Discounting and health benefits. *Health Economics,* 1(1), 71–6.

Pasta, D. J., Taylor, J. L. and Henning, J. M. (1999). Probabilistic sensitivity analysis incorporating the bootstrap: an example comparing treatments for the eradication of Helicobacter pylori. *Medical Decision-Making,* 19(3), 353–63.

Pauker, S. G. and Kassirer, J. P. (1987). Decision analysis. *New England Journal of Medicine,* 316(5), 250–8.

Paul, S. D., Kuntz, K. M., Eagle, K. A. *et al.* (1994). Costs and effectiveness of angiotensin converting enzyme inhibition in patients with congestive heart failure. *Archives of Internal Medicine,* 154(10), 1143–9.

Polsky, D., Glick, H. A., Willke, R. *et al.* (1997). Confidence intervals for cost-effectiveness ratios: a comparison of four methods. *Health Economics,* 6, 243–52.

Posnett, J. and Jan, S. (1996). Indirect cost in economic evaluation: the opportunity cost of unpaid inputs. *Health Economics,* 5(1), 13–23.

Pritchard, C. (1998). *Trends in economic evaluation.* Office of Health Economics Briefing Paper No. 36: London.

Raikou, M., Briggs, A., Gray, A. *et al.* (2000). Centre-specific or average unit costs in multi-centre studies? Some theory and simulation. *Health Economics,* 9(3), 191–8.

Raikou, M., Gray, A., Briggs, A. *et al.* (1998). Cost-effectiveness analysis of improved blood pressure control in hypertensive patients with type 2 diabetes: UKPDS 40. *British Medical Journal,* 317, 720–6.

Rittenhouse, B. E., Dulisse, B. and Stinnett, A. A. (1999). At what price significance? The effect of price estimates on statistical inference in economic evaluation. *Health Economics,* 8(3), 213–19.

Russell, L. B. (1986). *Is prevention better than cure?* The Brookings Institution, Washington, DC.

Ryan, M. (1999). Using conjoint analysis to take account of patient preferences and go beyond health outcomes: an application to in vitro fertilisation. *Social Science and Medicine*, 48(4), 535–46.

Sendi, P. P., Craig, B. A., Meier, G. *et al.* (1999). Cost-effectiveness of azithromycin for preventing Mycobacterium avium complex infection in HIV-positive patients in the era of highly active antiretroviral therapy. The Swiss HIV Cohort Study. *Journal of Antimicrobial Chemotherapy*, 44(6), 811–7.

Stinnett, A. (1996). Adjusting for bias in C/E ratio estimates. *Health Economics*, 5, 470–2. Stinnett, A. A. and Mullahy, J. (1998). Net health benefits: a new framework for the analysis of uncertainty in cost-effectiveness analysis. *Medical Decision-Making*, 18(2), S65-S80.

Stinnett, A. A. and Paltiel, A. D. (1997). Estimating CE ratios under second-order uncertainty: the mean ratio versus the ratio of means. *Medical Decision-Making*, 17(4), 483–9.

Stone, P. W., Chapman, R. H., Sandberg, E. A. *et al.* (2000). Measuring costs in cost-utility analyses. Variations in the literature. *International Journal of Technology Assessment in Health Care*, 16(1), 111–24.

Tambour, M. and Zethraeus, N. (1998). Bootstrap confidence intervals for cost-effectiveness ratios: some simulation results (comment). *Health Economics*, 7(2), 143–7.

Tambour, M., Zethraeus, N. and Johannesson, M. (1998). A note on confidence intervals in cost-effectiveness analysis. *International Journal of Technology Assessment in Health Care*, 14(3), 467–71.

Torrance, G.W. (1986). Measurement of health state utilities for economic appraisal: A review. *Journal of Health Economics*, 5, 1–30.

Wakker, P. and Klaassen, M. (1995). Confidence intervals for cost-effectiveness ratios. *Health Economics*, 4(5), 373–82.

Weinstein, M. C., Siegel, J. E., Garber, A. M., Lipscomb, J., Luce, B. R., Manning-W. G. and Torrance, G. W. (1997). Productivity costs, time costs and health-related quality-of-life: a response to the Erasmus Group. *Health Economics*, 6(5), 505–10.

Weinstein, M. C. (1995). From cost-effectiveness ratios to resource allocation: where to draw the line? In: F.A. Sloan, (ed.) *Valuing health care*. Cambridge University Press, Cambridge.

Weinstein, M. C. and Fineberg, H. V. (1980). *Clinical decision analysis*. W. B. Saunders Company, Philadelphia, PA.

Wennberg, J. and Gittelsohn, A. (1982). Variations in medical care in small areas. *Scientific American*, 4, 120–4.

Willan, A. R. and O'Brien, B. J. (1996). Confidence intervals for cost-effectiveness ratios: an application of Fieller's theorem. *Health Economics*, 5, 297–305.

Williams, A. (1985). Economics of coronary artery bypass grafting. *Br.Med.J.Clin.Res.Ed.*, 291(6491), 326–9.

Willke, R. J., Glick, H. A., Polsky, D. *et al.* (1998). Estimating country-specific cost-effectiveness from multinational clinical trials. *Health Economics*, 7(6), 481–93.

Zethraeus, N. and Löthgren, M. (2000). On the equivalence of the net benefit and the Fieller's methods for statistical inference in cost-effectiveness analysis. SSE/EFI Working Paper Series in Economics and Finance No.379. Stockholm School of Economics.

Zhou, X. H., Melfi, C. A. and Hui, S. L. (1997). Methods for comparison of cost data. *Annals of Internal Medicine*, 127(8 Pt 2), 752–6.

Chapter 9

Statistical considerations in analysing health care resource utilization and cost data

Joseph F. Heyse, John R. Cook and
George W. Carides

9.1 Introduction

Much attention has recently focused on statistical methods for assessing uncertainty in health economic evaluations. Uncertainty in the estimate of programme costs and effects arises from two primary sources. The first is uncertainty in assumptions about the form of the underlying economic model, including assumptions about key model parameters, such as the time horizon and discount rate. In other situations, economic models use point estimates for parameters relating to patient outcomes or cost. O'Brien *et al.* (1994) call this first type of evaluation a deterministic analysis and recommended that uncertainty be assessed by using a comprehensive sensitivity analysis. Briggs *et al.* (1994) discussed the different forms of sensitivity analysis that can be applied. These may include simple reporting of the results over a suitable range of parameters, analysis of extremes, or a threshold analysis. Probabilistic sensitivity analyses are also used in some studies.

The second source of uncertainty is the result of sampling variability in model parameter estimates, which are derived from studies of individual patients. This type of evaluation is called a wholly stochastic analysis, and formal statistical analysis can be used to estimate variability and 95 per cent confidence interval estimates of the key economic parameters. Specific hypotheses about treatment differences in economic outcomes can be tested within this sampling framework. Evaluations that involve uncertainty from both model parameters and sampling variability are called partially stochastic analyses.

This chapter will discuss the statistical considerations relating to evaluations of health care resource utilization and cost data. We will deal primarily with fully stochastic analyses arising from sampled data from randomized clinical trials, although similar issues arise in the analysis of administrative databases. In a randomized clinical trial, patients are randomly assigned to the candidate or a suitable control treatment. Candidate treatments can be a particular drug or vaccine under development or a defined programme of care. Control treatment is usually the existing standard of care or, in many clinical trials of pharmaceutical products, a placebo. Many modern clinical studies now also include an objective for conducting an economic evaluation of the candidate treatment. In these situations, the study will collect patient-level data on the amount and timing of health services used (e.g. hospitalizations, physician visits, medical procedures, diagnostic tests, drug utilization). It is usually recommended that data on health care resources be collected as part of the main clinical trial and that data on the cost of these services be determined outside of the trial. This allows the economic evaluation the flexibility to address the appropriate study perspectives. We acknowledge that there are important limitations to basing economic evaluations on clinical trial data (Drummond and Davies 1991; Powe and Griffiths 1995). However, randomized trials remain the standard design for evaluating the clinical effect of candidate treatments and many studies now include specific objectives to conduct economic evaluations.

A comprehensive economic evaluation includes analysis of patient health status, resource utilization, and cost. Statistical analysis of patient health status in terms of health outcomes and quality-of-life are beyond the scope of this chapter. We will first address the problem of analysing resource data and then focus on cost data, including complications caused by incomplete data due to patient censoring. Many of the statistical issues raised in the analysis of resource use and cost are common to both types of variables. Broadly, we will discuss methods of analysing count data for resource utilization and continuous data for costs. However, many of the methods described in this chapter can be used for either type of variable. We assume in our discussions that costs have been appropriately discounted to their present value. We will illustrate the methods using data from two randomized clinical trials.

In the first illustration, we consider the problem of estimating the effect of treatment on the expected costs due to AIDS-defining events among HIV patients with CD4 cell counts less than 200 cells/mm^3. A key feature of the analysis comes from the fact that the treatments differed in the proportions of patients that experienced an event. Also, since patients who do not have an AIDS-defining event have zero costs, there is no single statistical distribution that can be used. Non-parametric methods are described for this setting.

The second illustration considers resource utilization and cost within a long-term mortality study of patients with congestive heart failure. Patients in this analysis are not all followed for the same length of time, and some patients may have incomplete (censored) data. Appropriate longitudinal models of count data and censored data models are discussed as methods that can be used to deal with these real world complexities.

9.2 Resource utilization data

An economic evaluation based on clinical trial data should first determine whether the treatments differ in the actual resources (e.g. hospitalizations, number of bed days, procedures, drugs, physician visits) used to treat patients. We assume that patients are followed longitudinally in time and that data on health care resources are captured during the trial period. Patient follow-up time may be the completion of a fixed defined time interval for all patients, or it may vary among patients. The variation in follow-up time may be due to design considerations (e.g. a staggered study enrolment with fixed time study end) or patient dropouts and missing data. In this section, our interest is in comparing treatments based on the number of health care contacts a patient has during a defined period of time or, equivalently, on the rate of contacts per unit of time.

9.2.1 Poisson regression

Response variables Y that are based on counts or frequencies are often modeled with a Poisson distribution with rate parameter λ. One property of Poisson random variables is that the mean and variance of Y are both equal to λ. Poisson regression models can be used to relate the mean response to a log linear function of the covariables (e.g. treatment, patient characteristics, etc.) This log linear model has the form

$$\log \lambda = \alpha + \sum_{j=1}^{p} \beta_j x_j$$

where the β_j are the regression coefficients relating the p covariates $x_1, x_2, \ldots, x_p$ to $\log \lambda$. Parameters are estimated by using the method of maximum likelihood. For this model, the mean satisfies the exponential relationship

$$\lambda = \exp\left(\alpha + \sum_{j=1}^{p} \beta_j x_j\right) = e^\alpha \prod_{j=1}^{p} (e^{\beta_j})^{x_j}$$

which demonstrates the interpretation of the regression coefficient β_j. A one-unit increase in x_j has a multiplicative impact of e^{β_j} on λ. If $\beta_j = 0$, then the multiplicative factor is 1 and x_j has no effect on the mean of the response. Similarly, if $\beta_j > 0$, then the mean response increases as x_j increases. If $\beta_j < 0$, then the mean response decreases. When follow-up time (t) varies among patients, then the response rate y/t can be used. The expected value of the rate is λ/t, and the log linear model for λ/t is given by

$$\log(\lambda/t) = \alpha + \sum_{j=1}^{p} \beta_j x_j$$

which has the equivalent form

$$\log \lambda - \log t = \alpha + \sum_{j=1}^{p} \beta_j x_j$$

The offset term $(-\log t)$ is used to relate counts and rates by

$$\lambda = t \exp\left(\alpha + \sum_{j=1}^{p} \beta_j x_j\right)$$

Thus, the expected count for a patient (λ) is given by the follow-up time and the rate of services utilized per unit of time.

The Poisson model assumes that health care contacts accumulate at a constant rate over time. This assumption may be problematic if follow-up among the patients varies. For example, if the hospitalization rate is changing over time and not all patients are followed for the full duration of the study, then the overall estimate of hospitalization rate could be a biased estimate of λ. This would be even more troublesome if the patient follow-up time differed between two treatment groups. It is recommended that the utilization rates be plotted for distinct time periods over the entire follow-up period. This type of plot may also help identify differences between treatment groups that may exist at various points along the time horizon. When resource rates are not constant and patient follow-up is subject to censoring, then statistical methods for dealing with censored cost data (discussed below in Section 9.4) can be applied to resource data.

Another difficulty with the Poisson model is the property that the mean and variance are assumed to be equal. Often, other sources of variability are not accounted for by the covariables in the model, resulting in overdispersion (variance exceeding that assumed in a Poisson model). These other sources of variability may be due to individual demographic factors such as age and gender, patient differences in underlying disease severity, or differences in health care systems. Overdispersion can be readily detected by estimating the ratio O = (variance of the event frequency) / (mean of the event frequency) over selected subpopulations. If the values of O indicate substantial overdispersion, then an adjusted variance can be calculated by inflating the model-based estimated variance using an overall estimate of the overdispersion factor.

9.2.2 Longitudinal and random-effects models

Standard regression analysis assumes that all observations in the sample are independent. This is clearly not the case in longitudinal studies of patient outcomes in which the multiple observations on the same individual are typically correlated. Not accounting for this correlation usually leads to an underestimate of the variance and exaggerates the statistical significance of observed differences between treatments. Longitudinal models can be used to overcome some of these difficulties. Itzler *et al.* (1999) analysed health care contact data by creating distinct (weekly) time intervals for the follow-up period in a longitudinal clinical trial of adults with asthma. They computed the rate of health care contacts for each patient within each time interval. Contact rates were fitted to a Poisson regression model by using generalized estimating equations (Liang and Zeger 1986; Stokes *et al.* 1995) to account for the within-patient correlation between the multiple observations on the same subject. They showed that failing to account for the within-patient correlation between the multiple observations for each patient had the potential to exaggerate the statistical significance of the observed differences. Random-effects models (Liang and Zeger 1986) can also be used for regression analysis of correlated data.

9.3 Cost data

Computing patient cost data involves combining resource data with costs in a way that is consistent with the study perspective. Cost is considered a useful measure of total utilization because it is a common metric with which to value the resources used to treat patients over the time period of interest. This is particularly useful when comparing therapies because a candidate treatment may increase one type of resource but decrease another type. Patient cost is a unifying metric to allow a meaningful comparison.

The statistical analysis of cost data can present several potential challenges. The distribution of costs is typically right-skewed, with very few patients incurring very large costs. Use of summary measures that are insensitive to extreme values, such as the median, are usually not desirable to organizations attempting to manage total aggregate costs. Patients with high resource use are substantial contributors to aggregated treatment costs but have a small influence on the median.

Cost distributions also tend to exhibit large variability that can pose problems for the provision of accurate and precise estimates of cost differences with the appropriate level of statistical power. The variability in cost data often increases with mean cost to such a degree that the usual normalizing and variance stabilizing transformations may not be helpful. For these reasons, methods that assume a normal distribution and equal variances, such as Student's t-test, analysis of variance, or linear regression, may not be appropriate. Non-parametric methods, resampling methods (e.g. bootstrap methods), and permutation tests may be preferred to the parametric methods (Desgagne et al. 1998). Appendix 1 gives a brief description of the bootstrap resampling methods and permutation tests. We describe the use of these methods in the illustrations.

9.3.1 Transformations

When the analysis is performed by using a transformation, it is important to retransform the estimated means to the original scale. This helps to assure that the results can be interpreted with respect to units familiar to the investigators. When the log-transformation $\log(C_i)$ is used for the cost data C_i, then the retransformed mean value

$$\hat{M} = \exp\left[\frac{1}{n}\sum \log(C_i)\right] \tag{9.1}$$

is a biased estimate of the mean cost. When the C_i are sampled from a log-normal distribution, $\hat{M}$ estimates the median and

$$\hat{C} = \exp\left(\hat{M} + \frac{s^2}{2}\right)$$

is an unbiased estimate of the mean cost; s^2 is the sample variance of the $\log(C_i)$. Duan (1983) derived non-parametric retransformation methods based on smearing which can be used for other transformations. In a comparison of alternative models to predict the cost of stroke, Lipscomb et al. (1998) found that the use of a log-transformation $\log(C_i+1)$ improved the performance of the candidate models. The constant 1 was added to the cost data C_i to avoid the difficulties encountered when $C_i=0$.

9.3.2 Clumping at zero

A related problem encountered when analysing health care utilization and cost data occurs when a sizable proportion of patients have zero contacts. It is not necessarily the presence of zeros that causes problems because many models (e.g. Poisson regression and linear regression) can easily accommodate zeros. Also, as already discussed, a small constant can be added when a log-transformation is used to tighten up the heavy tails of skewed distributions. The issue of zero costs is more important when there are different underlying factors relating to: (1) whether a patient has any health care cost; or (2) the distribution of the costs incurred given that they are nonzero. This situation arises in prevention trials of interventions which may affect the likelihood that a patient experiences an event (and utilizes health care services) and/or the severity of the event given that it occurs.

Chang *et al.* (1994) proposed a burden of illness score that can be used to estimate the net cost in this situation. For two comparison groups with sample sizes N_1 and N_2 from which m_1 and m_2 patients have the event of interest, the burden of illness score (net cost) is given by

$$T = \left(\frac{1}{N_1}\right) \sum_{i=1}^{m_1} C_{1i} - \left(\frac{1}{N_2}\right) \sum_{i=1}^{m_2} C_{2i} \qquad (9.2)$$

where the C_{1i} and C_{2i} are the costs incurred by the patients in treatment groups 1 and 2 who experience the event. The proportions $\hat{p}_1 = m_1/N_1$ and $\hat{p}_2 = m_2/N_2$ estimate the probabilities that patients in each group will experience the event, and $\bar{C}_1$ and $\bar{C}_2$ are the average costs among those m_1 and m_2 patients who experience the event. Under the null hypothesis of no treatment effect, the variance of T is given by

$$\hat{V}(T) = \left[\bar{C}^2 \hat{p}(1 - \hat{p}) \left(\frac{1}{N_1} + \frac{1}{N_2}\right) + \hat{p} \left(\frac{s_1^2}{N_1} + \frac{s_2^2}{N_2}\right) \right]$$

where $\hat{p}$ is the overall proportion of the patients in both groups collectively who experience the event, $\bar{C}$ is the overall average cost, and s_1^2 and s_2^2 are the sample variances of costs in each group among those patients who had the event. The test statistic

$$Z = \frac{T}{[\hat{V}(T)]^{1/2}}$$

is approximately normally distributed and can be used for significance testing by comparing the computed value of Z with the appropriate critical value (Z_c) from the standard normal distribution. For a two-sided type I error of $\alpha = 0.05$, this would be $Z_c = 1.96$.

Duan *et al.* (1983) and Lipscomb *et al.* (1998) considered two-part models to address the problem generated by zero-cost observations. The first part fits a logistic or probit model to the dichotomous variable defined by whether the patient incurred costs. This essentially provides a model for the probability that the patient has any cost-generating events. The second part uses standard linear models to the cost data (possibly transformed) for patients who had costs greater than zero. Expected values for individual patients can be derived by multiplying the two components together. Two-part models are attractive because they allow the analyst to consider factors that may affect both parts of the expected cost. It is possible that a treatment may lower the probability that a patient has a resource-generating event but not the average cost given that an event occurs. In this situation, the overall mean costs would be reduced by the treatment. Modelling both components of costs allows a more thorough interpretation of the results.

Another related method is to explicitly model the complete data sample including the zero and nonzero data. Lachenbruch (1975) showed that the likelihood function for the combined sample can be factored, and that the maximum likelihood estimates of the parameters p_1 and p_2 are the observed proportions $\hat{p}_1 = m_1/N_1$ and $\hat{p}_2 = m_2/N_2$. The two treatment groups can be tested separately for the equality of the proportion of zeros between the two groups, and a test for equality of mean costs among the patients who actually incurred costs. Also, the mean and variance of the costs for patients who experience cost-generating events can be estimated directly from the patients who actually incurred costs. A suitable transformation can be applied to the cost data if needed. For log-normally distributed cost data, the parameters can be estimated by using $\hat{M}_1$, s_1^2 and $\hat{M}_2$, s_2^2 from Equation (9.1) using only the nonzero cost data.

Lachenbruch (1976, 1992) constructed a 2 degrees-of-freedom χ^2 test by combining the normalized test statistic from the separate analyses. In using this overall approach, it is important to be sure that the direction of the treatment differences is the same for both components. Otherwise, the proposed test may not recognize that the two components of cost could offset one another. Alternatively, the results of the separate tests could be interpreted by using a stepwise multiplicity procedure (Hochberg and Benjamini 1990). Recently, Tu and Zhou (1999) developed a Wald test based on the maximum likelihood estimates of the parameters for the combined data sample, assuming a log-normal distribution for costs among patients experiencing resource-generating events.

9.4 Censored cost data

One important complication that often arises in analysing cost data relates to the variable follow-up among patients. Censoring occurs whenever study data on patient outcomes collected over time are incomplete. This situation can arise because of study design considerations (e.g. a clinical trial uses a rolling enrolment period and a fixed study termination) or because a patient is lost to follow-up. The latter can occur for many reasons. For example, patients may transfer to other health care providers or drop out of the study because of the treatment's poor efficacy or adverse effects. Death is usually not considered a type of patient censoring in cost analyses. This position, however, is not universally held and depends to some extent on the purpose of the analysis. For example, Dudley et al. (1993) suggested that for cost studies of surgical procedures, deaths should be treated as censored observations so that hospitals with high mortality rates, and therefore lower costs, are not rewarded. However, patient death presents a well-defined endpoint for the accumulation of costs and therefore is uncensored.

Difficulties arise in the analysis of censored data because only partial data on the patient are available. Survival analysis techniques have been developed and are commonly used for time-to-event data that are subject to censoring. The most widely used estimator for survival time subject to censoring is the product-limit estimator (Kaplan and Meier 1958). The Kaplan–Meier estimator $\hat{S}(t)$ estimates the probability that the time-to-death (or time-to-event) T exceeds time t for any given value of t. Appendix 2 provides a brief overview of the Kaplan–Meier product limit estimator of the survival distribution.

Recently, health economists have shown interest in statistical methods to estimate mean costs when data for some patients are right censored. Quesenberry *et al.* (1989) applied the Kaplan–Meier estimator directly to the number of lifetime hospitalizations and inpatient days among patients with acquired immunodeficiency syndrome (AIDS). In that study, censoring occurred because of patients who were still alive at the time of the analysis. Dudley *et al.* (1993) compared several analytic models, including both parametric and non-parametric survival models, for estimating the effects of clinical factors on the hospital costs of coronary bypass graft surgery. Fenn *et al.* (1995) pointed out the biases that result when the censored observations are excluded from the calculations (the uncensored method) or included as complete observations (the full sample method). They suggested applying the Kaplan–Meier estimators to the individual patient cost data as a way to incorporate the censoring information. However, Carides and Heyse (1996) and Etzioni *et al.* (1999) showed that this approach can result in a substantial bias because the censoring is informative. The difficulty arises because different patients will typically accumulate costs at different rates over time. As a result, patients censored at the same time with different accumulated costs would be expected to ultimately have different total costs if they were followed for a long enough period of time. Carides (1998) showed that the Kaplan–Meier estimator of mean cost is unbiased only if there is a one-to-one correspondence in the rank ordering of survival time and total cost. Otherwise, and more typically, the method produces an over- or under-estimate of mean cost depending on whether cost at censoring time is positively or negatively correlated to cost accumulated to the time of death. Methods have been developed to overcome this difficulty.

9.4.1 Non-parametric methods for censored cost data

Lin *et al.* (1997) proposed a fully non-parametric method that first partitions the entire study period into a number of small intervals (e.g. weekly, monthly or yearly). The estimate of mean total costs essentially combines the Kaplan–Meier estimate of survival with average costs assigned to the distinct intervals. Two forms of the estimate are given depending on whether cost histories are available for individual patients.

Formally, the study period τ is divided into K distinct time periods $[a_k, a_{k+1}]$ for $k = 1, \ldots, K$ with $a_1 = 0$ and $a_{k+1} = \tau$. The time periods may be defined by weekly, monthly, or yearly intervals. If cost histories for individual patients are available, then the Lin *et al.* estimator of mean cost is given by

$$\hat{C} = \sum_{k=1}^{K} \hat{S}(a_k)\, \hat{C}_k \qquad (9.3)$$

where $\hat{S}(a_k)$ is the Kaplan–Meier estimator (Equation (A2.1) in Appendix 2) of the probability that a patient survives to time a_k or beyond, and $\hat{C}_k$ is the average costs incurred within interval k among patients who are under observation at the start of the interval. Etzioni *et al.* (1996) used this formulation to estimate the costs associated with ovarian cancer using Medicare claims data and the Surveillance, Epidemiology, and End Results cancer registry.

If only the total accumulated cost is available then mean cost is estimated by

$$\widetilde{C} = \sum_{k=1}^{K} \widetilde{C}_k \left[\hat{S}(a_k) - \hat{S}(a_{k+1}) \right] + \widetilde{C}_{K+1} \hat{S}(\tau) \tag{9.4}$$

where in this formulation $\widetilde{C}_k$, the total costs for patients who died within the kth interval, is multiplied by the Kaplan–Meier probability of death occurring within the kth time interval. The term $\widetilde{C}_{K+1} \hat{S}(\tau)$ estimates costs for patients who survive to the end of the final interval.

Standard errors of $\hat{C}$ and $\widetilde{C}$ are given in Lin et $al.$ (1997).

9.4.2 Two-stage estimate

One difficulty with the Lin et $al.$ method is the choice of interval length because the method assumes that censoring occurs at the start/end of the interval. If the censoring occurs in the middle of the interval, then the estimate is clearly biased. If the intervals are chosen to be fairly narrow, then the bias is reduced but there may not be enough patient deaths to provide a good estimate of mean cost for the interval. If the intervals are chosen to be wide, then the estimate will have more bias because more censoring occurs mid-interval.

Carides et $al.$ (2000) proposed a two-stage estimator when total accumulated cost is available. This method does not require the use of distinct time intervals. In the first stage, the relationship between total costs and follow-up time is estimated for uncensored patients by using a parametric regression model or a non-parametric smoother. Good choices for non-parametric smoothers include a cubic smoothing spline using the S-Plus function smooth: spline or a local regression using the S-Plus function loess. Eubank (1999) is an excellent reference for non-parametric regression and spline smoothing techniques. In the second stage, the expected total costs over time are combined with Kaplan–Meier estimates of survival to estimate mean total cost. The Carides et $al.$ (2000) two-stage estimator is given by

$$\hat{C}_{TS} = \int_0^\tau \hat{g}(t) \left| d\hat{S}(t) \right| + \hat{C}_{T>\tau} \hat{S}(\tau)$$

where $\hat{g}(t)$ is the estimated cost among patients who die at time t and $\hat{C}_{T>\tau}$ is an estimate of costs accumulated through time T for patients who survive past time τ. The integration is taken with respect to the probability of dying at time t and $\hat{S}(t)$ is the probability of surviving past τ. Since the Kaplan–Meier estimate of survival at the J distinct death times in the sample is used, the two-stage estimator can be calculated very simply by using

$$\hat{C}_{TS} = \sum_{j=1}^{J} \hat{g}(t_j) \left[\hat{S}(t_{j-1}) - \hat{S}(t_j) \right] + \hat{C}_{T>\tau} \hat{S}(\tau) \tag{9.5}$$

This method offers gains in efficiency over the Lin et $al.$ method in Equation (9.4) by modelling costs over time rather than by using interval-defined average costs. The standard error can be estimated by using the bootstrap (Efron and Tibshirani 1993). Extensive simulations by Lin *et al.* (1997) and Carides *et al.* (2000) show that these methods are consistent and overcome the bias in the Kaplan–Meier estimate of mean cost.

A final method proposed by Zhao and Tsiatis (1997) for estimating the distribution of quality-adjusted survival times can be modified to estimate the survival distribution for costs (see Bang and Tsiatis 2000). This method computes the weighted sum of the number of patients with costs exceeding a specific value y. The weights are inversely proportional to the probability of noncensorship with respect to y. The distribution can then be used to compute summary statistics such as the mean.

9.5 Illustration 1: HIV data

Alternative approaches to handling cost data that contain many zeros are illustrated by using data based on a randomized clinical trial among HIV-positive patients (Hammer *et al.* 1997). In this trial, patients with CD4 cell counts less than 200 cells/ mm^3 were randomly assigned to receive either triple antiretroviral therapy combining a protease inhibitor and two nucleoside reverse transcriptase inhibitors (nRTIs) or double antiretroviral therapy with two nRTIs. The primary endpoint was the rate of AIDS-defining events or death. Enrolment had reached 1156 patients when the trial was terminated early. The data safety monitoring board recommended termination because of a significant difference between treatments in disease progression.

Our interest is in estimating and comparing the average expected cost due to AIDS-defining events per patient-month. The cost per patient-month was estimated for each patient by obtaining the total cost due to AIDS-defining events by applying external cost estimates (Gable *et al.* 1996) to the specific types of AIDS-defining events observed and then dividing the patient's total cost estimate by the number of months the patient was followed. Summary statistics are provided in Table 9.1. Mean follow-up time was similar in the two treatment groups (7.9 months for the double-therapy group and 8.0 months for the triple-therapy group). Among the patients experiencing at least one AIDS-defining event during the trial, the average cost per patient-month of follow-up did not significantly differ between groups ($3222 for the double therapy group versus $3376 for the triple therapy group). However, the percentage of patients who experienced an AIDS-defining event significantly differed (9.0 per cent versus 4.7 per cent, respectively; $\chi^2 = 8.40$; $p = 0.004$). Consequently, the average cost per patient-month is estimated to be higher for patients assigned to double therapy ($289 per patient-month) than for those assigned to triple therapy ($158 per patient-month). On the basis of 1000 bootstrap replicates, bias-corrected and accelerated (BCa, see Appendix 1) 95 per cent confidence intervals were obtained for the average cost per patient-month for patients randomly assigned to double-therapy ($195 to $414) and to triple therapy ($93 to $264) and for the treatment difference ($3 to $270).

Treatment differences were first tested by using a permutation test in which each patient was randomly reassigned to either treatment, such that the original treatment sample sizes were maintained. For each replicate sample based on the reassignment,

Table 9.1 Summary statistics for economic evaluation of ACTG 320 based on average cost per month of follow-up

Variable	Double therapy	Triple therapy
No. of patients	579	577
Average follow-up time (months)	7.9	8.0
Patients with ADE(s)[a] (%)	9.0%	4.7%
Average cost per month for pts w/ ADE(s)	$3222 (sd = $3290)	$3376 (sd = $3178)
Average cost per month (all patients)	$289	$158
(95% confidence intervals – BCa percentiles)	($195; $414)	($93; $264)

Note: [a] AIDS defining event

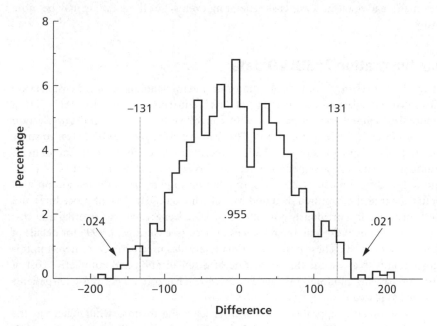

Fig. 9.1 One thousand permutation replicates of the treatment difference in the average AIDS-defining event cost per month for the ACTG 320 data under the null hypothesis (no treatment difference); horizontal dashed lines represent the observed difference ($131) and its negative; 24 of the 1000 replicates were less than −$131; 21 of the 1000 replicates were greater than $131

the treatment difference in the cost per patient-month was computed. This process was repeated 1000 times to obtain the distribution of the treatment cost difference, assuming that mean costs between the two treatments do not differ (see Figure 9.1). On the basis of this distribution, 45 of the 1000 differences were more extreme (positive or negative) than the observed cost difference of $131 per patient-month, yielding a two-sided *p*-value of 0.045.

Many patients did not experience an AIDS-defining event during the trial and thus did not incur any cost for AIDS-defining events during the trial. Because of the many patients with zero cost, one can use the methods that explicitly handle clumping at zero. By using the method of Chang *et al.* (1994), a burden-of-illness Z score of 1.89 is obtained ($p = 0.059$). The lack of significance is partly due to the large variability in the cost estimates among patients experiencing at least one AIDS-defining event. In contrast, a different picture emerges with the 2 degrees of freedom χ^2 test by Lachenbruch (1976). With this test, a significant χ^2 value of 8.40 ($p = 0.015$) is obtained. In this case, the highly significant difference in the percentage of patients who incur cost drives the test statistic. The lack of significance in the mean cost per patient among patients who experienced at least once AIDS-defining event reduces the significance of the test only by adding 1 degree of freedom. It is important to note that the direction of the treatment effect must be considered when this test is used. One treatment may result in fewer cost-generating events, but those events may be more costly.

9.6 Illustration 2: SOLVD data

Methods for assessing resource utilization data and for handling censored cost data are illustrated with data from the Study of Left Ventricular Dysfunction (SOLVD), a randomized clinical trial in patients with congestive heart failure and low ejection fractions (SOLVD Investigators 1991). The primary objective of SOLVD was to study the effect of enalapril on mortality. Patients receiving conventional treatment for heart failure were randomly assigned to either placebo ($n = 1284$) or enalapril ($n = 1285$) and followed for a mean of 2.7 years. In addition to obtaining information on vital status, the trial also captured data on hospital admission date, use of procedures and study drug use. In a previously published cost-effectiveness analysis, external unit cost estimates were used to value the resources utilized (see Glick *et al.* 1995 for details of the costing method). These unit cost estimates are also used here. Our interest in this illustration is to assess the three-year rate of hospitalization and cumulative cost of care for patients randomly assigned to receive enalapril versus those in-patients assigned to placebo.

To determine the appropriate method for assessing treatment differences in the hospitalization rate, we first examined the observed hospitalization rates over the period of interest (3 years in this example). We investigated this graphically by plotting the monthly crude hospitalization rate (number of hospitalizations during a given month divided by the total number of patient months of follow-up for patients randomly assigned to a given treatment) against the month of follow-up (Figure 9.2). A non-parametric regression line based on loess smoothing was fit to the monthly data for both treatment groups to help identify the general trend in the rates. According to the figure, the hospitalization rate seems to modestly decline among patients assigned to placebo. This trend appears to be driven primarily by the higher rate of hospitalizations during the first two months of follow-up. Nevertheless, the rates are fairly stable, with hospitalization rates for patients assigned to enalapril consistently lower than those for patients assigned to placebo.

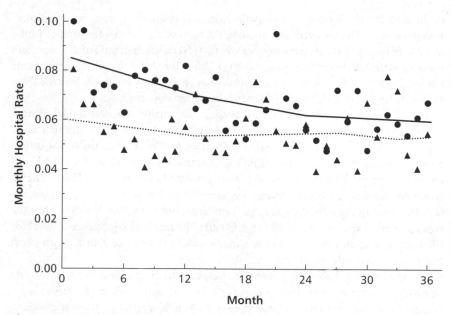

Fig. 9.2 Monthly hospitalization rate by month for SOLVD patients randomly assigned to placebo (●) or to enalapril (▲), with non-parametric regression lines based on loess smoothing for placebo (solid line) and enalapril (dotted line)

The crude hospitalization rate (total number of hospitalizations/total number of years of follow-up) was estimated for patients randomly assigned to enalapril (2054/3073 = 0.668 hospitalizations per year of follow-up) and for patients randomly assigned to placebo (2453/2934 = 0.836). The impact of treatment can be described by using either the absolute difference in the crude rate (0.168; 95% CI: 0.082, 0.239) or the relative reduction (20.1%; 95% CI: 11.7% to 28.2%), where the confidence intervals were obtained using the BCa percentiles based on 1000 bootstrap replicates.

The crude hospitalization rates were also obtained by using a simple Poisson regression model that was fit to two data points – one observation containing the total number of hospitalizations and follow-up time over the three years for the placebo recipients and the other containing the same summary information for the enalapril recipients. Application of Poisson regression to these data resulted in a treatment coefficient estimate of −0.2239 (s.e. = 0.0299), with the negative coefficient indicating that treatment with enalapril reduced the hospitalization rate. The equivalent relative rate reduction estimate of 20.1 per cent (= [1 − exp(0.2239)] 100%) is obtained. The 95 per cent confidence interval obtained with the parametric (Poisson) model (15.2 per cent to 24.6 per cent) is slightly tighter than those based on the non-parametric bootstrap.

One concern with the above approach which combines data across all patients within a treatment group, is the potential for the Poisson property (mean and variance are equal) to fail. Because some patients may have a higher propensity for hospitalizations than others receiving a given treatment, some degree of overdispersion is likely. Because of the differential follow-up among patients in each treatment group, the overdispersion parameter (O) was estimated by using the ratio of the mean and variance of the number of hospitalizations per year of follow-up (y/t) rather than ratio of the mean and variance of the number of hospitalizations (y). Values for O of 3.45 and 3.36 for patients randomly assigned to placebo and enalapril, respectively, were obtained. Because these values are large, it is likely that the Poisson assumption does not hold.

To overcome the problem of overdispersion, we refit the Poisson model using a generalized estimating equation with patient-level data. This should result in a more appropriate (larger) variance estimate for the treatment effect. Because of the differential follow-up among patients within each treatment group, we used a model with an offset term given by the natural log of the patient's follow-up time. The estimated treatment coefficient with this model was identical to that above (-0.2239), but the standard error of the estimate was 75 per cent larger (0.0524 versus 0.0299). While the treatment effect was still significant ($p < 0.0001$), the resulting confidence interval for the relative hospital rate reduction was much wider (11.4 per cent to 27.9 per cent) and comparable to the bootstrap interval.

The methods used above to analyse the hospitalization data assumed that the rate was roughly constant over time. Because of censoring, one could apply methods for censored cost data and relax the assumption. Rather than applying these methods to the hospitalization data, however, we used these methods to estimate the average three-year cost.

Approximately 20 per cent of the patients were censored by year 3, primarily because of the rolling enrolment period. We treated cost estimates for patients who died before year 3 as complete cases (not censored), since no cost was accumulated after death. Table 9.2 summarizes the three-year cumulative cost estimates for placebo and enalapril and the difference according to several methods. The Lin et al. (1997) estimator based on cost history was obtained by dividing each patient's follow-up time into monthly intervals. The average cost within each monthly interval for a given treatment group was multiplied by the survival probability at the start of the month and then accumulated over the 36 monthly periods. In an alternative approach, we obtained estimates of the three-year cost using the total cost observed for patients over the time horizon of three years (and ignored the timing of when the costs were incurred during the period). Table 9.2 also provides the cost estimates for the Lin total cost method (Lin et al. 1997) and the Carides two-stage method (Carides et al. 2000) using both a parameteric and a non-parametric method to estimate the cost function over time. These three methods are based on total cost and provide fairly similar results pointing to the potential downward bias associated with the cost history method proposed by Lin et al. (1997).

Finally, we use SOLVD to show the dramatic affect of censoring on the bias associated with the Kaplan–Meier estimator when applied to cost. Figure 9.3 shows the cumulative cost estimates among placebo recipients for increasing time horizons. While the estimates based on total cost (Lin and Carides's two-stage) are similar at each time point, the Kaplan–Meier estimate diverges as the amount of censoring rises. Even with censoring as low as 10 per cent at 2.5 years, one can begin to see the bias associated with the Kaplan–Meier estimator when applied to cost data.

Table 9.2 Three-year cumulative cost estimates for patients randomly assigned to placebo or Enalapril in SOLVD: comparison of alternative methods

	Placebo	Enalapril	Difference
No. of patients	1284	1285	
Percent censored (at 3 years) (%)	20.1	21.9	
Method of estimation			
Lin (cost history)[a]	$12,833	$10,991	$1842
Lin (total cost)[a]	12,881	11,306	1575
Carides two stage – parametric	12,852	11,378	1474
Carides two stage – non-parametric	12,904	11,203	1701

Notes: [a] based on dividing time into monthly intervals

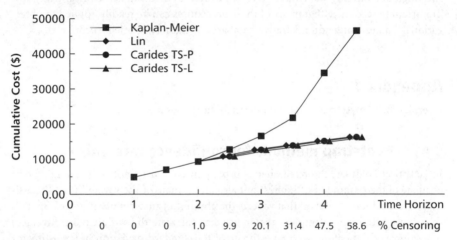

Fig. 9.3 Estimated cumulative cost for SOLVD patients randomly assigned to placebo for time horizons ranging from 1 year to 4.5 years for alternative estimators (Kaplan–Meier method applied to cost. Lin method based on total cost with monthly time intervals, Carides two-stage with parametric smoothing [TS-P] and Carides two-stage with non-parametric loess smoothing [TS-L]); with percentage of placebo patients censored at each time point

9.7 Concluding remarks

The concern over the costs of health care will continue to grow as more novel health care technologies and pharmaceutical products become available to a growing elderly population. In this environment, health care providers will attempt to identify and apply treatment programmes that offer the greatest benefit for society's investment in health care. Formal economic evaluations will be looked upon to help guide these decisions.

In this chapter, we considered statistical methods appropriate for the analysis of health care utilization and cost data. Many authors have dealt with the analytical issues relating to cost and utilization data as distinct. However, we have emphasized that the approaches share many common features. For example, methods for censored data have been developed for analysing survival data, quality-adjusted survival time and cost data. These same general approaches apply to data counting specific health care contacts, such as hospitalizations. The same generalization applies to longitudinal data models and random-effects models. In addition, the methods for analysing data clumping at zero are readily applicable to both cost and utilization data.

While both parametric and non-parametric methods can be used, we typically favour the non-parametric bootstrap and permutation methods for evaluating uncertainty in estimates of mean costs and in evaluating between treatment differences in mean costs. Those methods were illustrated with two examples from a clinical trial of HIV therapy and trial studying a drug used to treat congestive heart failure.

Our focus was entirely on evaluating uncertainty due to sampling variability. Although our development was mostly motivated by randomized clinical trials, it is important to recognize that many of these procedures can be readily applied to observational studies using administrative databases of claims or patient records.

Appendix 1

Overview of bootstrap estimation and permutation tests

9.A1.1 Bootstrap methods for confidence intervals

In statistical analyses, the researcher is usually interested in not only a single point estimate of the parameter of interest but also an estimate of the variability of the estimator. A confidence interval that reflects the amount of uncertainty in the estimate is thus constructed. For example, a researcher may calculate the sample mean (average) of a sample of data along with an estimate of the standard deviation of the estimator and a 95 per cent confidence interval.

When deciding on a method for confidence interval construction, we must consider both *exactness* and *accuracy*. Exactness refers to the property that the actual *coverage probability* is close to that which is stated; i.e. if the procedure were to be repeated many times, the percentage of intervals that would actually cover (contain) the true parameter value would be approximately the stated confidence level, say 95 per cent. Accuracy means that the length of the confidence interval is as small as possible for the given confidence level. Accuracy is alternatively referred to as precision. Thus, the narrower the confidence interval, the greater the accuracy and precision.

In some situations, researchers construct confidence intervals on the basis of normal theory. These intervals are nearly exact and accurate when the normal assumption holds. However, for many applications, including those in this chapter, the distributions are far from normal. Use of the usual normal-theory methods in these situations can result in confidence intervals that are neither exact nor accurate.

Bootstrap techniques provide valid methods for constructing confidence intervals for virtually any statistic, regardless of the distribution of the statistic or the population from which the data were drawn. The basic assumption is that the collected data are representative of the population. These data are repeatedly sampled to mimic the process of sampling from the population. In this way, we can 'pull ourselves up by our bootstraps', i.e., by the data. Specifically, we draw a sample *with replacement* of size equal to the number of observations in our dataset, and compute the statistic of interest using this resampled data. This process is repeated B times, where for confidence intervals B should be at least 1000. The following example illustrates this process and some of the alternative bootstrap confidence intervals available.

We have drawn five observations from a log-normal distribution (0.2, 0.4, 0.6, 3.8, 9.4) and we wish to construct a 95 per cent confidence interval for the mean. Of course, if it were known that the underlying population is log-normal, we could simply take the logs of each of the observations and construct the standard t-statistic confidence interval and then retransform the limits to the original scale. This interval would be the best in terms of both accuracy and exactness. In practice, however, we do not usually know what the underlying distribution is. A naive choice would be to compute a t-statistic confidence interval using the untransformed data. This would yield

$$\overline{X} \pm t_{0.025,4}(\cdot) \text{ (standard error)}$$

$$= 2.88 \pm 2.776 \, (1.76)$$

$$= 2.88 \pm 4.89 \tag{A1.1}$$

or $(-2.01, 7.77)$, where $\overline{X}$ is the sample mean. Note that the lower bound for this interval is negative, although the mean of a log-normal random variable must always be positive. This result is due to the incorrect normality assumption being made. As we will see, most bootstrap methods do not suffer from this phenomenon.

The following table shows some of the resampled data we used to construct the bootstrap confidence intervals:

Resample number	Resampled data					Bootstrap replicate of mean ($\hat{\theta}^*$)
1	0.6	0.4	9.4	0.6	0.2	2.24
2	0.6	3.8	9.4	3.8	0.2	3.56
3	0.4	3.8	9.4	0.6	0.6	2.96
.	.	.	.	.	.	.
.	.	.	.	.	.	.
.	.	.	.	.	.	.
999	0.4	0.6	0.6	0.2	0.6	0.48
1000	3.8	0.6	0.2	0.4	9.4	2.88

Note that for some resample sets, observations appear more than once. For example, for resample number 2, the value 3.8 appears twice. This is not unexpected because the sampling is done with replacement each time. The last column shows the *bootstrap replicates* of the mean for each resample set, i.e. the mean for each set. The bootstrap replicates are denoted with $\hat{\theta}^*$, where θ in this example denotes the population mean, the hat indicates an estimate based on a sample, and the asterisk indicates that the estimate is based on bootstrap resampled data. As illustrated in the chapter, the bootstrap method would also apply for statistics more complicated than the sample mean. In these situations resampling would simply be done on the subjects.

Various types of bootstrap confidence intervals can be constructed. In this Appendix we discuss the three most commonly used. The reader is referred to Efron and Tibshirani (1993) and Chernick (1999) for other variants. We will refer to the first method as the *bootstrap standard normal confidence interval*. This interval is the same as the *t*-statistic confidence interval discussed above except that the standard deviation of the bootstrap replicates is used in place of the standard error calculation. This method is useful when no standard error formula exists, as is the case for many statistics. The bootstrap standard normal confidence interval is both accurate and exact when the statistic $\hat{\theta}$ is normally distributed. When normality does not hold, however, this method will yield poor confidence intervals.

The second type of bootstrap confidence interval is called the *percentile method confidence interval*. This interval is constructed by taking the percentiles of the bootstrap distribution of replicates. For example, to construct a 95 per cent percentile method confidence interval for the above example, we take the 2.5th percentile (0.36) and the 97.5th percentile (6.44), yielding the interval (0.36, 6.44). Note that, unlike with the *t*-statistic confidence interval, the lower limit is positive rather than negative. One clear advantage of this method is that confidence intervals constructed in this manner never span values outside the range of possible values for the statistic

Unfortunately, the percentile method works well only when 50 per cent of the bootstrap distribution is less than the point estimate $\hat{\theta}$. The third method we will describe is a modification of the percentile method. This interval is called the *BCa (bias-corrected and accelerated) confidence interval*. The BCa method starts with the percentile interval and then shifts (bias correction) and either contracts or expands (acceleration) the interval to improve its accuracy and exactness. For the above example, the 95 per cent BCa confidence interval is (0.44, 6.52). This method yields good confidence intervals for most non-parametric applications and is currently recommended for general use. See Efron and Tibshirani (1993) for further discussion and details. The S-Plus computer package provides a function that can easily compute the bootstrap confidence intervals discussed in this appendix.

9.A1.2 **Permutation tests**

Randomization methods can also be used to test whether the parameter of interest (e.g. mean cost or rate of utilization) is significantly different between the two treatment groups. One approach is to conduct a permutation test. The key to this approach is approximating the distribution of the test statistic, say the mean difference, under the null hypothesis. The basic assumption of the permutation test is that if the two treatments do not differ (i.e. the null hypothesis is true), then the observed responses could have followed from either treatment (regardless of which treatment that patient had been randomized to receive). Consequently, a bootstrap sample is obtained by effectively randomly assigning the patients to their new treatment group. This is accomplished by randomly reallocating *without replacement* the responses into the two treatment groups while preserving the sample sizes. The resulting value for the test statistic from this bootstrap sample yields one possible realization under the null hypothesis. The null distribution for the test statistic can be approximated by repeating this process many times. The two-sided *p*-value is given by the proportion of test statistics from the permutation resamples that yield a more extreme value relative to the observed test statistics.

By reallocating patients to the treatment groups in each permutation replicate, one is assuming that the distribution of the responses (i.e. costs) are the same for the two treatment groups. This might not be the case, however, as a given treatment might yield more variable costs, but not differ in terms of the mean. If one only wants to assume that the parameter of interest (i.e., mean cost) is the same for the two treatment groups, then the replicates for generating the null distribution need to be obtained in a different manner. If the statistic of interest is the difference in the mean cost, this can be easily done by first subtracting the mean cost from each observation within each treatment group. With the centred observations, the bootstrap replicate is obtained by sampling with replacement within the treatment group. The test statistic is then computed and the process is repeated many times to approximate the distribution of the statistic under the null hypothesis. The two-sided *p*-value is then obtained in the same manner as with the permutation test.

Appendix 2

9.A2.1 Kaplan–Meier Estimator

The Kaplan–Meier estimator $\hat{S}(t)$ estimates the probability that the time-to-death (or time-to-event) T exceeds time t for any given value of t. For a random sample of N patients with ordered times of death, $t_1 < t_2 < \ldots < t_j$ the Kaplan–Meier estimator $\hat{S}(t)$ is given by

$$\hat{S}(t) = \prod_{j:t_j < t} \frac{n_j - d_j}{n_j} \tag{A2.1}$$

where d_j is the number of patients who died at time t_j and n_j is the number of patients who are at risk (i.e. alive and available for follow-up) just before time t_j. For example, suppose $N = 100$ patients are followed from time t_0; $d_1 = 1$ patient dies at time t_1 and no patient is lost to follow-up before t_1. $\hat{S}(t_1) = (100 - 1)/100 = 0.99$. Continuing to the next time a death occurs at t_2: suppose $d_2 = 2$ patients die and 1 patient is lost to follow-up, so that $n_2 = 98$ were alive and available at t_2. In this case, $\hat{S}(t_2) = \hat{S}(t_1)[(98 - 2)/98] = 0.970$. This process continues through all J death time. $\hat{S}(t)$ is typically plotted as a function of t over the observed range of event times and is called a Kaplan–Meier curve. It is a decreasing curve with $\hat{S}(0) = 1$ for time 0. The mean survival time is estimated numerically as the area under the Kaplan–Meier curve. With this approach, patients who are censored are considered at risk for the event at all times up until their censoring time. A key assumption of the Kaplan–Meier method is that of independent or noninformative censoring. This essentially means that the expected survival time is the same for censored patients as for uncensored patients.

References

Bang, H. and Tsiatis, A. A. (2000). Estimating medical costs with censored data. *Biometrika*, 87, 329–43.

Briggs, A., Sculpher, M. and Buxton, M. (1994). Uncertainty in the economic evaluation of health care technologies: the role of sensitivity analysis. *Health Economics*, 3, 95–104.

Carides, G. W. (1998). Estimation of mean treatment costs in the presence of right-censoring. Ph.D. dissertation, Temple University.

Carides, G. W. and Heyse, J. F. (1996). *Nonparametric estimation of the parameters of cost distributions in the presence of right-censoring*. Proceedings of the Biopharmaceutical Section, American Statistical Association Annual Meetings, 186–191.

Carides, G. W., Heyse, J. F. and Iglewicz, B. (2000). A regression-based method for estimating mean treatment cost in the presence of right-censoring. *Biostatistics*, 1, 299–313.

Chang, M. N., Guess, H. A. and Heyse, J. F. (1994). Reduction in burden of illness: a new efficacy measure for prevention trials. *Statistics in Medicine*, 13, 1807–14.

Chernick, M.R. (1999). *Bootstrap Methods: A Practitioner's Guide*. John Wiley & Sons, New York.

Desgagne, A., Castilloux, A. M., Angers, J. F. *et al.* (1998). The use of the bootstrap statistical method for the pharmacoeconomic cost analysis of skewed data. *Pharmacoeconomics*, 487–97.

Diehr, P., Yanez, D., Ash, A. *et al.* (1999). Methods for analyzing health care utilization and costs. *Annual Review of Public Health*, 20, 125–44.

Drummond, M. F. and Davies, L. M. (1991). Economic analysis alongside clinical trials: revising the methodological principles. *International Journal of Technology Assessment in Health Care*, 7, 571–3.

Duan, N. (1983). Smearing estimate: a nonparametric retransformation method. *Journal of the American Statistical Association*, 78, 605–10.

Duan, N., Manning, W. G., Morris, C. N. *et al.* (1983). A comparison of alternative models for the demand for medical care. *Journal of Business and Economic Statistics*, 1, 115–26.

Dudley, R. A., Harrell, F. E., Smith, L. R. *et al.* (1993). Comparison of analytic models for estimating the effect of clinical factors on the cost of coronary artery bypass graft surgery. *Journal of Clinical Epidemiology*, 46, 261–71.

Efron, B. and Tibshirani, R. (1993). An introduction to the bootstrap. Chapman & Hall, New York.

Etzioni, R. D., Feuer, E. J., Sullivan, S. D. *et al.* (1999). On the use of survival analysis techniques to estimate medical care costs. *Journal of Health Economics*, 18, 365–80.

Etzioni, R. D., Urban, N. and Baker, M. (1996). Estimating the costs attributable to a disease with application to ovarian cancer. *Journal of Clinical Epidemiology*, 49, 95–103.

Eubank, R. L. (1999). Nonparametric regression and spline smoothing, 2nd Edn. Marcel Dekker, New York, Chapters 1 and 5.

Fenn, P., McGuire, A., Phillips, V. *et al.* (1995). The analysis of censored treatment cost data in economic evaluation. *Medical Care*, 33, 851–63.

Gable, C. B., Tierce, J. C., Simison, D. *et al.* (1996). Cost of HIV/AIDS at CD4$^+$ counts disease stages based on treatment protocols. *Journal of Acquired Immune Deficiency Syndromes and Human Retrovirology*, 12, 413–20.

Glick, H., Cook, J. R., Binosian, B. *et al.* (1995). Costs and effects of enalapril therapy in patients with symptomatic heart failure: an economic analysis of the Studies of Left Ventricular Dysfunction (SOLVD) treatment trial. *Journal of Cardiac Failure*, 1, 371–80.

Hammer, S. M., Squires, K. E., Hughes, M. D., *et al.* for the AIDS Clinical Trials Group 320 Study Team. (1997). A controlled trial of two nucleoside analogues plus indinavir in persons with human immunodeficiency virus infection and CD4 cell counts of 200 per cubic millimeter or less. *New England Journal of Medicine*, 337, 725–33.

Hochberg, Y. and Benjamini, Y. (1990). More powerful procedures for multiple significance testing. *Statistics in Medicine*, 9, 811–18.

Itzler, R., Dasbach, E., Koch, G. *et al.* (1999). Using longitudinal models for the analysis of resource use data: the case of asthma. Economic Assessment in Clinical Trials, Drug Information Association Meeting, 11/99.

Kaplan, E. L. and Meier, P. (1958). Nonparametric estimation from incomplete observations. *Journal of the American Statistical Association*, 457–81.

Lachenbruch, P. A. (1975). Estimation of parameters of the Poisson with excess zeroes and negative binomial with excess zeroes distributions. *Biometrical Journal*, 339–44.

Lachenbruch, P. A. (1976). Analysis of data with clumping at zero. *Biometrical Journal*, 18, 351–6.

Lachenbruch, P. A. (1992). Utility of logistic regression in epidemiologic studies of the elderly. In: R. B. Wallace and R. F. Woolson, *The Epidemiologic Study of the Elderly*. Oxford University Press, New York, Oxford: Chapter 24:371–81.

Liang, K.Y and Zeger, S. (1986). Longitudinal data analysis using generalized linear models. *Biometrika*, 73, 13–22.

Lin, D. Y., Fewer, E. J., Etzioni, R. *et al.* (1997). Estimating medical costs from incomplete follow-up data. *Biometrics*, 53, 113–28.

Lipscomb, J., Ancukiewicz, M., Parmigiani, G. *et al.* (1998). Predicting the cost of illness: a comparison of alternative models applied to stroke. *Medical Decision Making*, 18 (suppl), S39-S56.

O'Brien, B.J. Drummond, M.F., Labelle, R.J. *et al.* In search of power and significance issues in the design and analysis of stochastic cost-effectiveness studies in health care. *Medical Care*, 32, 150–63, 1994.

Powe, N. R. and Griffiths, R. I. (1995). The clinical-economic trial: promise, problems, and challenges. *Controlled Clinical Trials*, 16, 377–94.

Quesenberry, C. P., Fireman, B., Hiatt, R. A. *et al.* (1989). A survival analysis of hospitalization among patients with acquired immunodeficiency syndrome. *American Journal of Public Health*, 79, 1643–7.

SOLVD Investigators (1991). Effect of enalapril on survival in-patients with reduced left ventricular ejection fractions and congestive heart failure. *New England Journal of Medicine*, 325, 293–302.

Stokes, M.E., Davis, C.S. and Koch, G.G. (1995). *Categorical data analysis using the SAS® system*. SAS Institute, North Carolina, USA.

Tu, W. and Zhou, X. H. (1999). A WALD test comparing medical costs based on log-normal distributions with zero valued costs. *Statistics in Medicine*, 18, 2749–61.

Zhao, H. and Tsiatis, A. A. (1997). A consistent estimator for the quality-adjusted survival time. *Biometrika*, 84, 339–48.

Chapter 10

Discounting in economic evaluation

John Cairns

10.1 **Introduction**

Discounting practices often play a central role in determining the relative cost-effectiveness of different interventions. If evaluations are undertaken on an incorrect basis the quality of decision-making will suffer and health service efficiency will be reduced. Moreover, confusion or lack of agreement over standard discounting practice potentially undermines the credibility and value of economic evaluation.

Time preference and discounting has a long history in economics (see for example, Rothbard (1990) and Loewenstein (1992)). With the rapid growth of interest in economic evaluation in the 1960s the choice of social discount rate became a topic of considerable interest. Emphasis on discounting and time preferences in health economics is rather more recent with most of the relevant studies appearing in the past decade. Much of this research has taken a decidedly empirical form. At one level such interest is readily explained by the twin concerns of understanding health-affecting behaviour and of informing discounting practice. But why is there a perceived need to inform discounting practice? Why are answers derived for the rest of the economy not adequate?

As with so much of health economics the starting point is the special nature of health and health care. As a result market equilibria are potentially less informative than elsewhere in the economy. This has fuelled the study of individual preferences rather than a reliance on market information. The individualistic and empirically-based research methodologies which have emerged as a result have provided a background making detailed consideration of individual inter-temporal preferences an obvious field of study. Given the focus on devising measures of the impact of interventions on individual health and to some extent the valuation of these outcomes it has proved natural to extend study to preferences over time rather than simply preferences over health states at a point in time.

10.2 **Theory**

10.2.1 **Rationale for discounting**

Generally three arguments are advanced why individuals might exhibit positive time preference. The first is a diminishing marginal utility argument placed in a temporal context. Diminishing marginal utility, coupled with the expectation that in the future consumption will be higher, provides grounds for discounting future gains depending on how far in the future they accrue. The second argument refers to the risk of death or more broadly the risk that, whether as a result of death or some other circumstances, future consumption opportunities may not be available. Finally it is suggested that individuals simply have a preference for earlier consumption compared to later consumption. This source of positive time preference is not infrequently described in terms of irrationality or a failure of the imagination, for example Pigou's oft-quoted 'defective telescopic faculty'. There is concern that this is an inappropriate element to take account of when determining a social discount rate. This is particularly the case when future generations are likely to be adversely affected by current decisions being informed by too high a discount rate as a consequence of permitting such 'inappropriate' preferences. Whether or not one subscribes to this view is a value judgement upon which little scientific discourse is possible.

Economists have for a long time favoured a specific model of inter-temporal preferences, namely the Discounted Utility (DU) model. Perhaps the most important assumption underlying this model is that of stationarity. This requires that preference between two outcomes depends only on the absolute time interval separating them. This implies that intertemporal preferences are not affected if the timing of all outcomes is incremented by a given constant amount. The preference for the DU model generally has a normative basis. It does not permit dynamic inconsistency in decision-making. However, the evidence that the DU model offers a good representation of individuals, intertemporal preferences is generally lacking. See Roelofsma (1996) for an extensive list of anomalies. Recently there has been increased interest shown by sections of the economics community in alternative models (Laibson 1997; O'Donoghue and Rabin 1999). There is still, however, a marked reluctance to adopt alternative models. Camerer (1999) has trenchantly observed that this results from '(i) ignorance about the overwhelming empirical superiority and parsimony of hyperbolic discounting; (ii) confusion about the normative versus descriptive appeal of dynamic consistency; and (iii) uncertainty about how to move away from the exponential model and still do analytical economics.'

10.2.2 **Individual time preferences and the social discount rate**

The main theme of this section is the relationship between individual time preferences and the discount rate to be applied when evaluating public or social investments. There are at least two issues with respect to determining a social discount rate for use in the evaluation of health care. One is the general (and traditional) question of the role of social time preference and social opportunity cost (Pearce and Nash 1981).

The other, assuming that time preferences will play some role with respect to the choice of social discount rate, is which time preferences are relevant.

Social time preference concerns society's preferences for consumption in one time period compared with another. The relationship of social to private time preferences is considered briefly below. The social opportunity cost approach emphasizes consistency in intertemporal decision-making. Resources should not be committed to marginal projects in the public sector when a greater social rate of return is available in the private sector. Under a fairly restrictive set of assumptions the economy will attain equilibrium where the social opportunity cost rate equals the social time preference rate. However, the consensus is that owing, for example, to imperfect capital markets the two rates are likely to diverge leaving the dilemma of which rate to use. After extensive debate in the economics literature there is support for an approach which combines both rates. The social opportunity cost rate is used to project forgone streams of consumption as a result of a particular investment and these streams can then be discounted using the social time preference rate. Olsen (1993) argues that the appropriate rate in a health care context is the time preference rate with respect to health. That is, he argues explicitly that the rate of discount need not be the same as that used elsewhere in the economy. Whether or not it is an empirical question.

However, before considering the empirical evidence regarding the rate of time preference for health, there is a prior question. Conceptually which is the relevant time preference for health? Gyrd-Hansen and Søgaard (1998) distinguish three different sets of preferences: individual preferences for private intertemporal choices, intertemporal social preferences and interpersonal social preferences which focus on interpersonal equity.

As emphasized in the introduction there are two distinct reasons for being interested in time preferences with respect to future health events. One is to obtain a better understanding of individual health-affecting behaviour, and the other is to inform the choice of social discount rate with which to evaluate competing uses of scarce health care resources. Clearly, in the former case the relevant preferences are those of the individual over their own future health. However, the appropriate preferences are less obvious in the case of social decision-making where there are a number of different time preferences which are potentially relevant. Parsonage and Neuburger (1992) consider the sources of positive time preference for individuals and assess their relevance for social choices. This leads them to question the relevance of individuals' pure time preference, and also the persuasiveness of the diminishing marginal utility and of the individual's risk of death arguments. Another argument against the relevance of private time preferences is that individuals may have preferences with respect to others' health that are different from those held with respect to their own health. For example, there is a long tradition of arguing that individuals might not want social decisions to be taken according to their private preferences (Sen 1967).

There is, however, a strong tradition in health economics to include individual preferences. A good illustration of this is the extensive research efforts with respect to valuing health states. Lipscomb (1989) suggests that given individual valuation of health it is anomalous not to incorporate individual time preferences. In a similar vein Gyrd-Hansen and Søgaard (1998) argue 'present value of life years gained or improved in the future is a matter of private consumption, and consequently it is not unreasonable that the present value of a life saved should be valued using individual time preferences' (p. 124).

Brouwer *et al.* (2000) argue strongly for the government to take a lead but they still leave the door open for the influence of approved private preferences when they concede that future effects might be adjusted 'in so far as this adjustment reflects a difference in the valuation of these effects by those receiving them.' (p. 117).

This lack of agreement over the appropriate basis for selecting a social discount rate re-emerges with respect to the specific question of whether or not health benefits should be discounted at the same rate as monetary costs.

10.2.3 How should health benefits be discounted?

The appropriate treatment of future health benefits has generated a considerable amount of interest in the past decade. While current practice and that generally recommended in guidelines suggests that future health benefits should be discounted at the same rate as future monetary costs, the answer to this question is rather more open than suggested by this uniformity of practice.

The orthodox view is based on two main arguments, one concerning eternal delay, and the other concerning consistency. Keeler and Cretin (1983) highlight a paradox that could arise if a lower discount rate were to be applied to health benefits than the one applied to monetary costs. A project could always be made to appear more attractive by delaying its implementation. Their solution is to require that costs and benefits are discounted at the same rate. This has provoked a number of responses. For example, van Hout (1998) has argued that the typical problem faced by decision-makers does not concern when to implement a particular policy but rather which of several projects to implement currently. More fundamentally, Gravelle and Smith (1999) argue that the Keeler and Cretin solution does not recognize that the underlying problem is that the CEA decision rule cannot cope with timing decisions.

The consistency argument was first made explicitly by Weinstein and Stason (1977) and has perhaps received more sustained support, for example, it has been endorsed in the recommendations of the Washington Panel (Gold *et al.* 1996). But it also has been questioned, specifically on the basis of a strong assumption regarding the future value of health benefits. Weinstein and Stason (1977) assume that 'life years are valued the same in relation to dollars in the present as in the future'. Without this assumption the consistency argument disappears (van Hout 1998). Gravelle and Smith (1999) argue that the value of health will increase over time as society becomes richer.

The monetary valuation of health effects, and specifically the difficulties encountered in achieving such valuations lies at the heart of the issue of appropriate discounting practice. If the stream of future health effects resulting from any particular intervention could be accurately represented in monetary terms there would surely be unanimity in the economics profession that the monetized streams of costs and benefits should be treated identically. There would be no grounds for using a lower rate of discount for those parts of these future streams that arise from changes in health.

Disagreement arises when the health effects are measured in physical non-monetary terms. This is not the place to explore issues such as whether health effects can be satisfactorily valued in monetary terms, or how such valuations should be made. For whatever reason, the monetary valuation of health effects is relatively uncommon in the extensive literature on the economic evaluation of health care. If an intervention results in increased survival should the life years gained be left undiscounted, be discounted at the same rate as used for future costs, or be discounted but at some rate lower than that applied to the costs?

The answer depends on what is to be assumed concerning changes in the shadow price of health. To see this, recognize that the present value (in money terms) of a future stream of life years gained is the sum of a series of products, each product has three elements – a discount factor, a marginal valuation of additional life years, and a quantity of additional life years. If the life years gained were to be left undiscounted and are simply summed, this is equivalent to assuming that the fall in the discount factor as the life years gained recede into the future is exactly balanced by a rise in the marginal valuation of life years gained. If the physical quantity of life years gained in any future year is weighted by the discount factor implied by the discount rate for costs, this is equivalent to assuming that the marginal valuation of life years remains constant over time. It appears plausible to suggest that neither practice will invariably yield the correct answer. Both will involve an element of approximation.

Encouraging explicitness is ultimately one of the major justifications for undertaking economic evaluation. In this spirit it would appear to be best to adjust explicitly the future stream of life years gained to take account of changes in the valuation of these life years and then apply a common discount rate to all the costs and benefits. There is a clear analogy here to the treatment of risk and uncertainty. While it has been suggested that discount rates could be adjusted using risk premia, the balance of opinion would suggest that this is unlikely to be a satisfactory means of taking risk and uncertainty into account. It doesn't make full use of the information available and it makes a highly restrictive assumption concerning the impact of risk and uncertainty.

But given the practical and possibly political difficulties in placing a monetary valuation on health effects is it really plausible that we could specify how this valuation is likely to change over time? The change in the marginal value of health benefits will depend primarily on the rate of growth of income and how the valuation of health changes *vis-à-vis* other goods as income rises. Also the valuation could be affected by shocks to health, for example, if new threats to health markedly reduce life-expectancy.

Clearly we have something of an impasse. If we can assume that the marginal valuation of life years will rise over time we should use a lower discount rate for unadjusted health effects. But if we had the information to enable us to identify how much lower the discount rate on health effects should be we might be better served by explicitly adjusting the future effects and using the common discount rate.

It is of course possible to make the unexceptionable suggestion that a variety of combinations of discount rates can be explored in the sensitivity analysis. But this possibly represents a slightly unsatisfactory failure to confront the issue. Such a resolution might further fuel doubts over the scientific basis of economic evaluation. It does suggest that there is a strong case for more research on the monetary valuation of health. The emphasis on cost-effectiveness analysis, and to a lesser extent on cost-utility analysis, has probably been important in winning acceptance of economic evaluation but has also slowed progress with respect to the monetary valuation of changes in health.

10.3 Evidence

10.3.1 Introduction

This section outlines the methods used to elicit time preferences for health events and summarizes the empirical evidence. First, however, it is necessary to note some differences in what different authors refer to as time preference, and to consider whether or not, in principle, time preferences for health events are measurable. Gafni and Torrance (1984) identify three distinct effects which make up an individual's attitude to risk in a health context: a quantity effect; a time preference effect; and a gambling effect. The time preference effect is sometimes described as *pure* time preference (or somewhat pejoratively as impatience). Other authors (for example, Olson and Bailey 1981) would argue that diminishing marginal utility (the quantity effect) and the risk attached to any future event are also elements of time preference.

Before anyone had attempted to measure time preferences for health events, Gafni and Torrance (1984) expressed some early optimism. They suggested that time preference could be 'measured by asking conventional time preference questions . . . but cast in the health, as opposed to financial domain' and claimed that it was not necessary to speculate on the nature of time preference '. . . since it is empirically determinable' (p. 449). However, drawing on Loewenstein and Prelec (1993) which highlighted the importance of another class of effects that affect inter-temporal choice – sequence effects, Gafni (1995) argues robustly that no measurement technique allows pure time preference to be distinguished. That the best that can be achieved is a measure of time preference for a given sequence of events. This may be true of preferences over one's own future health states. However, it is less clear that the sequence of events will be an important influence when considering preferences over life-saving profiles. In any case, Gyrd-Hansen and Søgaard (1998) argue that for economic evaluation we do not require a measure of pure time preferences but that we also wish to include diminishing marginal utility and uncertainty. It is thus an advantage if the method of eliciting time preferences doesn't capture only pure time preferences.

10.3.2 Methods for eliciting time preferences

Two broad approaches have been used to estimate time preference rates – revealed preference and stated preference. The distinction is that the former involves observing actual behaviour, specifically inter-temporal decisions, whereas the latter involves asking individuals what they would do in particular hypothetical circumstances. Despite a predisposition in favour of revealed preference, economists have in recent years shown an increasing willingness to explore the stated preference approach. Specifically, in health economics there is a recognition that the special nature of health and health care results in there being many fewer opportunities to obtain valuations from observed behaviour. There are still concerns about the validity of the information generated and the ideal corroborating evidence remains observed behaviour.

A wide range of behaviour has been studied including: the purchase of consumer durables (Hausman 1979); educational investment decisions (Lang and Ruud 1986); and labour market wage-risk choices (Viscusi and Moore 1989). These studies generally are based on larger sample sizes than those used in applications of the stated preference approach. Also the estimation of discount rates is relatively indirect and quite complicated. This results partly from the difficulty of using data collected primarily for some other purpose and the many more factors outwith the researchers control (as compared with an experimental approach).

The stated preference approach has also been applied in a wide range of settings. These have included: financial choices (Benzion et al. 1989); purchases of consumer durables (Houston 1983); saving lives; and non-fatal changes in health.

While there are, as noted below, many differences in design between studies the basic methods used to elicit preferences can be classified as either open-ended (or matching) methods or closed-ended (or choice) methods. As an example of a closed-ended approach consider Cropper et al. (1992). Individuals were offered a choice of two programmes. Programme A will save 100 lives now and programme B will save 200 lives 50 years from now. By varying the number of lives saved and how far in the future the lives are saved it is possible to identify the trade-off between delay and the number of lives saved. Whereas, in a typical example of an open-ended approach individuals are asked to identify the number of lives saved in five years time that would be equally good as saving 1000 lives one year in the future (Cairns 1994). The dichotomous choice is easier to answer but provides less information than its open-ended counterpart. One consequence is that implied discount rates are identifiable for the group rather than for the individual respondent.

There are numerous potential differences in design between studies. For example, in the case of non-fatal changes in health state with respect to: base health state; number of different health states; time horizon; and whether or not the comparison is between points in time or profiles. The base health state can be full-health and respondents make choices with respect to the consumption of ill-health (Redelmeier and Heller 1993) or the base health state is ill-health and respondents make choices with respect to the consumption of full-health (Chapman and Elstein 1995). Some studies consider only one ill-health state (Cairns 1992) others have considered more than one ill-health state (Dolan and Gudex 1995). A limited time period can be considered (Chapman 1996) (for instance five years), or a scenario can describe remaining life (Enemark et al. 1998). Respondents can be asked to consider two points in time or they can be presented with a profile. The standard approach has been the former, with few studies comparing profiles (Chapman et al. 1999).

In principle, open-ended studies could require respondents to specify: the *timing* of a given change in health; or the *magnitude* to be experienced at a certain point of time; or possibly the health-related *quality-of-life* to be experienced. Studies to date have asked individuals to specify the magnitude of the health benefit to be enjoyed at a particular point in the future either in terms of: lives saved (Olsen 1993); or duration of health state (Cairns and van der Pol 2000); or frequency of symptoms (Chapman *et al.* 1999). No study has asked individuals to specify timing or quality.

10.3.3 Estimates of time preference

The recent empirical work on time preference with respect to health states and with respect to lives and life years is summarized in Tables 10.1 and 10.2. The studies have been grouped into those using open-ended methods and those using closed-ended methods to elicit time preferences.

The most striking feature of these implied rates of discount is the wide range of estimates, particularly in the case of health states. It is important when considering any empirical estimates of time preference to note the period of delay with which these preferences have been elicited. Studies have repeatedly shown evidence of the implied rate of discount being a decreasing function of the period of delay. In Table 10.1 delay varies from one week to 25 years and in Table 10.2 from two years to 100 years. As a result it is impossible to draw any general conclusions. For example, at first sight studies reported in Table 10.2 using open-ended methods appear to have elicited higher rates of time preference than those using closed-ended methods but the periods of delay are typically longer for the latter group. In a similar fashion comparison of the rates in Tables 10.1 and 10.2 would be difficult if there are systematic differences between the time preferences of the general public and specific groups such as students since a higher proportion of the studies in Table 10.2 have used general public samples.

As noted above most studies have found evidence of an impact of the period of delay on the implied discount rate. Just under half of the studies have included variables to capture the characteristics of individual respondents. This has generally been done in an attempt to control for individual heterogeneity rather than as an explicit test of hypotheses regarding the determinants of time preference. The individual characteristic most commonly found to be significantly associated with the implied discount rate is the age of the respondent. As might be anticipated older respondents tend to have higher implied discount rates. There is limited evidence of significant associations between implied discount rates and a number of other variables including presence of young children in the household, ethnic group, smoking status and gender. To date an exploration of the factors which influence implied discount rates has not been a research priority, however, it may become more important in the future if the relationship between time preference and health-affecting behaviour continues to attract increasing attention.

Where predictions can be made about the impact of individual characteristics on implied rates of discount, successful prediction of the determinants of individual discount rates might be taken as indirect evidence of the validity of stated preference responses.

10.3.4 Limitations of the evidence

A central issue concerns the complexity of the questions used to elicit time preferences for health events. Thinking about your own or others' future health is difficult. Part of

Table 10.1 Studies of time preference with respect to health states

	Median r	Delay	Sample
Open-ended methods			
Cairns (1992)	−0.001–0.03[a]	10–28 yrs	29 economics students
Cairns and van der Pol (1999)	0.061	2–13 yrs	298 general public
Chapman (1996)	0.200–0.350	1–12 yrs	148 psychology students
Chapman and Coups (1999)	0.000	3 mths	409 corporate employees
Chapman and Elstein (1995)	0.360 and 1.000	1–12 yrs	104 psychology students
Chapman et al. (1999)	0.06–0.09[b]	1–6 mths	79 patients and 77 college students
Dolan and Gudex (1995)	0.000	9 yrs	39 general public
Lazaro et al. (2001)	0.149–0.213	2–15 yrs	203 law students
Lipscomb (1989)	–	1–25 yrs	52 students
Mackeigan et al. (1993)	–	1 wk–1 yr	108 university staff and hospital volunteers
Olsen (1993)	0.058–0.229	4–19 yrs	250 general public and 77 health planners
Olsen (1994)	0.02	5 and 20 yrs	90 economics students and 40 doctors
Redelmeier and Heller (1993)	0.023–0.041[a]	1 day–10 yrs	121 medical students, house officers and physicians
Closed-ended methods			
van der Pol and Cairns (1999)	0.032 and 0.086	5 and 13 yrs	158 general public
Cairns and van der Pol (2000)	0.038–0.066[a]	5–13 yrs	367 general public
Ganiats et al. (2000)	0.064–1.16	6 mths–20 yrs	169 patients

Notes: [a] mean r; [b] monthly not annual rate

Table 10.2 Studies of time preference with respect to lives and life years

	Median r	Delay	Sample
Open-ended methods			
Cairns and van der Pol (1997a, b)	0.160–0.410	2–19 yrs	473 general public
Cairns (1994)	0.160–0.380	4–19 yrs	223 general public
Enemark et al. (1998)	0.104	≈ 10 yrs	25 vascular surgeons
Lazaro et al. (2001)	0.199–0.204	2–15 yrs	203 law students
Olsen (1993)	0.058–0.229	4–19 yrs	250 general public and 77 health planners
Closed-ended methods			
Cropper et al. (1991)	0.027–0.086[a]	25–100 yrs	1600 general public
Cropper et al. (1994)	0.038–0.1688	25–100 yrs	3200 general public
Horowitz and Carson (1990)	0.045	5 yrs	75 economics undergraduates
Johannesson and Johansson (1996)	0.080–0.250	20–100 yrs	850 general public
Johannesson and Johansson (1997a)	0.013[a]	10–46 yrs	528 general public
Johannesson and Johansson (1997b)	0.010[a]	6–57 yrs	2577 general public

Note: [a] mean r

the problem is that most respondents are simply unused to thinking in the way required of them. A related difficulty is that of devising questions which are meaningful to the subject. It is quite evident that questions with respect to future financial events are easier to construct and are easier to answer. There exist many familiar financial instruments for postponing or expediting payment or consumption, the health analogue of which simply don't exist. The challenging nature of time preference questions is illustrated by the low response rates which are often achieved particularly when the subjects are members of the general public.

While the range of methods used to elicit time preferences is a sign of the vigour of this field of enquiry it does represent a major limitation of much of the empirical work. Comparison of the results is difficult when studies differ with respect to methods, subjects, health outcomes and delays.

This section has focused on studies adopting a stated preference approach. As argued earlier such approaches are unavoidable if significant progress is to be made with respect to understanding time preferences for future health events. However, there will always be doubts about the extent to which these methods have enabled researchers to accurately elicit time preferences. The ideal corroboration of findings using revealed preference methods will generally be unattainable. However, to the extent that different methods produce reproducible results confidence may be increased in the stated preference approach. Also studies which can link differences in implied time preferences with differences in behaviour would also increase confidence in the approach. The limited work of this type that has been undertaken so far is briefly reviewed in the next section.

10.4 Future developments

As noted in the introduction the exploration of the nature of time preferences for future health events is an exciting area of research with many issues unresolved. In this section four specific topics are outlined. These are: alternatives to the discounted utility model; time preferences and health affecting behaviour; time preferences for different health effects; and intra- and inter-generational discounting. Future developments can be anticipated with respect to each of these topics.

10.4.1 Alternative discounting models

There is an increasing body of evidence which questions the appropriateness of the discounted utility model as a description of intertemporal preferences. A detailed discussion of the numerous anomalies which have been identified with respect to the discounted utility model can be found in Loewenstein and Prelec (1992) and Roelofsma (1996).

Economists have generally used the Discounted Utility (DU) model to analyse intertemporal decision-making and continue to do so despite a growing body of evidence at odds with the predictions of the DU model. Loewenstein and Prelec (1992) identify four intertemporal choice anomalies that run counter to the predictions of the DU model. They describe these as: the common difference effect; the absolute magnitude effect; the gain–loss asymmetry; and the delay-speedup asymmetry. The last three are self-explanatory. The DU model assumes that the discount rate applied will not be related to the magnitude of the event which is subject to discounting, nor to whether the event represents a gain or a loss, nor to whether it is being brought forward or delayed. The common difference effect refers to the impact on choice between two delayed outcomes of a change in the delay applied equally to both outcomes. The DU model assumes that the choice depends only on the absolute interval between the two outcomes or in different language assumes that preferences obey the axiom of stationarity. These anomalies are explained by Loewenstein and Prelec in general terms with reference to future consumption, and supported by evidence from monetary choices. However, there is no reason to suppose that they are any less in evidence when the outcomes are in terms of health.

Stationarity is valued by economists because without it behaviour need not be dynamically consistent and preferences may reverse over time. However, as Loewenstein and Thaler (1989) memorably remarked:

'[B]ehavior will not generally be consistent over time. In the morning, when temptation is remote, we vow to go to bed early, stick to our diet, and not have too much to drink. That night we stay out until 3:30 a.m., have two helpings of chocolate decadence, and sample every variety of Aquavit at a Norwegian restaurant.' (p. 185)

Although many studies show evidence that discount rates decrease over time only a few studies have tested the axiom of stationarity explicitly. Green *et al.* (1994) and Kirby and Herrnstein (1995) found evidence of preference reversal as equal increments were added to the delays before the payment of hypothetical monetary rewards. Albrecht and Weber (1997) found that the stationarity axiom was violated when subjects had to *match* future risky monetary outcomes but not when they had to *choose* between risky future monetary outcomes.

Four studies have tested the stationarity axiom in a health context. Christensen-Szalanski (1984) tested whether women's preferences for avoiding anaesthesia reverse during childbirth. Cairns and van der Pol (1997a, 2000) investigated preferences for saving future statistical lives and for non-fatal changes in health respectively using data elicited using open-ended methods. A broadly similar approach was adopted by Bleichrodt and Johannesson (2001) but using dichotomous choice data derived from choices between different health profiles. All of these studies found that the stationarity axiom is violated.

This and other evidence has encouraged investigation of alternative models. To date efforts have concentrated on hyperbolic models. Most of the studies are to be found in the psychology rather than the economics literature. A number of studies have explicitly compared hyperbolic models with the exponential model (Meyerson and Green 1995, Kirby and Marakovio 1995, Ahlbrecht and Weber 1995). These studies generally involve hypothetical monetary choices but on occasion involve real rewards. Although they fit different hyperbolic models, each of them concludes that hyperbolic models fit the data better than the discounted utility model.

These studies are of relatively limited relevance to intertemporal preferences for health since the majority elicits intertemporal preferences for monetary awards. Also, the econometric modelling, especially in the instances where discounting functions are fitted on an individual basis, is hampered by the small number of observations.

Two studies have compared hyperbolic and exponential models in the context of saving future lives. Cropper *et al.* (1994) compared an exponential and a hyperbolic (Harvey) model when analysing their discrete choice data. The exponential function fitted the data better for delays equal to or smaller than 25 years while the hyperbolic function fitted the data better for delays greater than 25 years. Cairns and van der Pol (1997a) analyse open-ended data on preferences for future financial and health benefits. They compare the exponential model with two hyperbolic models: the Loewenstein and Prelec (1992) model and a special case of this model where $w_t = (1 + kt)^{-s}$ (Rachlin 1989). They found greater support for the hyperbolic models than for the exponential model.

To date, only one study has compared exponential and hyperbolic models using data on preferences over future health states. Cairns and van der Pol (2000) found that individuals' inter-temporal preferences are better represented by hyperbolic discounting models than by the discounted utility model.

However, while hyperbolic models accommodate non-stationarity there are other phenomena, such as magnitude and sign effects, which neither the DU model nor hyperbolic models can explain (Roelofsma 1996). Also, refinements of the DU model, for example incorporating habit formation (Wathieu 1997), may be able to account for several of the anomalies.

10.4.2 Time preference and health-affecting behaviour

One of the major reasons for being interested in time preferences is the potential role these preferences might play in terms of understanding individual health-affecting behaviour. Those with higher rates of time preference will be less willing to incur short-term costs in order to secure longer-term benefits. If this is the case there may be important implications for the design of policies to encourage healthy behaviour and to discourage unhealthy behaviour.

An early start was made by Fuchs (1982) in exploring the relationship between time preferences and health-affecting behaviour. Discount rates were estimated from answers to pair-wise choices offering the opportunity to delay the receipt of a money prize between one and five years in order to receive a larger prize. Five health behaviours were considered: smoking; weight; time since last dental check-up; frequency of exercise; and wearing of seatbelts. A significant positive association was found between time preference and smoking. However, there was little evidence of an association with the other health behaviours.

In subsequent years research has focused on the estimation of time preferences for health events rather than on the influence of time preference on behaviour. However, five further studies have recently examined the relationship between money time preferences and health-affecting behaviour. It is anticipated that individuals who discount the future more heavily may be more willing to engage currently in damaging activities than those with lower rates of time preference. Similarly, individuals with low rates of time preference may be more willing to incur short-term costs in order to secure longer-term benefits.

Madden *et al.* (1997) found that a sample of opioid-dependent patients discounted future hypothetical monetary rewards at a higher rate than non-drug-using controls (using a hyperbolic model). Additionally, the drug users revealed significantly higher rates of discount with respect to heroin than money (despite the scope for trading money for heroin). Kirby *et al.* (1999) also compared opioid-dependent individuals with non-drug-using controls using a hyperbolic model but offering real monetary rewards. They also found that the opioid-dependent group had higher discount rates.

Vuchinich and Simpson (1998) examined the time preferences of college students classified as light and heavy drinkers. Time preferences were elicited using questions involving the speeding up of the receipt of money over periods ranging from one week to 25 years. They found that a hyperbolic model fitted the data better than the exponential model and that heavy drinkers exhibited higher hyperbolic discounting than light drinkers.

Bretteville-Jensen (1999) estimated an annual and a weekly rate of time preference for injecting addicts, former users and non-users. Time preferences were elicited using questions concerning the speeding up of the receipt of money. Active drug users were found to have higher discount rates than former users, who in turn had higher rates than non-users.

Chapman and Coups (1999) investigated the time preferences of a workforce some of whom had accepted and some of whom had declined the offer of a free influenza vaccination. They elicited time preferences with respect to both a monetary and a health choice. The former involved delaying the payment of a fine and the latter delaying a period of ill-health for three months. A striking feature of this study was the very large proportion of respondents with a zero rate of time preference (greater than 80 per cent). Those expressing zero time preference for money were significantly more likely to have accepted a vaccination. No significant association was found in the case of health time preferences.

While all of these studies find some evidence of the expected association, in the case of smoking, drinking and injecting behaviour it is not possible to determine whether the health-affecting behaviour influences time preferences or whether time preferences influence health-affecting behaviour. However, in the case of flu vaccinations it seems implausible that causation could run from the vaccination decision to time preference.

The link between time preferences and health-affecting behaviour is likely to be a topic of increasing interest in the future, with the difficulties of establishing the direction of causation as an important research challenge. Also since there is relatively little evidence suggesting that health and money time preferences are closely related, the issue of which preferences to measure needs to be addressed.

10.4.3 Time preferences for different health effects

Since the discount rates elicited will not generally represent estimates of pure time preference they might be expected to differ across different types of health benefit. Also it is possible that there are framing effects such that hypothetical choices involving different types of health benefit give rise to different implied discount rates.

A further possibility is that there are real differences in time preferences over different health effects. At first sight the existence of long-run differences in implied discount rates might seem strange in that elsewhere in the economy we expect pressures equalizing rates of return on different assets. However, in the case of individual health the scope for such arbitrage is limited.

The empirical literature comprises two types of study: those involving the saving of statistical lives; and those examining non-fatal changes to health and saving life years. The studies of preferences with respect to saving future statistical lives clearly refer to the health of others. The majority of the studies of preferences with respect to non-fatal changes in health and saving life years have been posed in terms of the respondents' *own* health. Although, Mackeigan *et al.* (1993) while inviting respondents to consider their own health, asked respondents to imagine that they were 50 years old and married with children (none of whom lived with them). There have been four studies concerned with time preferences for the health of others. The scenarios used by Lipscomb (1989) invite respondents to consider 'A person in your community is now 25 years old'. Also as part of his life-saving study Olsen (1993) repeated the life-saving questions with 'a programme which improves the health of people in a chronic state of dysfunction and distress' substituted for 'a programme which saves human lives'. The study by Enemark *et al.* (1998) elicited the time preferences of vascular surgeons for their patients' future health. Finally, Cairns and van der Pol (1999) elicit preferences with respect to the future health of a group of middle-aged patients.

There does appear to be a broad pattern to the results in that studies concerned with own health report considerably lower estimated discount rates than do studies concerned with others' health. Although there are exceptions to this pattern (Chapman and Elstein 1995). However, there are too many differences between the studies with respect to design and methods for any strong conclusions to be drawn. The only study designed to examine whether preferences for own and others' health differ concluded that the implied discount rates for own and others' health are broadly similar (Cairns and van der Pol 1999).

10.4.4 Intra- and inter-generational discounting

A distinction can be drawn between intra-generational and inter-generational discounting. The use of any positive discount rate given a sufficiently long time horizon over which to operate will generate very small present values. It is often argued that this is unfair to future generations.

Collard (1978) made an early proposal for dealing with intergenerational equity and discounting but not in a health context. He suggested that the stream of benefits for each generation be discounted to their own present and that these present values be combined not by discounting to our present but by using weights which reflect our altruism towards the future generations. A broadly similar two-part approach has been suggested in the health economics literature (Lipscomb 1989; Gold *et al.* 1996). Individuals would use their own private rates to re-express the stream of benefits to them in present value terms and a social discount rate is then used to adjust this future stream of present values.

Brouwer *et al.* (2000), following a tradition stretching back at least to Pigou, ques-tion the use of individual values reflecting myopia and fear of death. They argue that the societal decision-maker should overrule such preferences and that 'the amount of future effects should only be adjusted for their timing when obvious differences between people at different points in time are present or can be rightfully expected' (p. 133). The differences that they have in mind are those that change the relative valua-tion of health effects.

A small number of empirical studies have considered periods of delay sufficiently long that the preference elicited is presumably an inter-generational one. For example, Cropper *et al.* (1991) and Johannesson and Johansson (1996) elicited preferences with respect to delays of up to 100 years. The period of delay over which to elicit preferences must be guided by the purpose for which a rate of discount is sought. Is a social rate of discount wanted for weighting future present values or is a private rate that an indi-vidual uses to re-express a stream of future benefits to themselves? To what extent is the widely observed inverse relationship between the implied rate of discount and the period of delay picking up preferences for inter-generational equity?

10.5 Discounting practice

From the preceding discussion it should be clear that there are several potential issues concerning discounting practice: which model to use; what rate to use; and whether or not to treat health benefits differently from monetary costs. There is no uniquely correct method for dealing with future streams of costs and benefits. Variations in practice are defensible.

Although there is considerable evidence that the exponential model does not provide a good representation of intertemporal preferences for health, most econo-mists are unwilling to discard such a tractable, familiar and (to some) normatively appealing model. To date there is rare unanimity across all jurisdictions for which guidelines have been developed regarding its use to discount future costs and benefits.

Less uniformity is apparent with respect to the discount rate (Gravelle and Smith 1999). However, most guidelines suggest the use of a number of alternative rates, frequently in the 3–5 per cent range. A key element in the recommendations of the Washington Panel is the Reference Case which is a 'standard set of methodologic prac-tices that an analyst would seek to follow'. The analyst would retain flexibility by being able to augment the Reference case but comparability would be secured across studies, at least via the Reference case. The discount rate is a prime candidate for inclusion in the Reference case. At first sight, the Reference case concept, that all evaluations should be in part conducted on a common basis so that different studies can be readily compared, is appealing. Whether in practice it performs well will depend on a number of factors. To what extent will varied approaches be discouraged by the introduction of a standard, and is more lost or gained by such standardization? Will the Reference case come to be regarded as the most appropriate indication of cost-effectiveness rather than simply facilitating comparison between studies?

Hillman and Kim (1995) suggest the use of undiscounted health outcomes as the base case and that when 'appropriate' discounted outcomes should also be included.

Their primary argument is that the lack of agreement among decision-makers over the values embedded in the discounting procedure means that the routine discounting of health benefits will introduce bias into allocative decisions. Thus they advocate discounting as the exception rather than the rule. However, their argument cuts both ways – if there is no agreement over values, failure to discount health outcomes can also be described as introducing bias.

Despite the many fascinating issues raised concerning the nature of intertemporal preferences for health, for many the central question is what rate of discount to use with respect to health benefits. Smith and Gravelle (2001) in a review of discounting practice in ten countries, found only one instance of an explicit recommendation to discount costs and health at different rates. The Department of Health (in England) in guidance issued in 1996, recommend a rate of between 1½ per cent and 2 per cent for health benefits (measured in physical as opposed to monetary units) and 6 per cent for costs (Department of Health 1996).

With respect to this central question of whether or not costs and health benefits should be discounted at a common rate, van Hout (1998) suggests that the debate can be recast in terms of believers and non-believers in market forces. This echoes the earlier remark of Redelmeier *et al.* (1994) that the constant marginal exchange rate between money and health is 'a matter of faith, not of science'. While this will necessarily remain the case, this chapter demonstrates that substantial progress has been made with respect to the science and also that there are many opportunities to further advance the scientific study of time preferences.

References

Ahlbrecht, M. and Weber, M. (1995). Hyperbolic discounting models in prescriptive theory of intertemporal choice. *Zeitschrift für Wirtschafts und Sozialwissenschaften*, 115(4), 535–68.

Ahlbrecht, M. and Weber, M. (1997). An empirical study of intertemporal decision-making in the case of risk. *Management Science*, 43(6), 813–26.

Benzion, U., Rapoport, A. and Yagil, J. (1989). Discount rates inferred from decisions: an experimental study. *Management Science*, 35(3), 270–84.

Bleichrodt, H. and Johannesson, M. (2001). Time preference for health: a test of stationarity versus decreasing timing aversion. *Journal of Mathematical Psychology*, 45(2), 265–82.

Bretteville-Jensen, A. L. (1999). Addiction and discounting. *Journal of Health Economics*, 18(4), 393–407.

Brouwer, W., van Hout, B. and Rutten, F. (2000). A fair approach to discounting future effects: taking a societal perspective. *Journal of Health Services Research and Policy*, 5(2), 114–18.

Cairns, J. A. (1992). Health, wealth and time preference. *Project Appraisal*, 7(1), 31–40.

Cairns, J. A. (1994). Valuing future benefits. *Health Economics*, 3(4), 221–9.

Cairns, J. A. and van der Pol, M. M. (1997a). Saving future lives: a comparison of three discounting models. *Health Economics*, 6(4), 341–50.

Cairns, J. A. and van der Pol, M. M. (1997b). Constant and decreasing timing aversion. *Social Science and Medicine*, 45(11), 1653–9.

Cairns, J. A. and van der Pol, M. M. (1999). Do people value their own future health differently rom others' future health? *Medical Decision-Making*, 19(4), 466–72.

Cairns, J. A. and van der Pol, M. M. (2000). The estimation of marginal time preference in a UK-wide sample (TEMPUS) project. *Health Technology Assessment*, 4, 1–73.

Camerer, C. (1999). Bounded rationality in individual decision-making. *Experimental Economics*, 1, 163–83.

Chapman, G. B. (1996). Temporal discounting and utility for health and money. *Journal of Experimental Psychology: Learning, Memory and Cognition*, 22(3), 771–91.

Chapman, G. B. and Coups, E. J. (1999). Time preferences and preventive health behavior: acceptance of the influenza vaccine. *Medical Decision-Making*, 19(3), 307–14.

Chapman, G. B. and Elstein, A. S. (1995). Valuing the future: temporal discounting of health and money. *Medical Decision-Making*, 15(4), 373–86.

Chapman, G. B., Nelson, R. and Hier, D. B. (1999). Familiarity and time preferences: decision-making about treatments for migraine headaches and Crohn's disease. *Journal of Experimental Psychology: Applied*, 5(1), 17–34.

Christensen-Szalanski, J. J. J. (1984). Discount functions and the measurement of patients' values. *Medical Decision-Making*, 4(1), 47–58.

Collard, D. (1978). *Altrusim and economy*. Martin Robertson, Oxford.

Cropper, M. L., Aydede, S. K. and Portney, P. R. (1991). Discounting human lives. *American Journal of Agricultural Economics*, 73, 1410–15.

Cropper, M. L., Aydede, S. K. and Portney, P. R. (1992). Rates of time preference for saving lives. *American Economic Review*, 82(2), 469–72.

Cropper, M. L., Aydede, S. K. and Portney P. R. (1994). Preferences for life saving programs: how the public discount time and age. *Journal of Risk and Uncertainty*, 8(3), 243–65.

Department of Health. (1996). *Policy Appraisal and Health*. Department of Health, London.

Dolan, P. and Gudex, C. (1995). Time preference, duration and health state valuations. *Health Economics*, 4(4), 289–99.

Enemark, U., Lyttkens, C. H., Troëng, T. *et al.* (1998). Implicit discount rates of vascular surgeons in the management of abdominal aortic aneurysms. *Medical Decision-Making*, 18(2), 168–77.

Fuchs, V. R. (1982). Time preference and health: an exploratory study. In: V.R. Fuchs (ed.) *Economics aspects of health*. The University of Chicago Press, Chicago.

Gafni, A. (1995). Time in health: can we measure individuals' 'pure time preferences'? *Medical Decision-Making*, 15(1), 31–7.

Gafni, A. and Torrance, G. W. (1984). Risk attitude and time preference in health. *Management Science*, 30(4), 440–51.

Ganiats, T. G., Carson, R. T., Hamm, R. M. *et al.* (2000). Population-based time preferences for future health outcomes. *Medical Decision-Making*, 20(3), 263–70.

Gold, M. R., Siegel, J. E. and Weinstein, M. C. (1996). *Cost-effectiveness in health and medicine*. Oxford University Press. Oxford.

Green, L., Fry, A. F. and Myerson, J. (1994). Discounting of delayed rewards: a life-span comparison. *Psychological Science*, 5(1), 33–6.

Gyrd-Hansen, D. and Sogaard, J. (1998). Discounting life years: whither time preference? *Health Economics*, 7(2), 121–7.

Hausman, J. A. (1979). Individual discount rates and the purchase and utilisation of energy-using durables. *Bell Journal of Economics*, 10(1), 33–54.

Hillman, A. L. and Kim, M. S. (1995). Economic decision-making in healthcare: a standard approach to discounting health outcomes. *PharmacoEconomics*, 7(3), 198–205.

Horowitz, J. H. and Carson, R. T. (1990). Discounting statistical lives. *Journal of Risk and Uncertainty*, 3(4), 403–13.

Houston, D. A. (1983). Implicit discount rates and the purchase of untried, energy-saving durable goods. *Journal of Consumer Research*, 10, 236–46.

van Hout, B. (1998). Discounting costs and effects. *Health Economics*, 7(7), 581–94.

Johannesson, M. and Johansson, P-O. (1996). The discounting of lives saved in future generations – some empirical results. *Health Economics*, 5(4), 329–32.

Johannesson, M. and Johansson, P-O. (1997a). The value of life extension and the marginal rate of time preference: a pilot study. *Applied Economic Letters*, 4(1), 53–5.

Johannesson, M. and Johansson, P-O. (1997b). Quality-of-life and the WTP for an increased life expectancy at an advanced age. *Journal of Public Economics*, 65(3), 219–28.

Keeler, E. B. and Cretin S. (1983). Discounting of life-saving and other nonmonetary effects. *Management Science*, 29(3), 300–6.

Kirby, K. N. and Herrnstein, R. J. (1995). Preference reversals due to myopic discounting of delayed reward. *Psychological Science*, 6(2), 83–9.

Kirby, K. N. and Marakovio, N. N. (1995). Modeling myopic decisions: evidence for hyperbolic delay discounting within subjects and amounts. *Organizational Behavior and Human Decision Processes*, 64(1), 22–30.

Kirby, K. N. and Marakovio, N. N. (1996). Delay-discounting probabilistic rewards: rates decrease as amounts increase. *Psychonomic Bulletin and Review*, 3(1), 100–4.

Kirby, K. N., Petry, N. M. and Bickel, W. K. (1999). Heroin addicts have higher discount rates for delayed rewards than non-drug-using controls. *Journal of Experimental Psychology: General*, 128(1), 78–87.

Laibson, D.I. (1997). Golden eggs and hyperbolic discounting. *Quarterly Journal of Economics*, 112, 443–77.

Lang, K. and Ruud, P.A. (1986). Returns to schooling, implicit discount rates and black-white wage differentials. *Review of Economics and Statistics*, 69(1), 41–7.

Lazaro, A., Barberan, R. and Rubio, E. (2001). Private and social time preferences for health and money: an empirical estimation. *Health Econ.*, 10(4), 351–6.

Lipscomb, J. (1989). Time preference for health in cost-effectiveness analysis. *Medical Care*, 27(3), S233-S253.

Loewenstein, G. (1992). The fall and rise of psychological explanations in the economics of intertemporal choice. In G. Loewenstein, and J. Elster (eds), *Choice over time*. Russell Sage Foundation, New York.

Loewenstein, G. and Prelec, D. (1992). Anomalies in intertemporal choice: evidence and an interpretation. *Quarterly Journal of Economics*, 107, 573–97.

Loewenstein, G. and Prelec, D. (1993). Preferences for sequences of outcomes. *Psychological Review*, 100(1), 91–108.

Loewenstein, G. and Thaler, R. H. (1989). Intertemporal choice. *Journal of Economic Perspectives*, 3(4), 181–93.

Mackeigan, L. D., Larson, L. N., Draugalis, J. R., *et al.* (1993). Time preference for health gains versus health losses. *PharmacoEconomics*, 3(5), 374–86.

Madden, G. J., Petry, N. M., Badger, G. J. *et al.* (1997). Impulsive and self-control choices in opiod-dependent patients and non-drug-using control participants: drug and monetary rewards. *Experimental and Clinical Psychopharmacology*, 5(3), 256–62.

Meyerson, J. and Green, L. (1995). Discounting of delayed rewards: models of individual choice. *Journal of the Experimental Analysis of Behavior*, 64(3), 263–76.

O'Donoghue, T. and Rabin, M. (1999). Doing it now or later. *American Economic Review*, 89(1), 103–24.

Olsen, J.A. (1993a). On what basis should health be discounted? *Journal of Health Economics*, 12(1), 39–53.

Olsen, J.A. (1993b). Time preferences for health gains: an empirical investigation. *Health Economics*, 2(3), 257–265.

Olsen, J.A. (1994). Persons vs years: two ways of eliciting implicit weights. *Health Economics*, 3(1), 39–46.

Olson, M. and Bailey, M. J. (1981). Positive time preference. *Journal of Political Economy*, 89(1), 1–25.

Parsonage, M. and Neuburger, H. (1992). Discounting and health benefits. *Health Economics*, 1(1), 71–6.

Pearce, D. W. and Nash, C. A. (1981). *The Social Appraisal of Projects*. Macmillan, London.

van der Pol, M. M. and Cairns, J. A. (1999). Individual time preferences for own health: an application of a dichotomous choice question with follow-up. *Applied Economic Letters*, 6, 649–54.

Rachlin, H. (1989). *Judgement, decision and choice*. Freeman, New York.

Redelmeier, D. A. and Heller, D. N. (1993). Time preference in medical decision-making and cost-effectiveness analysis. *Medical Decision-Making*, 13(3), 212–7.

Redelmeier, D. A., Heller, D. N. and Weinstein, M. C. (1994). Time preference in medical economics: science or religion? *Medical Decision-Making*, 14(3), 301–3.

Roelofsma, P. H. M. P. (1996). Modelling intertemporal choices: an anomaly approach. *Acta Psychologica*, 93(1), 5–22.

Rothbard, M. N. (1990). Time preference. In: J. Eatwell, M. Milgate and P. Newman (eds), *Utility and probability*. Macmillan, London.

Sen, A. K. (1967). Isolation, assurance and the social rate of discount. *Quarterly Journal of Economics*, 81(1), 112–24.

Smith, D.H. and Gravelle, H. (2001). The practice of discounting in economic evaluations of health care interventions. *International Joural of Technology Assessment in Health Care*, 17(2), 236–43.

Viscusi, W. K. and Moore, M. J. (1989). Rates of time preference and valuations of the duration of life. *Journal of Public Economics*, 38(3), 297–317.

Vuchinich, R. E. and Simpson, C. A. (1998). Hyperbolic temporal discounting in social drinkers and problem drinkers. *Experimental and Clinical Psychopharmacology*, 6(3), 292–305.

Wathieu, L. (1997). Habits and the anomalies in intertemporal choice. *Management Science*, 43(11), 1552–63.

Weinstein, M. C. and Stason, W. B. (1977). Foundations of cost-effectiveness analysis for health and medical practices. *New England Journal of Medicine*, 296(13), 716–21.

Chapter 11

Transferability of economic evaluation results

Michael Drummond and Francis Pang

11.1 Introduction

With the growing international literature on economic evaluation, there is a need to undertake, or at least interpret, economic evaluations on an international level. For example, health care decision-makers, especially in those jurisdictions having limited resources for health services research, may wish to reinterpret in their own setting the results of an economic evaluation done elsewhere.

Issues relating to the lack of generalizability of economic data have been widely discussed by health economists (Drummond *et al.* 1992; O'Brien 1997). The issues can relate to the problems of generalizing from data collected alongside clinical trials to regular practice, to the lack of generalizability of economic data over time, or the lack of generalizability from place to place. This chapter deals with the latter issue, which we call *transferability*.

Some of the jurisdictions requiring economic data in support of submissions for public reimbursement for pharmaceuticals or other health technologies, have pointed out that the data need to be relevant to the local setting (Commonwealth of Australia 1995; National Institute for Clinical Excellence 2001), but offer little advice on the approach to be adopted. Unless all data are to be generated for every setting, strategies for dealing with problems of transferability need to be developed.

However, whereas the clinical (i.e. effectiveness) data may be transferable from place to place, there are several prima facie reasons why the results of economic evaluations may not. For example, Späth *et al.* (1999) analysed the eligibility of published economic evaluations for transfer to the French health care system. They identified 26 published economic evaluations of adjuvant therapy in women with breast cancer. Of these, none were eligible for transfer to the French health care system, the main reason being that the cost data were not reported in a transparent way.

In addition, clinical trials are increasingly being mounted on an international basis in order to recruit sufficient numbers of patients or to satisfy the needs of different national regulatory agencies that like to see clinical evidence relating to their own patient population. Where data on resource use and cost are collected alongside these trials, a strategy for analysing these data is required. For example, can the data on resource use or cost-effectiveness be pooled, or should they be analysed by country or setting?

Therefore this chapter discusses the following issues:

- What factors limit the transferability of economic data?
- What analytic strategies have been employed to deal with issues of transferability?
- What are the implications for the design and analysis of economic evaluations in the future?

11.2 Factors limiting the transferability of economic data

11.2.1 Basic demography and epidemiology of disease

Countries differ in respect of the age structure of their population and the incidence of various diseases. In some cases this will affect the cost-effectiveness of health care programmes, particularly those delivered on the population level. For example, programmes of immunization or screening and treatment of disease are likely to be more cost-effective in populations where the incidence of the disease in question is high. Different age structures between countries are likely to lead to different levels of incidence in various countries and hence the size of the overall economic burden. The cost-effectiveness of treatment is also likely to vary by patient characteristics, including age, lifestyle, and medical history. Therefore, when discussing the cost-effectiveness of health care treatments and programmes, it is important to specify the patient population to which any statements apply.

11.2.2 Availability of health care resources and variations in clinical practice

Countries differ in respect of the range of treatments and health care facilities available to their populations. In the case of treatment for ulcer, the availability of surgery could vary from place to place. In some countries with national health care systems, such as Sweden and the UK, rationing takes place, with waiting lists for hospital admission. The availability of important diagnostic facilities, such as endoscopy, could also vary from one location to another. In turn, the availability of resources may affect the way medicine is practised. For example, if there are long waiting times for endoscopy, a clinician may try a therapeutic dose of a drug for a patient experiencing ulcer-type pain without waiting to confirm the diagnosis. Another difference between countries, more directly related to drug therapy, is the range of licensed products and availability of generic medicines.

Although clinical practice is partly constrained by the available alternatives, it is known that practice varies among clinicians in the same geographical area facing essentially the same range of treatment options. To the extent that clinical practice varies systematically between countries, this is likely to affect the relative cost-effectiveness of therapies.

11.2.3 **Incentives to health care professionals and institutions**

In some health care systems the level of remuneration of health care professionals and institutions is largely independent of the level of service delivered. For example, hospitals are given a global budget and physicians are paid by salary. In other systems physicians are paid by fee per item of service and hospitals reimbursed by the number of cases in each category treated.

It has often been suggested that physicians operating under a fee-for-service system are more likely to generate extra demand for their services, whereas those paid by salary or capitation are more likely to deter demand. This may affect the number of physician visits and diagnostic tests performed for a patient suffering from a given condition.

In the case of hospital treatment, the method of reimbursement could affect which services are delivered on an out-patient basis and also the length of stay for in-patients. A hospital being paid a fixed amount for treating a given case has more incentives to free the bed for the next patient than a hospital being funded through a global budget.

11.2.4 **Relative prices or costs**

It is well known that absolute price levels vary between countries. However, from the point of view of cost-effectiveness assessments, the critical issue is whether the *relative* prices of health care resources differ. Most obviously, if the relative prices of the main drugs for a given condition differ between countries, then their relative cost-effectiveness will differ.

Perhaps less obvious is the fact that the relative cost-effectiveness of drugs will differ if the relative prices of *other* health care resources differ between countries. For example, a drug with greater efficacy, a better side effect profile, or more convenient route of administration, will appear better value for money in a country where the costs of investigations, hospitalizations, surgery and physician visits are relatively higher, since consumption of these items is likely to be reduced.

However, it should also be remembered (as pointed out in Chapter 4) that the prices of health care resources do not always reflect costs, although it is often a tacit assumption of economic evaluations that they do. Therefore, in arguing that savings in other health care resources, such as surgical time, justify a more expensive but more efficacious drug, some consideration should be given to whether the prices of those resources really reflect their true opportunity costs.

In some cases the relative prices of medical procedures can affect the choice of clinical strategy. For example, Hull *et al.* (1981) found that the relative price of venography (a diagnostic test for deep-vein thrombosis) differed between the USA and Canada. This affected the relative cost-effectiveness of alternative diagnostic strategies for DVT in the two countries and would also affect the estimates of the value for money of drugs to prevent DVT. However, the size and direction of these changes are hard to predict. In a more recent study of diagnostic strategies for pulmonary embolism (PE), a condition related to DVT, van Erkel *et al.* (1999) found that while there were considerable differences in the costs of diagnostic and therapeutic procedures for PE among hospitals in the USA and five European countries, the differences did not affect the cost-effectiveness rankings of strategies.

11.2.5 Population values

The results of cost-benefit and cost-utility analyses depend on how the outcomes of treatments or interventions are valued by the general population. The values placed on health states could conceivably vary from place to place and the guidance for conducting economic evaluations issued by the National Institute for Clinical Excellence (2001) in the UK states that whatever method of health state preference valuation is employed, the onus is on the analyst to demonstrate that the values used in the economic evaluation reflect the preferences of the population of England and Wales.

There has been relatively little exploration of the extent to which health state preference values vary by geographical location and more research is required. However, the research to date on health 'utilities' suggests that the mean values for different health states does not very greatly (Johnson *et al.* 2000; Le Gales *et al.* 2000).

11.2.6 Summary

Whereas not every study shows that cost-effectiveness estimates vary by country or location, there is enough reason to suppose that they *may* vary. Therefore, when economic evaluations are required on a multinational level, methods are required to adjust for cross-national differences.

11.3 Analytic strategies to deal with issues of transferability

11.3.1 Modelling approaches

Modelling is frequently used in economic evaluations to explore the effects of varying key parameters. Therefore, it is not surprising that modelling approaches have been used to explore issues of transferability.

Modelling from the clinical data alone

Several studies have generated economic findings for different locations by modelling from the clinical data alone. The logic for this approach is that the clinical data may be generalizable and can be supplemented by local resource use and cost data in an economic model.

Drummond *et al.* (1992) drew together the findings of four national economic studies from Belgium, France, the UK and the USA, examining misoprostol in the prevention of NSAID-associated gastric ulcer in patients with osteoarthritis who experienced abdominal pain. All studies took endoscopically detected gastric ulcer rates from a US multicentre randomized, double-blind placebo-controlled trial, with a three month follow-up period. Using a decision-analytical framework, researchers

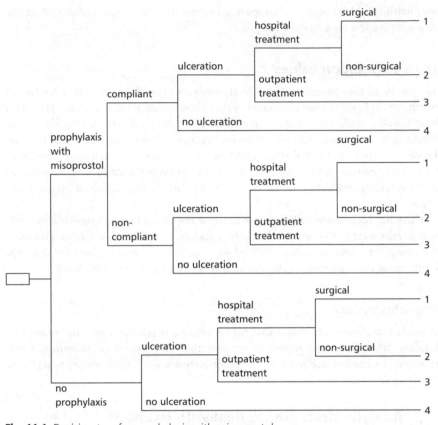

Fig. 11.1 Decision tree for prophylaxis with misoprostol
Source: adapted from Drummond et al (1992)

from each country estimated direct medical expenditures over a period of three months in their own settings (see Figure 11.1). Treatment efficacy was drawn from the trial, but compliance with therapy, detection rates and consequent use of healthcare resources were allowed to vary by country. Cost comparisons between countries were made by adjusting to US dollars using purchasing power parities.

The UK made the greatest use of ambulatory care, probably because of relatively well developed primary care services in that country. The acquisition cost of misoprostol was similar for the three European countries, but was higher in the USA. The four countries differed both in the percentage of patients who were hospitalized with ulcer and the percentage who underwent a surgical operation. Duration of hospital stay was shortest in the USA, but the cost of surgical care was by far the highest. The estimated net costs of three months' misoprostol prophylaxis showed surprisingly similar results, despite differences among the countries' clinical practice patterns and cost components.

The main problems encountered in this study related to the availability and type of data found in each country, a common problem in modelling studies. Data on ambulatory care were sparse and had to be obtained by structured interviews with physicians. For France and Belgium, hospital utilization statistics were based on all peptic ulcers rather than just gastric ulcer. Availability of hospital cost data varied greatly between countries. In the UK, where disease-related hospital cost data were not available, locally based costing studies were required. The Belgian study used diagnostic-related group (DRG) data based on charges. (Issues relating to the availability of cost data in different countries are discussed below.)

Arikian et al. (1994) conducted a cost-effectiveness analysis for the treatment of onchymycosis. A decision-analytic modelling approach was used comparing four oral therapies (griseofulvin, itraconazole, ketoconazole and terbinafine) for onchomycosis of fingernails and toenails in 13 countries; Austria, Belgium, Canada, Finland, France, Germany, Greece, Italy, Netherlands, Portugal, Spain, Switzerland and the UK. Clinical data on success rates, relapse rates and side-effect rates were taken from a worldwide meta-analysis of randomized controlled trials and combined with resource for the implementation of therapy and the management of adverse events devised around patient profiles and treatment algorithms. It was demonstrated that terbinafine was the most cost-effective therapy for both infections despite its higher acquisition cost in all countries in the study.

The reliability of studies that model from the clinical data depends on two factors. First, they assume that the clinical data are, indeed, transferable from one setting to another. This assumption is likely to be more justifiable for drug therapy than (say) surgery, where the success of surgery may be very dependent on the skill of the surgeon and the availability of other facilities.

However, differences in clinical outcome across settings may even be found for drug therapies. For example, some economic evaluations of chemotherapy for cancer consider the rates of adverse events, such as neutropenia, since these are costly to treat. It is possible that the reported rates of these events could vary from place to place, even within a given clinical trial, if physicians in some locations monitor their patients more closely, or make greater efforts to maintain the chemotherapy dose schedule.

The other major factor affecting the reliability of studies that model from the clinical data is the more general problem of data availability and the need for assumptions. In this respect these studies are no better or worse than other modelling studies (Sheldon 1996).

For example, in the study by Drummond et al. (1992) it was assumed that 40 per cent of the ulcers detected by endoscopy were 'silent' (i.e. not likely to be bothersome enough to be noticed by patients or their physicians). Subsequent studies (Maetzel et al. 1998) have shown that this assumption was rather optimistic, in that as many as 85 per cent of endoscopically-detected ulcers are 'silent'.

Applying this rate, rather than 40 per cent, in the decision analysis by Drummond et al. (1992) would make use of misoprostol considerably less economically attractive. Of course, this issue has nothing to do with transferability per se, beyond the fact that, in international studies, estimates of the key parameters are needed for more than one setting.

Adapting data from an economic clinical trial

In certain countries, such as the USA and Japan, regulatory authorities demand evidence of safety and efficacy in their own populations and therefore trials are usually conducted in these localities, many including economic data capture. However, although economic data may have been collected in a prospective clinical trial in one country (e.g. the USA), economic evaluations may also be required for other settings. In this case, the analyst has two options. The first option is to undertake a modelling study using the clinical data alone, as above. The second option is to adapt the resource data in some way to make it relevant to another country or setting, using local knowledge of factors likely to cause variation in cost-effectiveness results.

Menzin *et al.* (1996) attempted to determine the expected impact of recombinant human deoxyribonuclease (rhDNase) therapy on the costs of treating respiratory tract infections (RTIs) among cystic fibrosis patients in France, Germany, Italy and the UK. However, economic data were only available for patients in a US phase III trial comparing two different doses of rhDNase with vehicle (placebo). In the trial patients were treated for 24 weeks and the outcome measures included change in pulmonary function (FEV1) and incidence of respiratory tract infections (RTIs) requiring parenteral therapy. In terms of economic endpoints, data on hospital admissions, inpatient days and days of oral and intravenous antibiotic therapy were collected.

The US trial demonstrated a significant reduction in RTI-related hospital admissions with rhDNase (0.41 versus 0.56 for placebo; $p < 0.05$) and in days of RTI-related

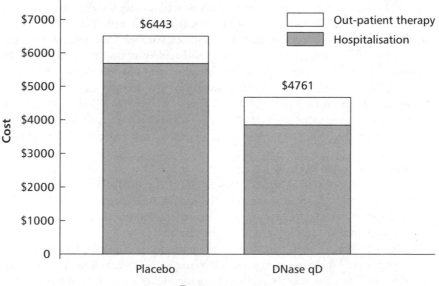

Fig. 11.2 Economic evaluation of DNase therapy in the USA. Mean total costs of care related to respiratory tract infection over 24 weeks by treatment group
Source: Oster *et al.* (1995)

Table 11.1 Difference in mean cost of RTI-related care (placebo minus rhDNase) excluding cost of study medication over 24 weeks in local currencies and US dollars, by country

Component of cost	Country			
	France (FF)	Germany (DM)	Italy (L)	UK (£)
Costs in local currency				
Inpatient care:				
Days in hospital	4540	711	982,000	300
Antibiotic therapy	806	1259[a]	122,000	50
Outpatient care	1665	—[a]	181,000	84
Total	7011	1970	1,285,000	434
Costs in US$[b]				
Inpatient care:				
Days in hospital	693	337	660	477
Antibiotic therapy	123	607[a]	82	79
Outpatient care	254	—[a]	122	134
Total	1070	934	864	690

Notes:
[a] A detailed breakdown of inpatient and outpatient antibiotic costs was not available.
[b] Calculated using 1990 Purchasing Power Parities. Organization for Economic Cooperation and Development (OECD): OECD Health Data File, 1992.

outpatient intravenous antibiotic therapy (2.9 versus 4.4; $p < 0.05$). Compared with placebo, the cost of treating RTIs over 24 weeks was $1682 less among patients receiving rhDNase once daily, primarily due to reductions in the cost of hospitalization (see Figure 11.2). However there was interest in determining the economic impact of the therapy in France, Germany, Italy and the UK.

A simple approach would be to price the US resource use observed in the trial in local currency, effectively ignoring differences between the countries in clinical conventions and resource use. When this approach was used, savings ranged from £434 ($711) in the UK to 7010 FF ($1064) in France (see Table 11.1).

However, it is likely that there are differences in clinical practice and that hence the US trial-based resource estimates would be misleading. Therefore, adjustments had to be made for resource use and cost. Adjustments were made by seeking expert opinion on the likely treatment patterns for RTI and by analysing a series of patient case notes (charts) to estimate the length of hospital stay and resource use for treatment of RTI. In the UK no adjustments were considered necessary, but in Germany the length of stay was considered to be longer (14.4 days versus 12.3 days) and in France and Italy, both the rate of hospitalization and the length of stay were adjusted. The overall effect was to reduce slightly the estimates of savings in Italy (from $908 to $607) and in France (from $1064 to $850). In Germany, there was a very small increase in savings from treating RTI.

The main discretionary factor in the adjustment approach is the identification of the factors likely to impact on the generalizability of the results observed in the trial. Therefore, there is a danger that analysts could be accused of bias. Analysts wishing to make adjustments to trial-based data are therefore advised to specify the adjustments in the analysis plan prior to seeing the data. The factors that need to be adjusted can be identified through prior expert opinion, or a thorough review of the literature to identify the major cost drivers, or other parameters, likely to impact on the results. In recent years, there has been increasing use of pre-trial modelling from Phase II data and the literature, which could potentially assist the analyst in identifying the adjustments to be made. However, when adjustments are made, the trial-based estimates should also be reported, so that the reader can assess the impact on the results of the economic evaluation.

11.3.2 Analysing multinational clinical trials

Multicentre clinical trials have been carried out for a number of years and an increasing number are now being conducted on a multinational basis. The main motivation for the development of multinational trials is that larger sample sizes can be assembled in a shorter period, thus allowing a quick, precise estimate of treatment effect. In addition, because these trials enrol patients from a wide range of treatment settings and countries, they may increase the representativeness of the study sample and promote interest among clinical opinion leaders in several countries.

Although practice patterns and patient characteristics may differ among centres in clinical trials, it is generally believed that the clinical effect of a health technology or treatment should not differ greatly across centres. Consequently, one should be able to pool the clinical data across centres to assess the effect of treatment on clinical outcomes. While tests of homogeneity for estimates of the relative effects of new therapies are usually undertaken before the data are pooled, statistically significant treatment effect-by-country interactions for these estimates are rarely observed with clinical outcomes. Even if an interaction exists, it may go undetected because of the small sample sizes of some centres, which provide only modest statistical power for the tests of differences in treatment effect by centre.

Because of the increased interest in the cost-effectiveness of health care interventions, resource use data are now more often being collected alongside multinational trials. Given the threats to transferability outlined in Section 11.2 above, it is therefore less likely that there are no treatment effect-by-country interactions for the economic data. Thus the prior assumption is that, unlike the clinical data, the economic data cannot be pooled and that new analytic strategies need to be devised.

Several analysts have proposed approaches for analysing economic multinational trials. Jönsson and Weinstein (1997), in an evaluation of a medicine used in the treatment for myocardial infarction, argued that there would be a difference between countries in the baseline level of resource utilization (e.g. revascularization procedures), since this had been seen in earlier studies (Mark *et al.* 1995).

Therefore, they suggested calculating the pooled proportional difference in resource allocation across all countries and then applying this proportional reduction to country-specific baseline costs. Unfortunately, the study itself was never undertaken as the medicine concerned did not complete its clinical development. However, the approach proposed is analogous to the one used in interpreting the results of clinical studies, where it is usually argued that the relative risk reduction from a given therapy is fairly constant across different study populations. Nevertheless, more empirical evidence is required, to assess whether the 'relative resource reduction' is constant across different health care systems, before this method can be recommended.

Cook *et al.* (2001) have proposed an approach for analysing multinational economic clinical trials based on testing for homogeneity in the data. The general idea was to follow the approach used in the analysis of the clinical data from such trials, where tests of homogeneity are typically performed before pooling the data.

The example used was the Scandinavian Simvastatin Survival Study (4S), a controlled trial of simvastatin versus placebo for hypercholesterolaemic patients with existing coronary heart disease. The 4S trial was a randomized, double-blind, placebo-controlled study of 4444 patients from Denmark ($n = 713$), Finland ($n = 868$), Iceland ($n = 157$), Norway ($n = 1025$) and Sweden ($n = 1681$). Data on hospitalizations were collected during the trial and unit costs (prices) obtained external to the study (Scandinavian Simvastatin Survival Study Group 1994).

Cook *et al.* were interested in the possibility of a country-by-treatment interaction in the effect of treatment on the measure of effectiveness, cost, or cost-effectiveness. Gail and Simon (1985) describe a framework for characterizing the nature of potential interactions in more detail. A *qualitative*, or crossover, interaction occurs when the treatment effect is positive for the patients in some countries and negative for those in other countries. A non-crossover interaction occurs when the magnitude, but not the direction, of treatment effect varies. (Cook *et al.* refer to this as a *quantitative* interaction.)

The results of the test for mortality (the effectiveness measure used) and hospitalization rates showed no evidence of a country-by-treatment interaction, indicating that the data could be pooled. However, separate evaluations of homogeneity among countries for treatment effects in clinical outcomes and utilization variables are not adequate to ensure homogeneity in the cost-effectiveness ratios. For example, models used to evaluate treatment effects often use relative measures such as the odds ratio, or percentage reduction, whereas incremental cost-effectiveness ratios use the ratio of absolute differences in costs and effects.

Therefore, heterogeneity in absolute treatment effects (measured as a difference) can occur when there are large country-to-country differences in baseline rates coupled with a constant multiplicative treatment effect. In addition, matters are further complicated by the fact that costs and effects are not independent and that prices can significantly affect health care utilization. Thus the correct approach would be to estimate separately the country-specific cost-effectiveness ratios and then to evaluate the heterogeneity of ratios among countries. A pooled (average) ratio could then be estimated for the overall study if no country-by-ratio interaction is seen.

Because estimates of the cost-effectiveness ratios may vary widely, especially when the denominator of the ratio is numerically close to zero, Cook *et al.* applied an angular transformation of the incremental cost-effectiveness ratio (Cook and Heyse

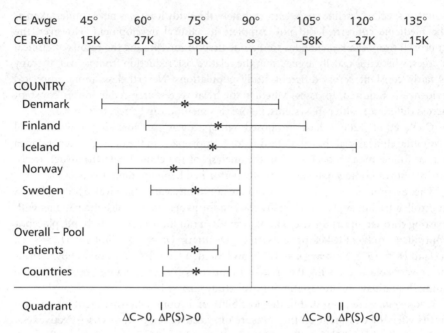

Fig. 11.3 Ninety-five per cent confidence intervals for the incremental cost per additional survivor in the Scandinavian Simvastatin Survival Study by country and for the overall country average. CE = cost-effectiveness
Source: Cook et al. (2001)

2000). Essentially, this method transforms cost-effectiveness ratios in the four quadrants of the cost-effectiveness plane (Drummond *et al.* 1997) to angles in the range of 0 to 90 degrees (quadrant I), 90 to 180 degrees (quadrant II), and so on. Such a transformation provides a stable estimate of variance for ratios throughout the cost-effectiveness plane.

The results are shown in Figure 11.3. Unfortunately, unit cost data were only available for Sweden, so this may have reduced the overall variability in the cost-effectiveness estimates. (The Swedish prices were converted to US dollars.) However, although the estimates of the cost-effectiveness ratio for the five countries differed, the Gail and Simon test indicated no evidence of a quantitative interaction.

The assessment for qualitative interaction depends on the specification of an 'acceptable' threshold for cost-effectiveness (e.g. $50,000 per additional survivor). That is, one would need to assess whether any of the country-specific estimates exceeds the threshold where the others do not. However, in this case no evidence of qualitative interaction was found, no matter which threshold was specified.

Given the lack of evidence of treatment-by-country interaction, Cook *et al.* suggest that the data across countries can be pooled to improve the precision of the estimated cost-effectiveness ratio. One method would be to ignore country and pool all patients to estimate the cost-effectiveness ratio. This gives a pooled ratio of $59,364 per additional survivor. Alternatively, one can pool the data by giving equal weight to each country. This gives a pooled ratio of $62,653 per additional survivor. Therefore, an approach based on testing for homogeneity may be useful in analysing multinational economic clinical trials, since those data can be pooled if no treatment-by-country interactions are found. However, as mentioned earlier, such tests for interaction typically have low statistical power. Also, the relative similarity of the five countries in the 4S study and the lack of unit costs for all the countries may have led to a bias towards homogeneity that may not be found in other situations.

In situations where treatment-by-country interactions are more likely to exist, it would be useful to understand the nature of those interactions. For example, the treatment may directly affect cost by changing resource use independent of the clinical outcome, or it may indirectly affect it by modifying the clinical outcome (which in turn may affect costs).

In a thoughtful exploration of the problems in analysing multinational economic clinical trials, Willke et al. (1997) used a regression approach to analyse costs and outcomes for a drug treatment in five countries. The approach assumed that the costs of an episode of care for an individual patient are determined by the treatment the patient receives, a series of exogenous variables (e.g. disease severity, etc.), the health outcome of the episode, and country-by-treatment and country-by-outcome inter-action terms.

This model specification allows treatment to affect the cost independent of outcome (i.e. for two identical individuals who experience the same outcome, one with the study treatment and the other with usual care, the study treatment may cause the cost of care to differ). (The authors called this the *net treatment effect* on cost.) It also allows the outcome to affect the cost of care, independent of treatment (i.e. two identical individuals may experience different outcomes due to the study treatment and thus different costs). (The authors called this the *outcome effect* on cost.) It also differentiates these independent effects by country.

Willke et al. drew their data from a randomized, double-blind, placebo-controlled trial of tirilazad mesylate for the treatment of aneurysmal subarachnoid haemorrhage. (The trial was conducted in 11 countries and data from the five countries was used in the analysis reported here.) Follow-up was for three months or until death, whichever came first. Most of the utilization data and all of the outcome data were collected prospectively as part of the clinical trial. Unit cost data were collected in a separate study, by Schulman et al. (1998). (This is discussed later in this chapter.)

The univariate analysis of mortality and cost is given in Table 11.2. It can be seen that the proportion who died and the average hospital cost per patient both vary by country. The results of the regression analyses showed that the full treatment effect on cost ranged from $-$4812 in Country 5 to $5845 in Country 2 and that the statistical test for the country-by-treatment interactions tended towards significance (F test, $p = 0.088$). The net treatment effect on cost ranged from $-$5041 in Country 5 to $4543 in Country 2. In this case these differences were statistically significant ($p = 0.046$). The outcome effect on cost was negative in all countries but also tended towards significant differences between countries. Finally, the country-specific effects of mortality were not statistically different from one another ($p = 0.64$).

Willke et al. then used the regression estimates to calculate the cost-effectiveness ratios for tirilazad treatment in three ways: (i) using own-country costs and mortality

Table 11.2 Mean variations in total cost and mortality rate by country for trial patients

	Average hospital cost per patient ($)	Mortality rate
Country 1	18,180	0.200
Country 2	14,476	0.206
Country 3	14,007	0.111
Country 4	19,561	0.257
Country 5	41,258	0.084
Test of equality of country means	$F = 66.6, p < 0.0005$	$\chi^2 = 23.6, p < 0.0005$

effects; (ii) using own-country costs and the trial-wide mortality effect; and (iii) using own-country prices, but trial-wide utilization and mortality effect. As one might expect, the greatest variation in the country-specific ratios was in case (i), where country-specific resource utilization, unit prices and outcome levels were all taken into account.

In case (ii), the ratios still varied considerably, although in three of the countries the ratios were quite similar, suggesting similar resource utilization patterns. In case (iii), when only prices were country-specific, there was much less variation in the cost-effectiveness ratios, suggesting that country-specific utilization differences, controlling for outcome, clearly contribute to the variation in the cost-effectiveness ratios.

The authors concluded that, while they found no significant country-specific differences in outcome (and hence outcome results are transferable from place to place), simple transfer of trial-wide cost results to specific countries would have been inappropriate in their study. However, the proposed strategy for making regression-based adjustments should provide results that are more applicable to the costs and resource utilization patterns observed in the individual countries.

11.3.3 Costing methods for multinational studies

Both modelling studies and those that involve the analysis of data from multinational trials require data on the unit costs of key resource items in various countries. It was mentioned earlier that accounting practices vary greatly between countries, so it is often a challenge to generate a comprehensive and consistent set of unit costs or prices to be applied to the resource use estimates.

Despite the importance of this issue and the fact that costs are required in every multinational study, relatively few analysts have explored the theory and practice of multicountry costing.

In one of the few published papers addressing this topic, Schulman *et al.* (1998) explain how attempts were made to develop a standardized costing methodology in seven countries and to apply it in the costing of treatments for subarachnoid haemorrhage. The collection of cost data was structured through the use of worksheets to provide accurate and efficient cost reporting. Total average costs were converted to

Table 11.3 Relative medical cost indices of the study countries

Index	Germany	Italy	France	Sweden	UK	Australia	Spain
Germany	1.00	1.35	1.35	2.64	2.41	2.03	1.92
Italy	0.74	1.00	1.33	1.96	1.79	1.51	1.43
France	0.56	0.75	1.00	1.47	1.34	1.13	1.07
Sweden	0.38	0.51	0.68	1.00	0.91	0.77	0.73
UK	0.42	0.56	0.75	1.10	1.00	0.84	0.80
Australia	0.49	0.66	0.88	1.30	1.19	1.00	0.95
Spain	0.52	0.70	0.93	1.37	1.25	1.06	1.00

average variable costs and then aggregated to develop unit costs for the relevant resource items.

Despite the detailed approach adopted, there were still several resource items for which unit costs were unavailable for certain countries. For these items the analysts developed an index table (Table 11.3), based on a market-basket approach. To estimate the cost of a given procedure, the market-basket estimation process required that cost information be available for at least one country. Where cost information was unavailable in all countries for a given procedure, costs were estimated using a method based on physician-work and practice-expense resource-based relative value units. It can be seen from Table 11.4 that a substantial number of unit cost items were unavailable for some countries, and had to be imputed. This study shows that little attention has been paid to the availability of cost data in different countries. The derivation of standard unit costs is important, both for modelling studies and the analysis of multinational clinical trials.

11.3.4 Undertaking systematic overviews of economic evaluations

In the clinical literature, systematic overviews of individual studies have been used to produce an estimate of the clinical effect of a given intervention. The motivations of systematic overviews are twofold. First, by combining data from a number of studies, a more precise estimate of the clinical effect can be obtained. Second, by using data from studies conducted in a range of settings, the estimate produced will reflect the size of clinical effect that is likely to be obtained on average.

Often the effect size is presented as a relative risk reduction, which can then be applied to patient populations with different baseline risks, to generate the absolute risk reduction likely to be obtained in a given clinical setting.

Several organizations, including the Cochrane Collaboration (1996), have put forward standard steps for systematic overviews of clinical studies. These are outlined in Box 11.1. In particular, emphasis is placed on undertaking a thorough literature search (including the grey literature) to minimize the effects of publication bias, and on critically appraising the quality of studies to be included in the overview.

Table 11.4 Reported procedure and per diem costs for study countries

	Costs (US$)						
	Germany	Italy	France	Sweden	UK	Australia	Spain
Procedure costs							
Burr holes	130	77	216	*372*	365	711	72
Chest tubes	87	210	*150*	175	*201*	120	93
Central nervous system shunt	1148	1749	617	371	357	699	*526*
Craniofacial procedures	*350*	*471*	*628*	693	*843*	888	*673*
Cranioplasty	*590*	794	*1059*	*1557*	*1420*	*1197*	*1134*
Debridement of brain	824	357	740	1386	2247	717	552
Dialysis	*153*	206	*275*	*404*	*368*	*310*	294
Elevation of skull fracture	367	357	483	693	377	*505*	336
Evacuation of lesion	506	357	493	1386	476	*722*	705
Filtration for renal failure	*248*	*334*	*441*	*655*	597	759	234
Gastroscopy	*106*	245	63	347	*256*	156	*204*
Gastrostomy (procedure)	79	*148*	361	*290*	*264*	*223*	95
Humeral shaft fracture	*287*	*386*	106	*757*	1904	*582*	21
Intracranial drainage	273	432	*340*	175	365	389	259
Laparotomy (exploratory)	130	209	301	866	462	573	492
Lobectomy	*544*	830	*977*	1040	569	2251	705
Peritoneal lavage	*38*	117	*69*	*102*	*93*	23	34
Removal of bone flap	506	357	411	175	408	1650	332
Replacement of bone flap	809	604	524	*1203*	526	1308	616
Shunt placement	*642*	1749	*1152*	260	2087	*1302*	580
Spine operation	*1125*	1515	*2019*	2970	2708	2283	2164
Splenectomy	249	389	*483*	*711*	648	*547*	*518*
Swan–Ganz monitor	*207*	335	*371*	*546*	*498*	420	317
Superficial laceration	16	31	20	175	154	*68*	36
Tracheostomy	151	120	301	347	256	1105	132
Per diem costs							
Daily intensive care unit	445	601	774	1231	1159	945	876
Daily intermediate care unit	*169*	304	301	573	315	207	*324*
Daily routine care unit	134	187	350	267	173	159	236
Daily rehabilitation unit	140	324	210	336	*384*	186	464

Note: Actual costs are in plain text; market-basket imputed costs are in italic text.

Box 11.1 **Standard steps involved in conducting a meta-analysis**

(i)   Development of study protocol
(ii)   Formulation of the problem
(iii)   Location and selection of studies
(iv)   Critical appraisal of studies
(v)   Analysis and presentation of results
(vi)   Interpretation of results

Source: Cochrane Collaboration (1996)

There has been recent interest in the systematic overviews of economic evaluations as a way of handling the issue of transferability. That is, a structured review of results from previous studies could potentially provide an overall summary of cost and effectiveness and allow for the exploration of reasons for inconsistencies and variability. In practical terms, performing a systematic overview could be potentially less costly and less time-consuming than performing further primary economic studies in yet further locations (Jefferson *et al.* 1996).

Also, there are situations when decisions need to be made based on limited information, if there are no resources available to conduct a further economic evaluation for the setting concerned. Systematic overviews may give decision-makers confidence that they are making the best use of what economic evidence is available at the time. The use of systematic overview in the reimbursement approval process of drugs represents a potential application. Currently assessments are based on one or more primary economic evaluations. However, as more studies are published, systematic overviews could potentially assist the reimbursement authorities in their decision through summarizing the available economic evidence at the time alongside the clinical evidence. Further, systematic overviews may provide a stimulus for updating knowledge in a particular disease area and providing guidance concerning the design of future economic studies.

The science of systematic overviews of economic evaluations is still in its infancy. Jefferson and colleagues (Jefferson and Demicheli 1996; Jefferson *et al.* 1996) attempted a systematic overview of epidemiological and economic variables for the prevention and treatment of influenza, incorporating most of the standard steps in their study. Their primary research objective was to summarize the evidence about the cost and cost-effectiveness of influenza vaccine from published and unpublished studies. To protect against bias and to ensure that all relevant data were included, Jefferson and Demicheli (1996) conducted a rigorous literature search. A MEDLINE CD-ROM search in all European languages was conducted for the period January 1966 to 1 May 1995, using the keywords: vaccine, influenza, prevention, cost-benefit, cost-effectiveness, economic evaluation, cost. This was extended with searchers of biographies of retrieved studies, handsearches of the journal *Vaccine* from 1983 to 1994 and through dialogue with the manufacturers of the vaccines and researchers active in the field of the economics of prevention of communicable diseases. After the studies were retrieved, the authors reviewed the studies against broad inclusion criteria and classified the economic evaluations according to standard definitions.

Studies were included if they contained:

- clear aim, viewpoint and time span;
- design consistent with study aim(s);
- coherent methods, results and conclusions;
- itemized costs;
- marginal and sensitivity analysis; and
- all the above clearly and unequivocally stated in the text.

Thirty-one studies in total were retrieved, but 17 studies were excluded on the basis of their inclusion criteria and on methodological grounds. Studies using resource or cost estimates derived from other works were excluded in order to avoid double-counting, as well as studies which did not contain a clear separation between resources used and unit costs. At this stage, the authors did not proceed to score the quality of economic evaluations, as might typically be done in the case of clinical studies. Hence the implicit assumption is that each economic evaluation in their review had equal weighting. If scoring for quality assessment had been done, it would have required several further decisions to be made. One prime consideration would have been the nature of the quality assessment scoring system for economic evaluation. Another consideration for scoring would have been the number, skills and experience of assessors, and the need to mask certain information in the studies such as the identity of the authors and the institutions at which a study was conducted.

Jefferson and Demicheli proceeded to construct a secondary economic model using a 'resource costing' approach. This model derived data on resource inputs from existing studies and estimated costs and cost-effectiveness from unit cost data specific to a particular setting. They reviewed the methods and results sections of all studies and extracted the following data: influenza attack rate; vaccine effectiveness; direct costs; indirect costs; vaccine cost per dose; cost per avoided cases; cost per healthy life-year gained and cost to benefit ratio; medication consultations; hospital admissions per 1000 cases; length of hospital stay per hospitalized patient (Days); working days lost per employed case. Study authors were not contacted to provide supplementary information, as it was the intention to attempt a review from published data only. Costs from the studies for resource inputs were standardized to 1994 US dollars using official exchange rates and the US Consumer Price Index. Through pooling, ranges of resource estimates were constructed, to which standard costs from a cost of illness study (which had been previously carried out in a region of Italy) were attached. These were then used in a series of evaluations performed on a hypothetical cohort of 1,000,000 individuals to determine benefit to cost ratios (BCRs), maintaining the efficacy of the vaccine at 80 per cent throughout.

Finally, a sensitivity analysis was performed by varying the costs and influenza attach rates to assess the robustness of the BCRs. The number of doctor–patient consultations and work days lost did not substantially affect the BCR, whereas the model was sensitive to the length of hospital stay. The BCRs ranged from 0.3 to 1.2 for the low-attach scenarios and 1.1 to 3.6 for the high attach rate scenarios. Jefferson and Demicheli concluded that their overview was consistent with the currently available reliable literature, in that prevention of influenza by vaccination is efficient, especially in high incidence scenarios (intra- or interepidemic).

This overview highlighted several difficulties in applying systematic overview methodology to economic data. A majority difficulty in conducting a systematic overview of economic studies can be attributed to the current, rather poor, 'transparency' of economic studies. There is a need for clearer guidance for what should be expected in the reporting of future economic studies. Perhaps an approach would be to standardize the reporting along the lines of the BMJ guidelines for economic publication (Drummond and Jefferson 1996).

It is common practice in clinical systematic overviews to assess the quality of the studies being considered for inclusion. This is because one might wish to use study quality as part of a weight assigned to each study in the analysis, as a way of excluding poor quality studies, or as a stratification factor for allowing the separate estimation of good quality and poor studies. In a systematic overview of economic evaluations, an economist has two distinct components to assess: the clinical data and the economic data. Whilst several checklists for economic studies have been published in recent years, no one has attempted to develop a reliable quality assessment scoring system. This perhaps is due to the state of the art of economic evaluation at the present time, with several methodological issues remaining unresolved. With regard to the clinical data, a number of scoring systems exist, but these may not be sensitive enough for the needs of economic analysts. The effectiveness data on which economic models are based are occasionally derived from a mixture of clinical study designs (i.e. RCTs and observational studies) in an informal literature review/meta-analysis. A related, but important, point is that several economic studies, which may be included in an economic systematic overview, may contain effectiveness data drawn from the same source. This may introduce potential bias in quality assessment as the same clinical data is included more than once. Hence the development of quality assessment scoring systems for economic evaluations should be part of the future research agenda.

While there are no easy answers to many of these questions, it is known that systematic overview will play an increasingly important role in making treatment and policy recommendations. Therefore, the quality of the systematic overviews performed is of the utmost importance; the quality of such analyses depends upon not only the methodology of the systematic overviews themselves, but also on the data from the individual studies used.

11.4 Conclusions: implications for the design and analysis of economic evaluations in the future

It is clear that there are several threats to the transferability of economic evaluation results. This chapter has discussed several of the analytic strategies that have been employed to date and several conclusions can be drawn. First, models can be constructed using the clinical data alone, or the results of an economic clinical trial conducted in one country can be adapted for other settings. Analysts following these approaches should be aware of good practices in modelling (Consensus Conference on Guidelines on Economic Modelling in Health Technology Assessment 2000), many of which relate to transparency in methods and the reporting of results.

Second, the strategies for analysing data for multinational clinical trials proposed by Willke et al. (1997) and Cook et al. (2001) offer a partial solution, but suffer from limitations owing to lack of power of some of the statistical tests performed and ideally require country-specific unit costs (prices) as well as data on resource utilization. Schulman et al. (1998) describe a method for generating country-specific unit costs.

Third, the lack of standardization in the methods of economic evaluation, and lack of transparency in reporting, seriously limits the potential to undertake systematic overviews of economic evaluations. If economists are to satisfactorily develop methods of systematic overview, as has been done for clinical studies, several difficulties will have to be overcome.

Therefore, several recommendations can be made, relating both to the design and analysis of economic evaluations. In respect of the design of studies, more consideration could be given to the economic characteristics of the settings used for multinational economic clinical trials (Ellwein and Drummond 1996). Should more homogeneous settings be selected? Can settings or countries be selected so that they can be grouped some way in the subsequent analysis? Can more data be collected on the economic characteristics of the settings (analogous to the patient characteristics recorded in trials) for potential use in any subsequent multivariate analysis? In addition, attempts should be made to standardize the collection of resource use and price data across countries, in order to make the process less costly and to avoid some of the problems experienced in the Schulman et al. (1998) study.

In respect of the analysis of data from multinational economic trials, approaches based on multilevel modelling and cluster analysis have been proposed (Pang 1999), but as yet few if any full analyses have been published. However, multilevel modelling has already been applied to administrative data sets in managed care (Carey 2000). Several applications to clinical trial data sets are now under way and will be published in the near future.

References

Arikian, S. R., Einarson, T. R., Kobelt-Nguyen, G. et al. (1994). A multinational pharmacoeconomic analysis of oral therapies for onychomycosis. British Journal of Dermatology, 130(S43), 35–44.

Carey, K. (2000). A multilevel modelling approach to analysis of patient costs under managed care. Health Economics, 9, 435–46.

Cochrane Collaboration. (1996). Cochrane databases of systematic reviews. Version 2. Oxford Update Software.

Commonwealth of Australia. (1995). Guidelines for the pharmaceutical industry on preparation of submissions to the Pharmaceutical Benefits Advisory Committee: including economic analyses. Department of Health and Community Services, Canberra.

Consensus Conference on Guidelines on Economic Modelling in Health Technology Assessment. (2000). Consensus statement and background papers. *PharmacoEconomics*, 17(5), 443–513.

Cook, J. R., Drummond, M. F., Glick, H. *et al.* (2001). Analysing economic data from multinational clinical trials. (*Mimeo.*)

Cook, J. R. and Heyse, J. F. (2000). Use of an angular transformation for ratio estimation in cost-effectiveness analysis. *Statistics in Medicine*, 19, 2989–3003.

Drummond, M. F., Bloom, B. S., Carrin, G. *et al.* (1992). Issues in the cross-national assessment of health technology. *International Journal of Technology Assessment in Health Care*, 8(4), 671–82.

Drummond, M. F. and Jefferson, T. O. for the BMJ Working Party. (1996). Guidelines for authors and peer reviewers of economic submissions to the BMJ. *British Medical Journal*, 313, 275–83.

Ellwein, L. B. and Drummond, M. F. (1996). Economic analysis alongside clinical trials: bias in the assessment of economic outcomes. *International Journal of Technology Assessment in Health Care*, 12, 691–7.

van Erkel, A. R., van den Hout, W. B. and Pattynama, P. M. T. (1999). International differences in health care costs in Europe and the United States: do these affect the cost-effectiveness of diagnostic strategies for pulmonary embolism? *European Radiology*, 9, 1226–931.

Gail, M. and Simon, R. (1985). Testing for qualitative interactions between treatment effects and patient subsets. *Biometrics*, 41, 361–72.

Hull, R. D., Hirsh, J., Sackett, D. L. *et al.* (1981). Cost-effectiveness of clinical diagnosis, venography and non-invasive testing in patients with symptomatic deep-vein thrombosis. *New England Journal of Medicine*, 304, 1561–7.

Jefferson, T. O. and Demicheli, V. (1996). Economic evaluation of influenza vaccination and economic modelling. Can results be pooled? *PharmacoEconomics*, 9(3), 67–72.

Jefferson, T. O., Mugford, M., Gray, A. *et al* (1996). An exercise on the feasibility of carrying out secondary economic analyses. *Health Economics*, 5, 155–65.

Johnson, J. A., Ohinmaa, A., Murti, B. *et al.* (2000). Comparison of Finnish and US-based visual analog scale valuations of the EQ-5D measure. *Medical Decision-Making*, 20(3), 281–9.

Jönsson, B. and Weinstein, M. C. (1997). Economic evaluation alongside multinational clinical trials. Study considerations for GUSTO IIb. *International Journal of Technology Assessment in Health Care*, 13(1), 49–58.

Le Gales, C., Buron, C., Costet, N. *et al.* (2000). The French Health Utilities Index Mark 3 (Abstract). *Value in Health*, 3, 103.

Maetzel, A., Ferraz, M. B. and Bombardier, C. (1998). The cost-effectiveness of misoprostol in preventing serious gastrointestinal events associated with the use of nonsteroidal anti-inflammatory drugs. *Arthritis and Rheumatism*, 41, 16–25.

Mark, D. B., Hlatky, M. A., Califf, R. M. *et al.* (1995). Cost-effectiveness of thrombolytic therapy with tissue plasminogen activator as compared with streptokinase for acute myocardial infarction. *The New England Journal of Medicine*, 332(21), 1418–24.

Menzin, J., Oster, G., Davies, L. *et al.* (1996). A multinational economic evaluation of rhDNase in the treatment of cystic fibrosis. *International Journal of Technology Assessment in Health Care*, 12(1), 52–61.

National Institute for Clinical Excellence. (2001). *Health technology assessment: guidance for manufacturers and sponsors*. NICE, London, February.

O'Brien, B. J. (1997). A tale of two (or more) cities; geographic transferability of pharmacoeconomic data. *American Journal of Managed Care*, 3, S33–9.

Pang, F. (1999). The application of multilevel modelling and cluster analysis to multinational economic evaluation data. (Abs.) *Value in Health*, 2(3), 138.

Scandinavian Simvastatin Survival Study Group. (1994). Randomised trial of cholesterol lowering in 4444 patients with coronary heart disease: The Scandinavian Simvastatin Survival Study (4S). *The Lancet*, 334, 1383–9.

Schulman, K., Burke, J., Drummond, M. *et al.* (1998). Resource costing for multinational neurological clinical trials: methods and results. *Health Economics*, 7, 629–38.

Sheldon, T. A. (1996). Problems of using modelling in the economic evaluation of health care. *Health Economics*, 5(1), 1–11.

Späth, H.-M., Carrère, M.-O., Fervers, B. and Philip, T. (1999). Analysis of the eligibility of published economic evaluations for transfer to a given health care system. *Health Policy*, 49, 161–77.

Willke, R. J., Glick, H. A., Polsky, D. *et al.* (1997) Estimating country-specific cost-effectiveness from multinational clinical trials. *Health Economics*, 7, 481–493.

Index